Peter Petros

The Female Pelvic Floor

Function, Dysfunction and Management According to the Integral Theory

Second Edition

Peter Petros

The Female Pelvic Floor

Function, Dysfunction and Management
According to the Integral Theory

With 237 Figures and 3 Tables

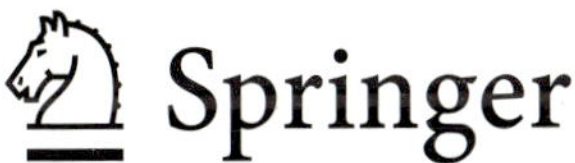

Springer

PE Papa Petros MB BS (Syd) Dr. Med Sc (Uppsala) DS (UWA) MD (Syd) FRCOG FRANZCOG CU
Dept of Gynaecology
Royal Perth Hospital
Western Australia

ISBN 978-3-540-33663-1 Springer Medizin Verlag Heidelberg

Cataloging-in-Publication Data applied for
A catalog record for this book is available from the Library of Congress.

Bibliographic information published by Die Deutsche Nationalbibliothek
Die Deutsche Nationalbibliothek lists this publication in the Deutsche Nationalbibliografie;
detailed bibliographic data is available in the Internet at http://dnb.d-nb.de.

Springer Medizin Verlag
springer.com
© Springer Medizin Verlag Heidelberg 2007
Printed in Germany

SPIN 11740940
Cover Design: deblik Berlin, Germany
Typesetting: TypoStudio Tobias Schaedla, Heidelberg, Germany
Printer: Stürtz GmbH, Würzburg, Germany

Printed on acid free paper   18/3160/yb – 5 4 3 2 1 0

Cover Idea by Sam Blight, Rangs Graphics

The three arrows represent the three major force vectors featured in the Integral Theory which control the
tensioning of ligaments and membranes in the pelvic floor.

The enclosing circular brush stroke is inspired by the traditional 'enso' character in Zen calligraphy which
represents non-duality or wholeness. This is to evoke the integrated approach covered in this book.

The butterfly represents the 'butterfly effect' concept from Chaos Theory, also known as 'sensitive
dependence on initial conditions', which describes how small variations in a dynamic non-linear system (such
as the pelvic floor) can produce a 'cascade' of events leading to a major change in the state of the system.

It also represents the freedom which this technology will give to women suffering from the many pelvic
floor dysfunctions which can be cured by applying the Integral Theory System.

ὃ βίος βραχὺς
ἣ δὲ ἣ τέχνη μακρή

Life is short,
But the craft is long

Hippocrates 460-377 BC

Science is the father of knowledge, but opinion breeds ignorance.

Hippocrates 460-377 BC

Preface to 2nd Edition

I would like to express my gratitude to my colleagues around the globe for the overwhelming support given to the first edition of 'The Female Pelvic Floor'. The publishers inform me that Spanish, Japanese, and Chinese translations are underway, an indication, perhaps, of the increasing acceptance of at least some of the concepts within the book.

Since the release of the first edition in September 2004, many new surgical techniques have been developed. These have extended the concepts of suspensory slings to replace and to reinforce damaged vaginal fascia. New insights have been gained from further application of the Tissue Fixation System. Its use in anterior and posterior wall prolapse repair has unlocked new anatomical concepts concerning the relationship between the cervical ring and cardinal ligaments; also, uterosacral ligaments and rectovaginal fascia.

These advances have necessitated some further additions in Chapter 2, and extensive additions in Chapter 4, so as to better explain the anatomical basis for these recent surgical advances, and hopefully, for the newer techniques which will inevitably emerge in the coming years.

Notwithstanding the immense progress achieved since the 1990 publication of the Integral Theory, three important challenges remain: finding methods to more accurately assess the degree of damage in the various connective tissue structures; continuing to develop understanding of the interactions which lead to abnormal symptoms in the individual patient; and further minimizing the need for surgical operations.

A central focus for these challenges is to apply them to those most in need of assistance, that is, the frail and the elderly, for example, Nursing Home patients.

In this context, the 2nd edition of this book is presented as an invitation to colleagues to participate in the further development of this methodology, surgical technique and technology.

Peter Petros, Royal Perth Hospital, Perth Western Australia, June 2006

Preface

I first encountered the Integral Theory system in the early 1990's at the Royal Perth Hospital laboratory in Western Australia where I was working on laparoscopic colposuspension. Even in prototype form, the IVS operation was so simple and effective that I adopted it immediately. Subsequently, based on my experiences, I wrote the following in the Medical Journal of Australia in October 1994:

> *(the operations) promise a new era for women, virtually pain-free cure of prolapse and incontinence without catheters, and return to normal activities within days.*

Now, ten years later, more than 500,000 'tension-free' anterior or posterior sling operations have been performed.

One case in particular stands out from those early years. A woman patient in her mid-50's came to see me with a five year history of urinary retention which required an indwelling catheter. This woman had consulted more than a dozen medical specialists who had told her the same story: no cure was possible. Using the Structured Assessment of the Integral Theory it was deduced that she had a posterior zone defect. I performed a Posterior IVS. The next day the patient was voiding spontaneously with low residuals, and she has remained well since.

At first I was sceptical about some of the other predictions of the Integral Theory, in particular, surgical cure of nocturia, frequency, 'detrusor instability', chronic pelvic pain, intrinsic sphincter defect and 'idiopathic faecal incontinence. However, the high cure rate obtained by following the diagnostic system described in this book soon convinced me that the Integral Theory framework had much wider applications than those predicted in the original publications.

It is self-evident that the Integral Theory has now matured into an important medical Paradigm, every aspect of which is outlined in this book.

The original work on the Integral Theory was done at Royal Perth Hospital, Western Australia and the University of Uppsala, Sweden. However, the defining concepts concerning management and surgery were done at Royal Perth Hospital. It was here that the biomechanical and fluid dynamic principles developed at the University of Western Australia's Department of Mechanical and Materials Engineering and Fluid Dynamics were applied in practical form. For these works, Professor Petros received his Doctor of Surgery degree in 1999.

It should be emphasized that this book is mainly clinically based. Using the Diagnostic Algorithm and 'simulated operations', techniques which are thoroughly described herein, it is possible for the generalist to achieve a high degree of diagnostic accuracy and high cure rates. Furthermore most conditions can be treated at the clinical level without the use of expensive diagnostic equipment or surgical facilities. This means that the methods described in this book can be accessed by medical professionals in less developed countries where resources and equipment may not be readily available.

Peter Richardson FRCOG, FRANZCOG
Immediate Past Chairman, National Association of Specialist Obstetricians and Gynaecologists of Australia (NASOG).

Acknowledgments

It is now almost twenty years since the first threads of the Integral Theory arrived in my consciousness. This book brings together these and all the other threads which have materialized over these years. Throughout this time, I have had the unflinching support of my family, my wife Margaret, and children Eleni, Angela and Emanuel, my brother, Dr Sid Papapetros, my co-director of the Kvinno Centre, Dr Patricia M. Skilling, and the staff at the Kvinno Centre, Carole Yelas, Linda Casey, Maria O'Keefe, Margeurite Madigan and Joan McCredie.

No enterprise can be achieved without passion, the interest of other colleagues, and above all, teamwork. My hospital, Royal Perth Hospital, has been immensely supportive. Much of the experimental work was done with internal hospital support. I am especially indebted to Dr Bill Beresford, Director of Medical Services, Drs Jim Anderson and Richard Mendelson, Department of Radiology, Mr Ed Scull and Dr Richard Fox Department of Medical Physics, Professor Mark Bush, Department of Mechanical and Materials Engineering, University of Western Australia (UWA), Professor Yianni Attikiouzel, Centre for Intelligence Processing, UWA, Professor Byron Kakulas from the Department of Neuropathology, Professor John Papadimitriou and Dr Len Matz from the Department of Pathology, Dr Ivor Surveyor from the Department of Nuclear Medicine, Mr Terry York Director of the animal laboratory, personnel from the Departments of Pathology, Morbid Anatomy, Bacteriology and Biochemistry, Dr John Chambers, Emeritus Gynaecologist, and Dr Graham Smith, Head of Department Gynaecology, colleagues from the Department of Surgery, UWA, in particular Professor Bruce Gray, and Dr G Hool.

Several colleagues played a seminal role in the late 1980s and early 1990s. In Australia, Dr Peter Richardson, Chairman of the National Association of Specialist Obstetricians and Gynaecologists and Dr Colin Douglas Smith Emeritus Consultant from King Edward Hospital who made a prospective case by case assessment of 85 patients on behalf of the Hospital Benefits Fund of Western Australia. His conclusion that the surgical operations had largely fulfilled the predictions of the Integral Theory was a key factor in the wider propagation of the surgery. Since 1995, an ever-growing group of Gynaecological Surgeons belonging to the Association of Ambulatory Vaginal and Incontinence Surgeons (AAVIS) have used the Integral Theory diagnostic system and have learnt the various operations derived from the theory. I am indebted to the AAVIS President, Dr WB Molloy, Secretary, Dr Bruce Farnsworth, and Treasurer, Dr Laurie Boshell for their invaluable advice and assistance. I acknowledge a major intellectual debt to Dr Robert Zacharin whose 1961 anatomical works provided an inspirational starting point for the Integral Theory.

In December, 1989 I met the late Professor Ulf Ulmsten from the University of Uppsala. We began a close and productive collaboration lasting some years. During this time we published the 1990 and 1993 publications of the Integral Theory, and in time I became Associate Professor in his department. Coming from a clinical surgical background, it was a revelation for me to work in Uppsala in an environment which gave such emphasis to basic science, and I hungrily absorbed this scientific milieu until it became part of my being. Ulf Ulmsten opened the door to many Scandinavian works on urodynamics, to which he himself had made some major contributions. I maintain a strong interest in urodynamics to this day. Through Ulf Ulmsten I met Professor Ingelman -Sundberg, the father of Urogynaecology whose writings I studied. In 1994 I met Professor Michael Swash who encouraged my interest in faecal incontinence, and with whom I later collaborated in studies of myogenic changes in patients with urinary incontinence. Another major intellectual influence in the development of the anatomically-based surgical techniques described in this book was the late Professor David Nichols, whom I knew and with whom I corresponded. Nichols in turn acknowledged his debt to major English, American, German and Austrian anatomists and surgeons, as do I. Over the years I have travelled widely in Europe, Asia, North and South America, teaching and being taught. To all these colleagues, I express my gratitude for affording me that privilege.

In particular, I would like to thank Dr Victoria D'Abrera, FRCPath FRCPA and Carole Yelas for their invaluable scrutiny of the final text. The process of writing this book was managed by Mr Gary Burke. His insights have given the book a coherence which I hope translates into readability. Mr Sam Blight has added his creativity to the basic diagrams. Finally a special thanks to Yvonne Bell from Springer, whose assistance made this book possible.

Peter Papa Petros
Perth, 2004

Foreword

The initial objective of this work was to reduce stress incontinence surgery from a major surgical procedure (requiring up to ten days in hospital) to a minor day-care operation. From the beginning it was clear that the two major impediments to achieving this goal were post operative pain and urinary retention. Addressing these problems became a long and winding road and culminated in the Integral Theory.

The IVS 'tension-free' tape operation was inspired by Dr Robert Zacharin's anatomical studies. Though Zacharin suggested that the ligaments and muscles around the urethra were important for urinary continence control, he did not say how. The observation that implanted foreign materials created scar tissue led to the hypothesis that a plastic tape inserted in the position of the pubourethral ligament, would leave behind sufficient scar tissue to reinforce that ligament, which would then anchor the muscles for urethral closure.

In September 1986, two prototype Intravaginal Sling operations were performed. A Mersilene tape was inserted with neither tension nor elevation, in the position of the pubourethral ligament. Restoration of continence was immediate and both patients were discharged on the day following surgery without requirement for catheterization. There was minimal pain, and immediate restoration of continence. After six weeks the tapes were removed. Both patients were still continent at last review 10 years later. The results appeared to confirm the importance of a midurethral anchoring point. Furthermore, as there was no elevation of the bladder neck, the results cast doubt on the validity of the prevailing 'pressure equalization theory' of Enhorning.

In 1987, with Professor John Papadimitriou and colleagues from Royal Perth Hospital, a series of experimental animal studies was performed to scientifically analyse the safety, efficacy and modus operandi of a tape implantation. Tape implantation was found to be safe and it worked by creating a linear deposition of collagen in the position of implantation.

The first of 30 operations were performed at Royal Perth Hospital, Western Australia, between 1988 and 1989. An adjustable intravaginal Mersilene sling was sited at midurethra. The sling was set in an elevated position but this caused urgency and obstructed flow post-operatively. As the sling was lowered, these symptoms disappeared, yet most of the patients remained cured of their stress incontinence.

On comparing the pre-operative and post-operative x-rays, no elevation of bladder base was evident. This appeared to invalidate the 'Pressure Equalization Theory' for maintenance of urinary continence. Furthermore, when the midurethral tape was anchored by grasping it with a haemostat, the distal urethra was seen to move forward, but the Foley balloon catheter moved backwards and downwards around the midurethral point. From these observations the concept of two separate closure 'mechanisms' emerged. Over the space of a year, a theoretical framework that integrated these disparate findings with known anatomy was developed (the Integral Theory 1990). The key concepts were that the suspensory ligaments were essential for normal bladder function, and that bladder dysfunction occurred because of connective tissue damage within these same ligaments.

In 1990 a collaboration with Professor Ulf Ulmsten began. Further studies were performed, and the first formulation of the Integral Theory was published:

For different reasons, stress and urge derive mainly from laxity in the vagina or its supporting ligaments, a result of altered collagen/elastin.

Separate urethral and bladder neck closure mechanisms were described. Abdominal ultrasound studies in 1990 demonstrated that the urethra was closed from behind by the hammock closure mechanism. Bladder instability in the non-neurological patient was defined as a premature activation of the micturition reflex.

In 1993 the second exposition of the Integral Theory presented radiological and urodynamic studies and brought a higher level of proof.

Five prototype suburethral sling operations for stress incontinence were analysed with reference to *modus operandi* and surgical methodology (1993 Integral Theory). A problem that remained was the relatively high rate of Mersilene tape erosion. This was largely solved in 1996 by Professor Ulmsten's Scandinavian group (Ulmsten et al. 1996) through use of a polypropylene mesh tape. The 'posterior fornix syndrome' was described (1993 Integral Theory). Reconstruction of the posterior ligaments improved symptoms of urge, nocturia, abnormal emptying and pelvic pain. These findings were seminal in the construction of the Pictorial Diagnostic Algorithm.

The ten years to 2003 has seen a consolidation and international acceptance of many parts of the Integral Theory, in particular, the treatment of stress incontinence with a midurethral sling. The Theory framework has expanded to include faecal incontinence, abnormal emptying, and some types of pelvic pain. New ultrasound and urodynamic techniques promise to improve diagnostic accuracy, especially when used with the 'simulated operations' technique described later in this book. Improvements in surgical methodology have been running on a parallel path with the expansion of the Integral Theory. These new methods were developed because traditional vaginal surgery methods of excision and approximation were unable to restore tissue strength sufficiently to restore structure, as described by the Integral Theory system. To overcome this deficiency, double layered techniques such as the 'bridge' repair, which recycles excess vaginal tissue (Petros 1998), and the Posterior IVS (Petros 2001) were developed. Tightening the suburethral hammock in addition to a midurethral sling has increased the cure rate for stress incontinence and intrinsic sphincter defect (Petros 1997). The posterior sling has been further improved and simplified.

In particular, the new tissue fixation system (TFS) appears to be a major advance on the existing 'tension-free tape' slings in that it is possible to repair *any* ligament or fascial defect in the pelvic floor. The TFS operations are more anatomical, far less invasive, and they are able to be performed *under direct vision*.

This book has been written in the hope that it will further clarify and disseminate the ideas of the Integral Theory and help provide the basis required for further advances in theory, diagnosis and surgical techniques to alleviate problems in the female pelvic floor.

Chapter 1 is an introduction and overview of the Integral Theory. It outlines the 'problem' being addressed, that is, the various symptoms of pelvic floor dysfunction, current knowledge and treatments. The overview explains normal function, and introduces the causes of dysfunction, diagnosis of damaged structures and the principles of minimally invasive surgical repair according to the Integral Theory.

Chapter 2 aims to familiarize the reader with the roles of ligaments and muscle forces and describes how they work synergistically to maintain form and function of the pelvic organs. It describes the anatomy of the pelvic floor, the interrelated roles of bone, muscles, ligaments and organs in the context of structure, form and biomechanics. It describes the static and dynamic anatomy of the pelvic floor and the seminal role played by connective tissue in function and dysfunction. It introduces the concept of the 'three zones' of the vagina, which is a central part of the Integral Theory diagnostic system, surgical anatomy and techniques.

Chapter 3 describes the Integral Theory system for diagnosis of connective tissue damage in the three zones of the vagina. Two diagnostic pathways are discussed in detail: the Clinical Diagnostic pathway, suitable for the general clinician, and the Structured Assessment pathway for use in specialist pelvic floor clinics. The components of these pathways and their role in the diagnostic process are described thoroughly. The concept of the 'simulated operation', used for verification of diagnosis, is introduced. This is an invaluable part of the Integral Theory system. It is used for preoperative direct testing of the zone of diagnosed anatomical damage.

Chapter 4 discusses the conceptual basis for minimally invasive pelvic floor surgery and introduces a new perspective on the surgical anatomy of the three zones of the vagina. It presents the minimally invasive surgical techniques developed for addressing anatomical defects in each of the zones, in particular the 'tension-free' tape anterior and posterior slings, and introduces the tissue fixation system.

Chapter 5 explains the pelvic floor rehabilitation exercises that were developed from the Integral Theory approach. Originally these exercises were designed as an alternative to surgery, but it has been found that they also assist the patient in maintaining the benefits they have attained from surgery.

Chapter 6 gives an anatomical basis for the 'mapping' of connective tissue dysfunction and the anatomical basis for urodynamics is explained. Many of the internal contradictions within conventional urodynamics are explained using the Chaos Theory framework, non-linear methodology and Boolean algebra. Boolean algebra is used to explain the concept of switching between the closed and open phases of the bladder. There are descriptions of the expanded use of transperineal ultrasound to the middle and posterior zones.

Chapter 7 discusses current and emerging issues related to further enhancement of the Integral Theory system, in particular, faecal incontinence. The potential of the new scientific concepts, methodologies and technologies in making the diagnostic process more efficient is discussed. The Integral Theory Diagnostic System (ITDS), a computer based diagnostic system, incorporating the potential of a large data base developed across the internet is presented.

Chapter 8 is the conclusion. It briefly tracks the evolution of the Integral Theory from theory to working system and discusses the future importance of the internet for this new direction for pelvic floor science.

The questionnaire and other tools used in the diagnostic process are included and described in Appendix 1. References and further reading are included in Appendix 2.

Contents

Contents

List of Frequently Used Abbreviations and Acronyms

A	anus
AAVIS	Association of Ambulatory Vaginal and Incontinence Surgeons
ATFP	arcus tendineus fascia pelvis
BN	bladder neck
BNE	bladder neck elevation
C	closure phase of the bladder/urethra
CL	cardinal ligament
CP	closure pressure
CT	connective tissue
CX	cervix
CTR	cough transmission ratio
DI	detrusor instability
EAS	external anal sphincter
EUL	external urethral ligament
F	fascia
FI	faecal incontinence
GAGS	glycosaminoglycans
GSI	genuine stress incontinence
H	suburethral vagina (hammock)
ICS	International Continence Society
IS	ischial spine
ISD	intrinsic sphincter defect
ITDS	Integral Theory Diagnostic Support System
IVS	Intravaginal slingplasty
LA	levator ani - anterior portion of PCM
LP	levator plate
LMA	longitudinal muscle of the anus
MUCP	maximal urethral closure pressure
N	nerve endings/stretch receptors
O	opening phase of the bladder/urethra
PB	perineal body
PM	perineal membrane
PAP	post-anal plate
POPQ	The ICS prolapse classification
PCF	pubocervical fascia
PCM	pubococcygeus muscle
PNCT	pudendal nerve conduction times
PofD	Pouch of Douglas
PS	pubic symphysis
PRM	puborectalis muscle
PUL	pubourethral ligament
PUSM	periurethral striated muscle
PVL	pubovesical ligament
RVF	rectovaginal fascia
R	rectum
S	sacrum
SI	stress incontinence
T	Tapes
TFS	tissue fixation system
U	urethra
USL	uterosacral ligament
UT	uterus
V	vagina
ZCE	zone of critical elasticity

Nocturia

Nocturia is defined as a problem when it occurs more than two times per night. Causation is mostly unknown and it is treated with drugs or bladder training, both of which are not effective in the longer term.

Bowel Dysfunction

Bowel dysfunction has two elements, difficulty with evacuation ('constipation') and incontinence, involuntary loss of wind or faeces (FI). FI causation is unknown, but is thought to be due to anal sphincter or pelvic muscle damage. The prevalence of all bowel dysfunctions in women varies between 10 and 20%. Treatment usually consists of drugs to slow down the bowel action, diet and operations such as levatorplasty. None of these treatments are particularly effective.

Abnormal Bladder Emptying

Abnormal bladder emptying can be defined as difficulty in bladder evacuation. It has specific symptoms and can present as chronic urinary infection due to a high residual urine. Conventionally it is treated with urethral dilatation, even though there is no obstruction and the treatment is not very effective.

Chronic Pelvic Pain

Chronic pelvic pain is characterized by a one-sided 'dragging' pain, of varying severity. The incidence can be as high as 20% of women. The cause is unknown but is thought to be psychological.

Other Problems

'Interstitial Cystitis' is a debilitating condition. The cause is unknown and no long term effective treatment is known. 'Vulvodynia' may occur in 10% of women. Symptoms can be severe in affected women. Causation is unknown. Treatment is empirical, and not always effective.

1.1.2 The Integral Theory - A New Perspective

In the pages that follow, the scientific framework and contemporary practical applications of the Integral Theory approach to improving the above problems are presented. For some practitioners, it will be a new way of looking at anatomy and incontinence problems. It has been the aim of the author to present explanations for the specialist, general practitioner, and even the general public who may have a specific interest in understanding the origins and curative options for these pelvic floor disorders.

1.1.3 A Guide to the Diagrams Used in this Book

Many diagrams are used in this book to illustrate the components of various aspects of pelvic floor function and dysfunction. The purpose of the following series of diagrams is to familiarize the reader with the anatomical structures as well as the abbreviations and acronyms used. It is hoped that the reader will spend a few minutes contemplating these generic diagrams so that the general flow of the text can be more easily followed as the diagrams become more complex.

Series 1 Static Anatomy

Figures 1-01 to 1-04 illustrate the organs and connective tissue structures.

Fig. 1-01 (right) Pelvis with organs: urethra and bladder are green, vagina is blue and rectum is brown.

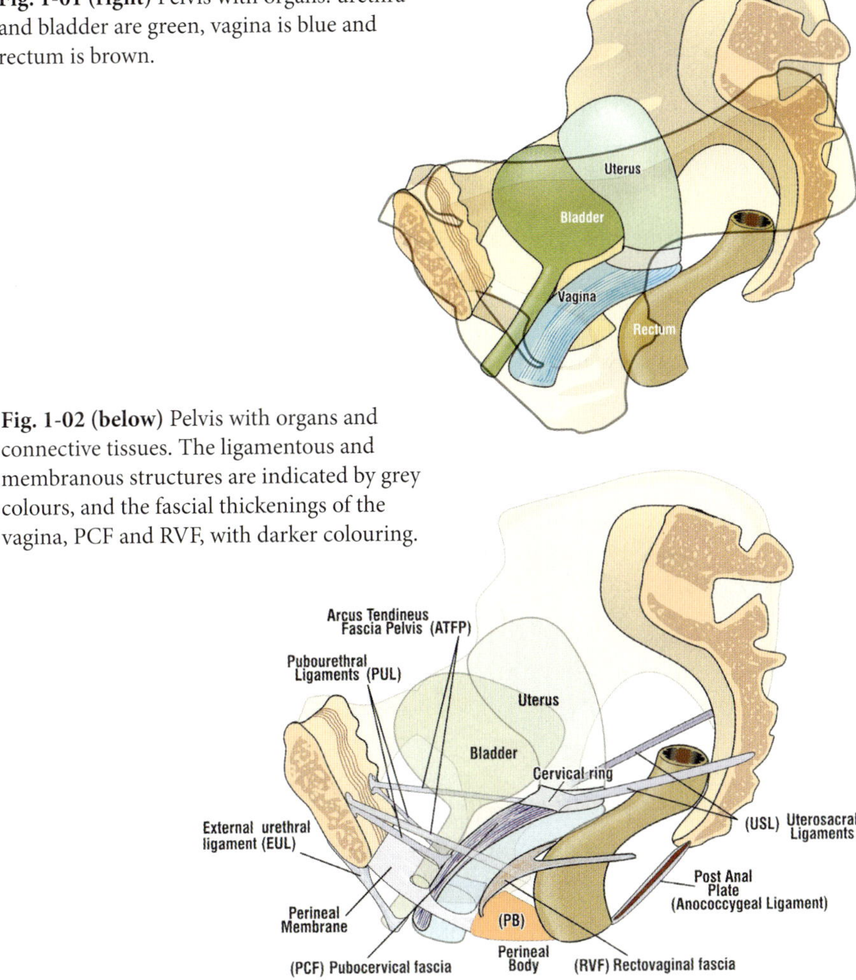

Fig. 1-02 (below) Pelvis with organs and connective tissues. The ligamentous and membranous structures are indicated by grey colours, and the fascial thickenings of the vagina, PCF and RVF, with darker colouring.

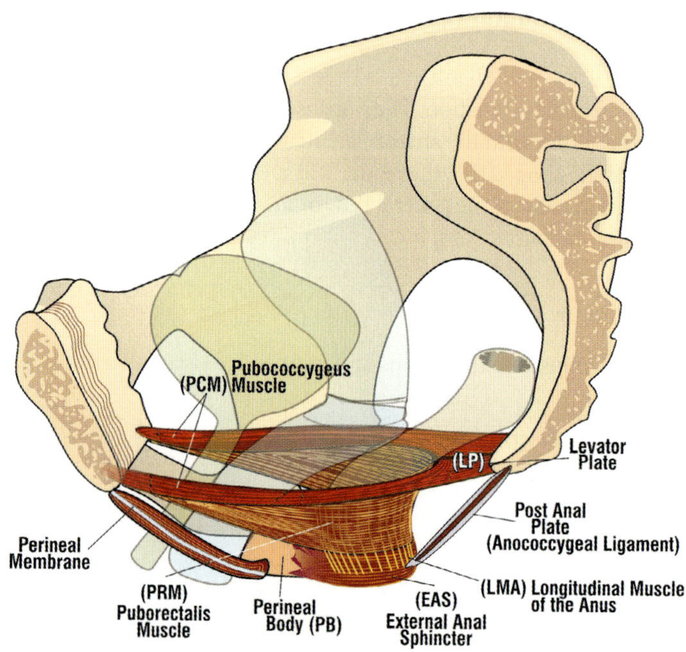

Fig. 1-03 Pelvis with organs and muscles – Muscles are brown colours with striations.

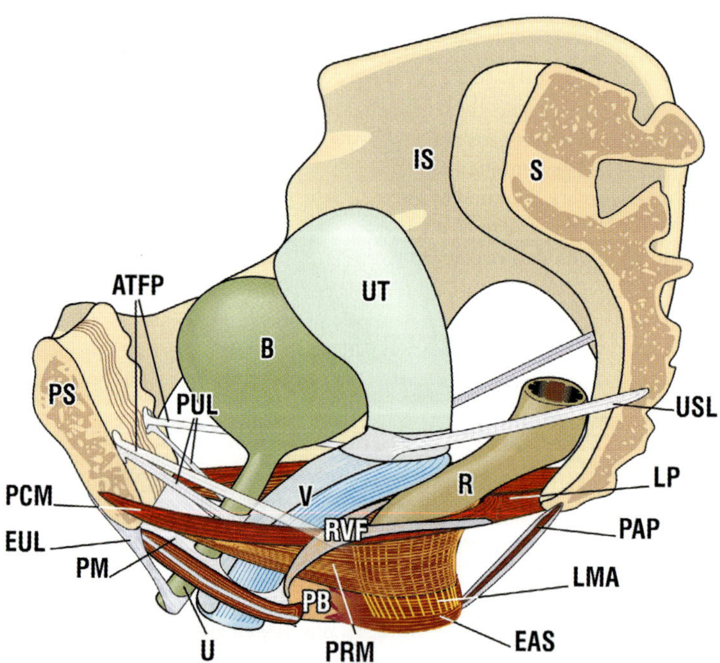

Fig. 1-04 The relationship of the pelvic muscles to organs, ligaments and fascia

Series 2 Dynamic Anatomy

Figure 1-05 shows the components involved in the transition from static to dynamic anatomy.

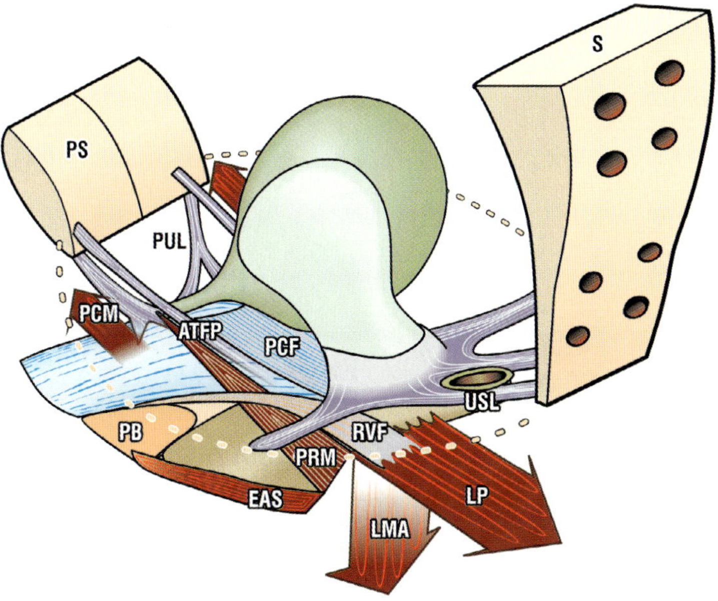

Fig. 1-05 Transition diagram, from static to dynamic - The arrows represent the directional closure forces and are marked according to their derivation. These forces act against the suspensory ligaments PUL, ATFP and USL to stretch the three organs.

Bone:

  PS = pubic symphysis;

  S = sacrum.

Suspensory ligaments:

  PUL = pubourethral ligament;

  ATFP = arcus tendineus fascia pelvis;

  USL = uterosacral ligament.

Muscle forces:

  PCM = pubococcygeus muscle;

  LP = levator plate;

  LMA = longitudinal muscle of the anus;

  PRM = puborectalis muscle.

Supporting fascia:

  PCF = pubocervical fascia;

  RVF = rectovaginal fascia.

Perineal anchoring structures:

  PB = perineal body;

  EAS = external anal sphincter.

Series 3 Functional Anatomy

Figures 1-06 and 1-07 illustrate the transition from dynamic to functional anatomy. They show three pelvic muscle forces acting during normal closure (fig 1-06), and two pelvic muscle forces acting during normal opening (micturition) (fig 1-07).

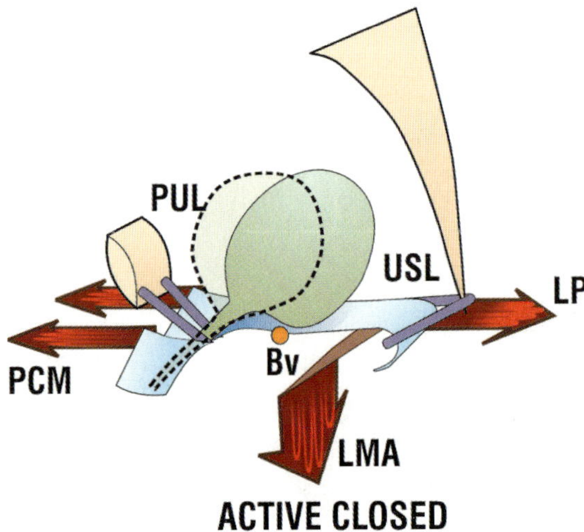

Fig. 1-06 Active Closure. This diagram shows how three muscle forces stretch and close the urethra and bladder neck. Arrows = muscle forces. Blue = vagina; green = bladder and urethra; yellow = bone. Bv = attachment of bladder base to vagina.

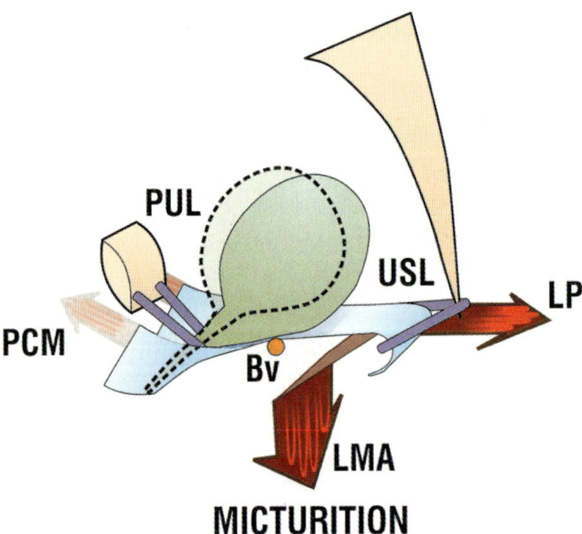

Fig. 1-07 Micturition. This diagram shows how two muscle forces (red arrows) open out the urethra once the anterior muscle force (PCM) relaxes.

1.2 Overview of Pelvic Floor Function and Dysfunction According to the Integral Theory

As the name suggests, the Integral Theory is an interrelated and dynamic anatomical framework for understanding pelvic floor function and dysfunction. The pelvic floor is an interrelated system where the whole is greater than the sum of the parts. The fundamental principle of the Integral Theory is that the *restoration of form (structure) leads to restoration of function*. Although 'form' and 'structure' are used interchangeably throughout the book, they are slightly different. 'Structure' is a static concept. 'Form' is a dynamic concept and carries the connotation that damaged connective tissue structures may cause loss of form (shape) and therefore, function. Hence the importance of an accurate diagnosis of the location of the damaged structure prior to surgery. The Integral Theory may be stated thus:

> *Symptoms of stress, urge, and abnormal emptying mainly derive, for different reasons, from laxity in the vagina or its supporting ligaments, a result of altered connective tissue.*

More recently, the Theory has been expanded to include idiopathic faecal incontinence and some types of pelvic pain.

1.2.1 Basic Tenets of the Integral Theory

The Integral Theory emphasizes the role of the connective tissue of the vagina and its supporting ligaments in both function and dysfunction, as well as in surgical correction. The Integral Theory views normal pelvic floor function as a balanced, interrelated system composed of muscle, connective tissue (CT) and nerve components, with connective tissue being the most vulnerable to damage.

To help explain the Integral Theory, two key analogies are used, the suspension bridge analogy for structure, and the trampoline analogy for function.

The clinical application of the Integral Theory culminates in the Pictorial Diagnostic Algorithm (fig. 1-11). This algorithm provides the surgeon with a guide to the anatomical causes of dysfunction and the damaged structures that may need repairing. The surgical techniques developed from the Integral Theory focus on reinforcing damaged ligaments and fascia with polypropylene tapes, and preserving vaginal tissue and elasticity, especially in the bladder neck area of the vagina. This approach reduces pain and urinary retention and allows the surgery to be performed on a day-care or overnight stay basis with early return to normal activities.

The Integral Theory System, when applied to pelvic floor rehabilitation, focuses on strengthening structures of the pelvic floor - muscle, nerve and connective tissue – all of which work synergistically as a dynamic system.

Form and Structure: The Suspension Bridge Analogy

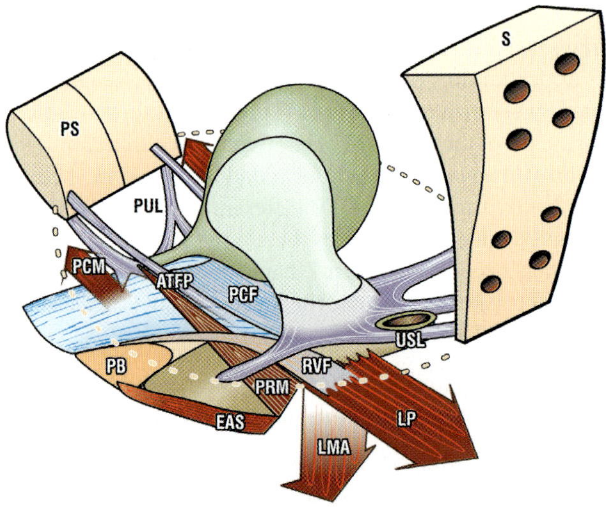

Fig. 1-05 Form – This diagram illustrates the synergism of the pelvic floor structures. It shows how the organs are suspended by ligaments and stretched by muscle forces acting against these same ligaments to create form and strength.

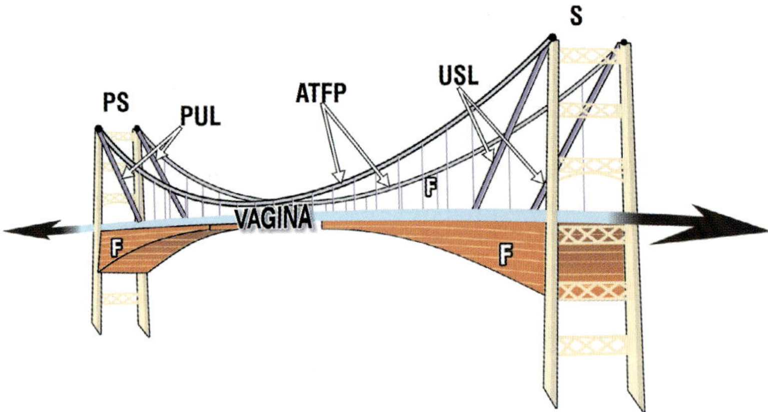

Fig. 1-08 Structure - The suspension bridge analogy. The suspension bridge analogy illustrates how the pelvic structures are interdependent. In a suspension bridge strength is maintained through tensioning of suspensory steel wires (arrows). Weakening any one part of the structure may disturb the equilibrium, strength and function of the whole. Relating the analogy to figure 1-05, form (ie shape and strength) is achieved because the vagina and bladder are suspended from the bony pelvis by ligaments (PUL, USL, ATFP) and fascia (F). The structural dimension develops when these are stretched by muscle forces (arrows).

Structure and Form

Structure and form in the pelvic floor arise from the interaction of muscles, nerves and ligaments acting on the pelvic organs. The vagina and ligaments must be stretched to their limit of extension to attain the strength required to carry loads. Unequal balance of the forces may stretch the system one way or the other, thereby affecting opening or closure. The 'suspension bridge' analogy (figs 1-05 and 1-08) is used to illustrate how structure and form (and thereby function) arise from a system in balanced tension.

Function and Dysfunction

The Integral Theory describes normal bladder function as having two stable states: closed (continence) and opening (micturition). These states are deemed to be stable because they are the resultants of a balance of forces.

Three muscle forces interact during closure (fig 1-06) and two muscle forces interact during opening (fig 1-07). If the efficacy or balance of these muscle forces is disrupted through damage to their ligamentous anchoring points (fig 1-09), dysfunction may result in *both* closure (incontinence) or opening (abnormal emptying).

Causes of Dysfunction - Delineating the Zones of Damage

The damaged suspensory ligaments and associated fascia are sited in three zones: anterior, middle and posterior (fig 1-09). The anterior zone extends from the external urethral meatus to the bladder neck, and contains *three structures* which may be damaged: the pubourethral ligament (PUL), the suburethral hammock, and the external urethral ligament (EUL) (see figs 2-03 and fig 2-04).

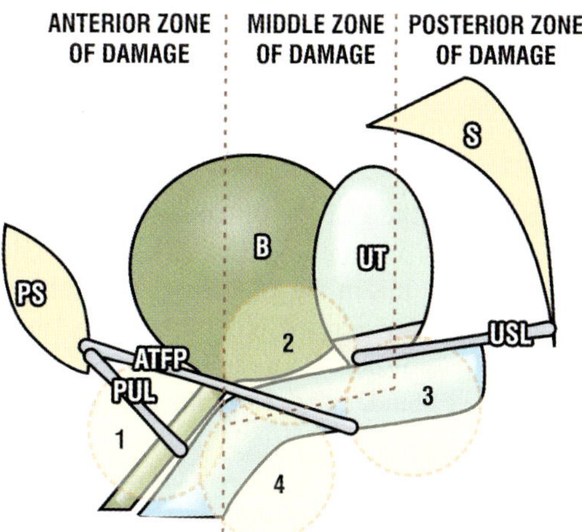

Fig. 1-09 The causes of dysfunction: the zones of damage. The circles represent the foetal head descending through the birth canal. Damage to one or more ligaments leads to imbalance of the system and hence dysfunction. Congenitally defective collagen may also cause dysfunction.

The middle zone extends from the bladder neck to the cervix or hysterectomy scar. It contains *three structures* which may be damaged: the pubocervical fascia (PCF), the arcus tendineus fasciae pelvis (ATFP), and the anterior cervical ring.

The posterior zone extends from the cervix or hysterectomy scar to the perineal body. The uterosacral ligaments (USL), rectovaginal fascia (RVF) and perineal body (PB) are the key posterior zone structures which may be damaged.

Locating the damaged structures within the zones

Within each zone are key structures which facilitate normal pelvic floor function. If any of these is damaged, dysfunction may result. The Integral Theory delineates nine key structures in which damage may occur. The three zones each contain three main stuctures which may be damaged (fig 1-10). They are:

Anterior Zone

Excess Laxity

1. External urethral ligament (EUL)
2. Suburethral vagina (hammock)
3. Pubourethral ligament (PUL)

Middle Zone

Excess Laxity

4. Arcus tendineus fascia pelvis (ATFP)
5. Pubocervical fascia (PCF) (midline defect - cystocoele)
6. Cervical ring attachment of PCF (high cystocoele)

Excessive tightness

'ZCE' - Excessive tightness in the 'Zone of critical elasticity' (ZCE) (cause: excess scarring; excess elevation with colposuspension)

Posterior Zone

Excess Laxity

7. Uterosacral ligaments (USL)
8. Rectovaginal fascia (RVF)
9. Perineal body (PB).

Note that the ZCE is part of the PCF. It is included here as a separate structure to emphasize the importance of maintaining elasticity at the bladder neck area of the vagina (ZCE) during surgery. It is in the ZCE where the 'tethered vagina syndrome' originates. The 'tethered vagina syndrome' is described fully later in this book. Briefly, it is caused by loss of elasticity at ZCE from vaginal or bladder neck elevation surgery due to scarring or excessive bladder neck elevation. It is entirely iatrogenic.

Diagnosis of Damage

The Pictorial Diagnostic Algorithm (fig 1-11) provides an efficient method for locating and remedying structural damage or pelvic floor dysfunction. It summarizes in graphical form the relationship between structural damage in the three zones and symptoms of dysfunction. By using the 'simulated operations' technique (described later) and other

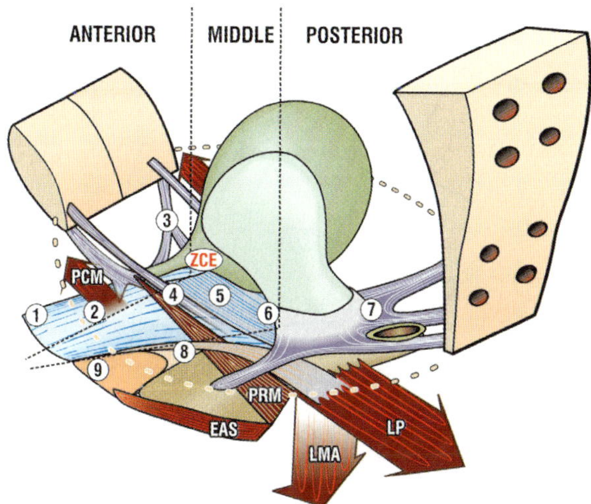

Fig. 1-10 The nine main connective tissue structures potentially needing surgical repair.

empirical research, it has been found that certain symptoms occur more frequently in one zone than another. The Pictorial Diagnostic Algorithm illustrates these varying probabilities. Most importantly, it shows that *almost any symptom may be caused by dysfunction in any zone*, even if the probability is very small. The Pictorial Diagnostic Algorithm is the key to the clinical application of the Integral Theory system.

Surgical Repair of Connective Tissue Structures

Reconstructive pelvic floor surgery according to the Integral Theory differs from conventional surgery in four ways:

1. It is minimally invasive (day-care).
2. It is based on specific surgical principles which minimise risk, pain and discomfort to the patient.
3. It takes an holistic approach to pelvic floor dysfunction by isolating the contribution(s) of each zone of the vagina to dysfunction.
4. It has a symptom-based emphasis (the Pictorial Diagnostic Algorithm) which expands the surgical indicators to include cases with major symptoms and only minimal prolapse.

In keeping with the overall framework of the Integral Theory, the surgical techniques are organised by zone. The zones consist of nine key structures which potentially need repair in pelvic reconstructive surgery (fig 1-10). Using a special delivery system, polypropylene tapes are inserted as an anterior sling at midurethra, a posterior sling in the position of the USLs, and other positions according to which structure in which zone has been damaged (fig 1-12).

The uterus needs to be conserved wherever possible. It is the central anchoring point for the posterior ligaments (USL), the rectovaginal fascia (RVF) and the pubocervical fascia (PCF). The descending branch of the uterine artery is a major

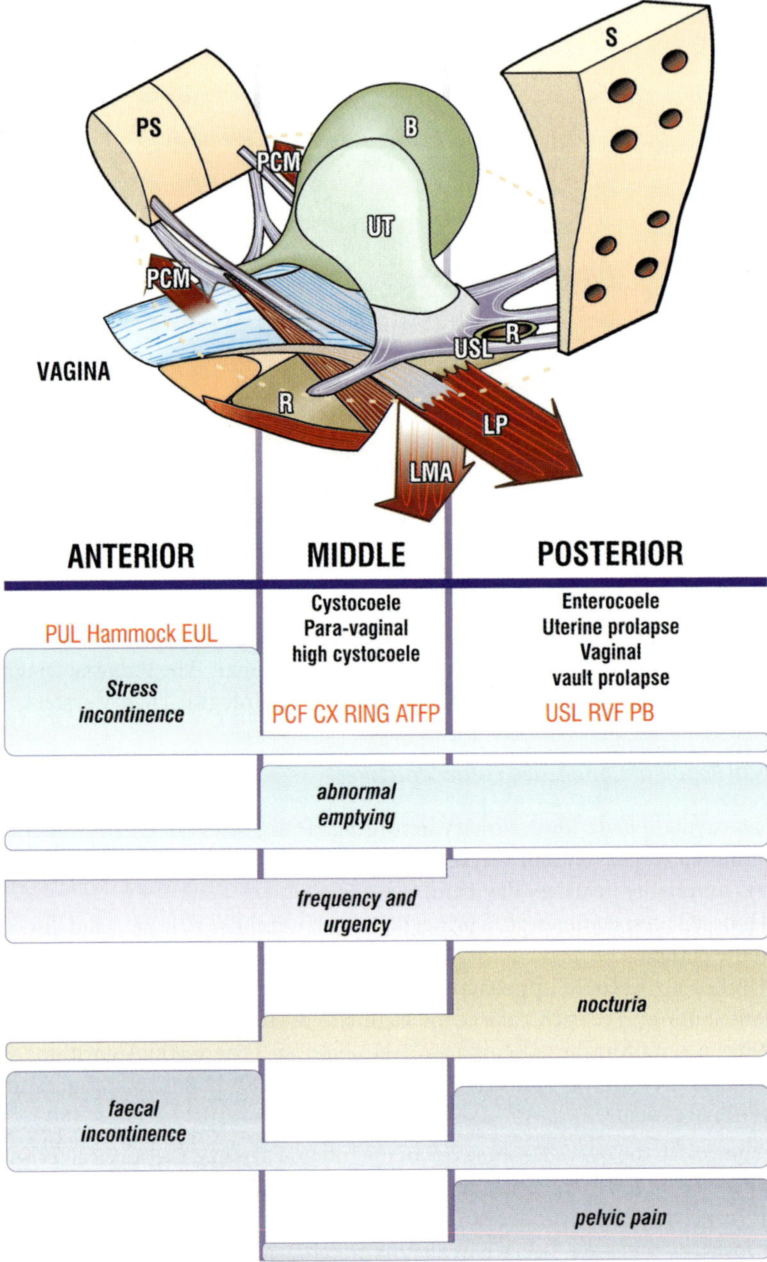

Fig. 1-11 The Pictorial Diagnostic Algorithm summarizes the relationships between structural damage in the three zones and symptoms. The size of the bar gives an approximate indication of the prevalence (probability) of the symptom. The same connective tissue structures in each zone (red lettering) may cause prolapse and abnormal symptoms.

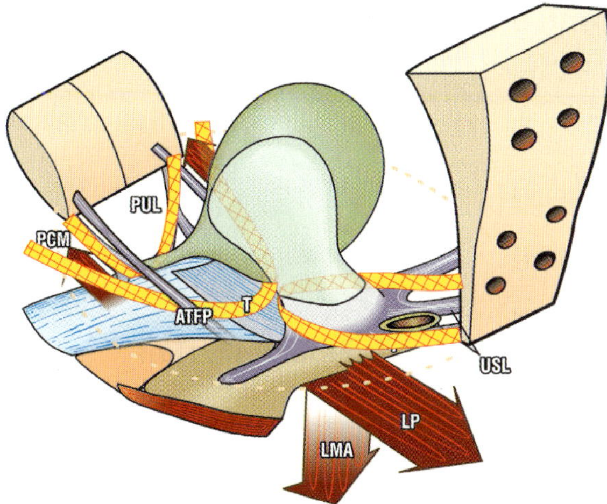

Fig. 1-12 Polypropylene tapes 'T' may be used to reinforce the three main suspensory ligaments – pubourethral (PUL), uterosacral (USL) and arcus tendineus fascia pelvis (ATFP).

blood supply for these structures, and should be conserved where possible even if subtotal hysterectomy is performed.

1.3   Summary Chapter 1

The pelvic floor consists of an interrelated system of muscles, ligaments and nerves, with connective tissue being the most vulnerable to damage.

The Integral Theory specifies that damaged connective tissue in the suspensory ligaments or fascia may cause the following symptoms:

- stress incontinence
- urge incontinence
- frequency
- nocturia
- abnormal emptying
- faecal incontinence
- pelvic pain.

The Pictorial Diagnostic Algorithm is based on a relationship between specific symptoms and connective tissue damage in three zones of the vagina. It indicates which connective tissue structures have been damaged. The main structures damaged are the pubourethral ligament in the anterior zone, pubocervical fascia and ATFP in the middle zone, and uterosacral ligaments in the posterior zone. Minimally invasive surgical operations repair the damaged ligaments and abnormal symptoms by precise insertion of polypropylene tapes in the position of the damaged ligaments. This is based on the surgical principle that restoration of form leads to restoration of function.

The Anatomy and Dynamics of Pelvic Floor Function and Dysfunction

2.1 The Anatomy of Pelvic Floor Function

2.1.1 Introduction

Pelvic anatomy may be defined as those bones, muscles, ligaments and organs which contribute to normal pelvic floor function.

Ligaments, muscles and fascia constitute a musculo-elastic system which gives form and function to the organs of the pelvic floor.

Connective tissue is a generic term generally applied to tissues which contain collagen, proteoglycans and sometimes elastin.

Fascia is defined as that fibromuscular tissue which suspends or strengthens the organs, or connects them to muscles. Fascia is composed of smooth muscle, collagen, elastin, nerves and blood vessels and may form part of the wall of the vagina. Fascia is the main structural component of the vagina. Discrete thickenings may be termed ligaments.

The organs of the pelvis are the bladder, vagina and rectum. None of these has any inherent shape or strength (fig 2-01). While the role of fascia is to strengthen and support the organs, the role of the ligaments is to suspend the organs and act as anchoring points for the muscles. Muscle forces stretch the organs to contribute to their shape, form and strength.

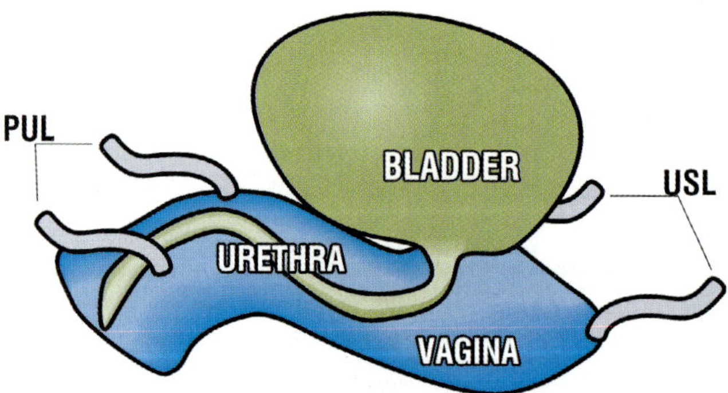

Fig. 2-01 Vagina and urethra have no inherent shape or strength when the suspensory ligaments are severed. Likewise, loose ligaments weaken the muscle forces which provide form and function to healthy organs. PUL = pubourethral ligament; USL = uterosacral ligament.

2.1.2 The Role of Ligaments, Muscles and Fascia in Creating Form, Strength and Function

The pelvic organs, urethra, vagina and rectum, have no inherent form, structure or strength. Form, structure and strength are created by the synergistic action of ligaments, fascia and muscles. *Normal* function of these pelvic organs is directly dependent on the integrity of the pelvic floor structure.

2.1.3 The Role of Connective Tissue Structures

Bones and connective tissue are the main structural components of the pelvis. The connective tissue consists of ligaments and fascia. The critical elements of connective tissue are collagen and elastin, both of which are changed during pregnancy, childbirth and ageing. These changes may weaken the ligaments and fascia, thereby affecting the structural integrity of the pelvic floor. This may result in prolapse and affect organ function. Connective tissue structures are classified in three levels (fig 2-02).

Level 1: Uterosacral ligaments (USL), pubocervical fascia (PCF).
Level 2: Pubourethral ligaments (PUL), rectovaginal fascia (RVF).
Level 3: External urethral ligament (EUL), perineal membrane (PM), perineal body (PB).

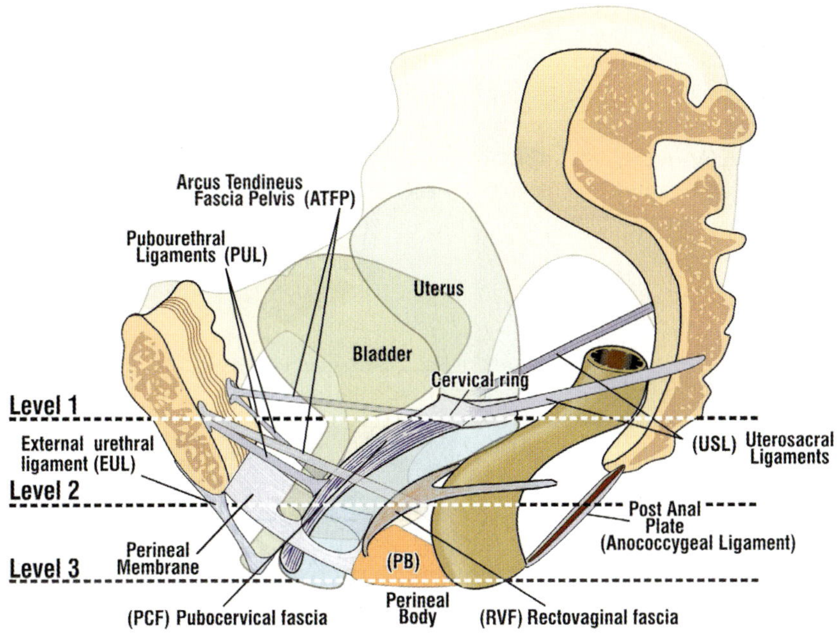

Fig. 2-02 Connective tissue levels - This is a schematic 3D sagittal section of the main connective tissue structures of the pelvis, showing their relationship to the organs and pelvic bones.

2.1.4 The Key Ligaments of the Pelvic Floor Structure

The key ligaments of the pelvic floor are the external urethral ligament (EUL), which is sited anterior to the perineal membrane, the pubourethral ligament (PUL), which lies behind the perineal membrane (urogenital diaphragm), the arcus tendineus fasciae pelvis (ATFP), the cardinal and uterosacral ligaments (USL) and the pubovesical ligament (PVL). The composition of all the suspensory ligaments and fascia is similar (fig 2-05). The presence of nerves (N), smooth muscle (Sm) and blood vessels (Vs) indicates that ligaments are active contractile structures, as is the fascial layer of the organs. The perineal body also contains striated muscle.

The Pubourethral Ligament (PUL)

The pubourethral ligament (PUL) (figs 2-03 & 2-04) originates from the lower end of the posterior surface of the pubic symphysis and descends like a fan to insert (fig 2-03) medially (M) into the midurethra and laterally (L) into the pubococcygeus muscle and vaginal wall (Zacharin 1963, Petros 1998).

The external urethral ligament (EUL) (fig 2-03 and fig 2-04) anchors the external urethral meatus to the anterior surface of the descending pubic ramus. It extends upwards to the clitoris and downwards to PUL. It is approximately equivalent to Robert Zacharin's anterior pubourethral ligament.

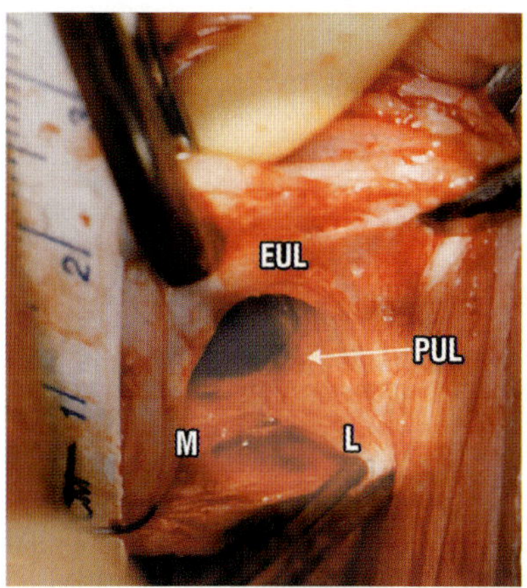

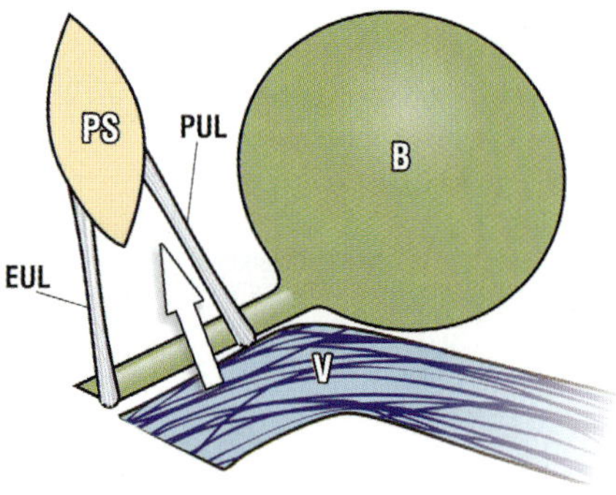

Fig. 2-04 Sagital view of fig 2-03.
Arrow = muscle force

Fig. 2-03 (Above) The suspensory ligaments of urethra - a live anatomical study. Perspective: Looking into the vagina. Incision: left paraurethral sulcus.
EUL = external urethral ligament;
PUL = pubourethral ligament;
M = medial part; L = lateral part.
Fig. 2-05 (Right) Biopsy of a pubourethral ligament. Cn = collagen; E = elastin; Vs = vessel; Sm = smooth muscle.

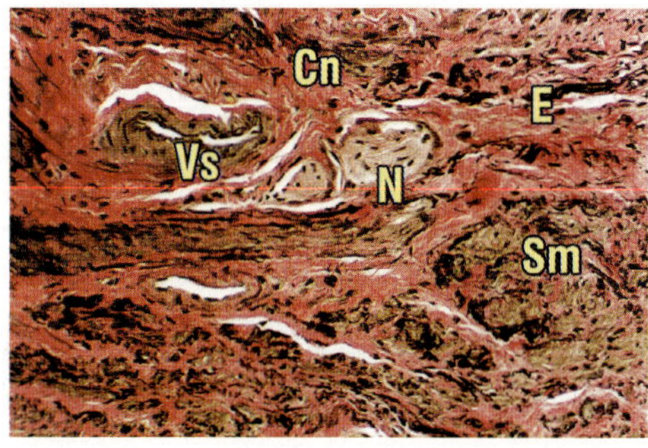

The Arcus Tendineus Fascia Pelvis (ATFP)

The ATFP (fig. 2-02) are horizontal ligaments which arise just superior to the pubourethral ligament (PUL) at the pubic symphysis and insert into the ischial spine (IS). The vagina is suspended from the ATFP by its fascia, much like a sheet slung across two washing lines (Nichols 1989). The muscle force of the levator plate and adjacent muscles tension the ATFP ligament and the vagina itself.

The Uterosacral Ligaments (USL)

The uterosacral ligaments (USL) (fig. 2-02) suspend the apex of the vagina and are the effective insertion points of the downward muscle force, the longitudinal muscle of the anus (LMA). The USL arises from the sacral vertebrate S2,3,4 and attaches to the cervical ring posteriorly. Its main vascular supply is the descending branch of the uterine artery.

The Pubovesical Ligament (PVL)

The pubovesical ligament (PVL) was described by Ingelman-Sundberg (1949) as the main structural support of the anterior wall of the bladder. It inserts into the transverse precervical arc of Gilvernet, a stiff fibromuscular structure on the anterior bladder wall (fig 2-06). PVL brings rigidity to the anterior wall of bladder.

During effort, pubococcygeus muscle (PCM) contraction stretches the hammock forwards. This anchors the urethra, and helps create the internal urethral meatus at 'O'–'O'. Levator plate (LP) and longitudinal muscle of the anus (LMA) vectors rotate the upper vagina and trigone in a plane ('O'–'O') around PVL insertion point like a ball valve, to create bladder neck closure. As this ligament is sited well away from the passage of the head in childbirth, it is rarely injured.

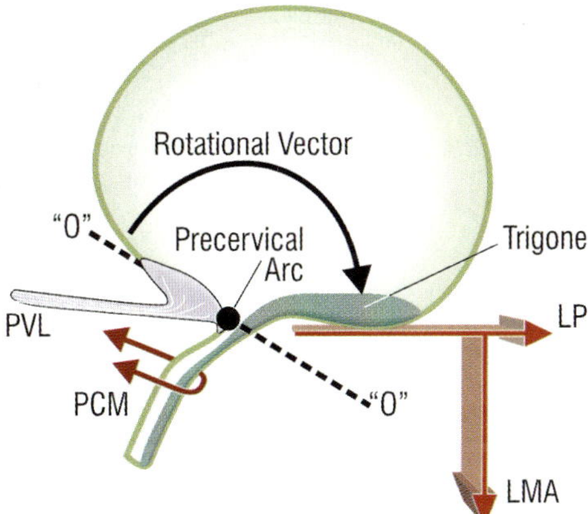

Fig. 2-06 The role of the trigone and precervical arc (PVL) in bladder neck closure. Sagittal section. Arrows represent the directional closure forces. Relaxation of PCM allows the LP/LMA vector to open out the outflow tract.

The Precervical Arc of Gilvernet

The precervical arc of Gilvernet (fig 2-06) is essentially a thickened insertion of PVL in the anterior wall of the bladder. This structure limits posterior displacement of the anterior bladder wall. It prevents inward collapse of the anterior bladder wall during micturition and it is rotated downwards to close off the bladder neck during stress.

The Trigone

The trigone (fig 2-06) forms part of the bladder base and is composed mainly of smooth muscle. It extends down the posterior wall of the urethra to the external meatus. Although it is not a ligament, it behaves like one. The trigonal extension creates a 'backbone' for the hammock muscles to pull forward in order to close off the urethra from behind. During micturition, the trigone splints the posterior urethral wall facilitating the backward stretching by LP and LMA that is required to expand the outflow tract.

Fascial attachment of the vagina to ATFP

The vagina is suspended like a trampoline between the two Arcus tendineus Fascia Pelvis (ATFP) ligaments, by lateral fascial extensions (fig 2-07). These lateral extensions fuse with the pubocervical fascia superiorly, and the rectovaginal fascia inferiorly (fig 2-08).

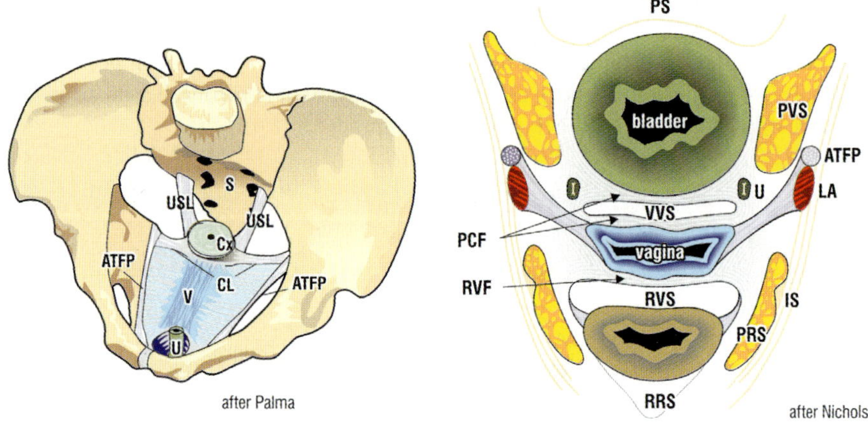

Fig. 2-07 (Above left): Vaginal attachments to ATFP. The vagina is suspended like a trampoline membrane between the Arcus Tendineus Fascia Pelvis (ATFP) ligaments laterally, the anterior part of the cervical ring, and its collagenous extensions onto the cardinal ligament (CL).

Fig. 2-08 (Above right): The connective tissue spaces. Perspective: transverse section, horizontal part of vagina just anterior to cervix. PVS = paravesical space; VVS = vesicovaginal space; RVS = rectovaginal space; RRS = retrorectal space; RVF = rectovaginal fascia; U = ureter; PCF = pubocervical fascia; ATFP = Arcus Tendineus Fascia Pelvis; IS = ischial spine; LA = m. levator ani.

Organ Spaces

The fascial components of the organs are separated from each other by spaces (fig 2-08), and these spaces allow the organs to move independently of each other during organ opening, closure and especially, during intercourse. These spaces provide an avascular dissection plane during surgery.

The Pubocervical Fascia

The pubocervical fascia (PCF) stretches from the lateral sulci to the anterior part of the cervical ring (fig 1-05). The anterior part of the cervical ring in turn fuses with the cardinal ligament. Separation of the fascia from the ring may cause a high cystocoele, or even an anterior enterocoele.

The Rectovaginal Fascia

The rectovaginal fascia or Fascia of Denonvilliers, extends as a sheet between the lateral rectal pillars, from the perineal body below to the levator plate above (fig 1-05). It is attached to the uterosacral ligaments (USL) and the fascia surrounding the cervix.

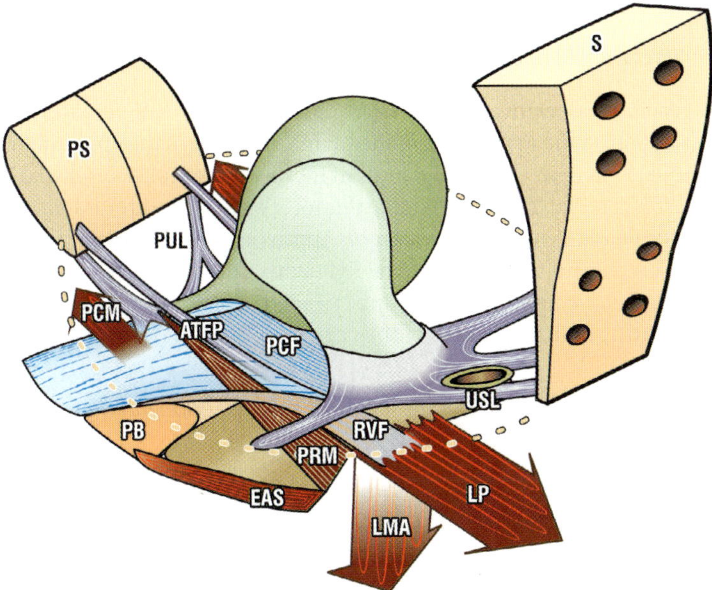

Fig. 1-05 Fascial attachments and tensioning mechanism. Anteriorly, the fascia connects the vaginal membrane to the pubourethral ligaments (PUL) laterally to the Arcus Tendineus Fascia Pelvis, posteriorly to the cardinal/uterosacral ligament complex (USL) and inferiorly, to the perineal body (PB) and its tensor, the external anal sphincter (EAS). The pubocervical fascia (PCF) and rectovaginal fascia (RVF) are tensioned by the three directional muscle forces (PCM, LP and LMA arrows) to provide structural support to the vagina.

The Cervical Ring

The cervical ring surrounds the cervix and acts as an attachment point for the cardinal and uterosacral ligaments, and also, the pubocervical and rectovaginal fascia. It consists mainly of collagen.

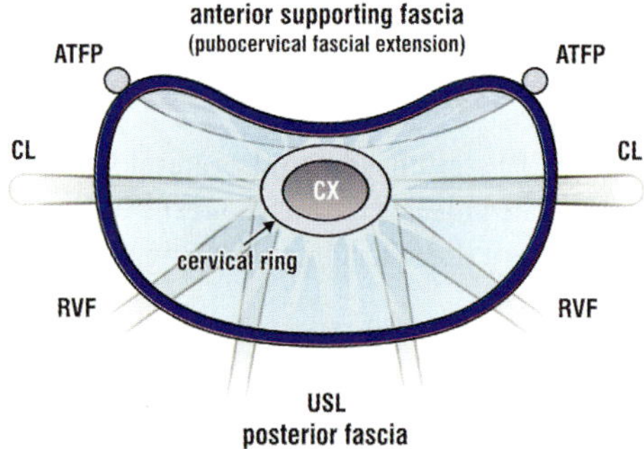

Fig. 2-09   Role of the cervical ring in the connectedness of pelvic fascia. All fascial and ligamentous structures insert directly or indirectly into the cervical ring. Perspective: 3D view, looking into the posterior fornix of the vagina. CL = Cardinal ligament, RVF = rectovaginal fascia, USL = uterosacral ligament, and ATFP = Arcus Tendineus Fascia Pelvis.

The Role of Proximal Cervical Ring Fascia in Preventing Everting Vaginal Prolapse

The pubocervical and rectovaginal fascia around the cervical ring act as an adjunctive structural support to the upper walls of the vagina. Collapse of the upper vaginal walls is an essential element in the pathogenesis of uterovaginal prolapse, which is really a type of intussusception. Therefore simple reinforcement of the uterosacral ligaments may not be sufficient to restore the prolapse. Approximation of the laterally displaced fascia below and lateral to the uterosacral ligaments inferiorly, and above and lateral to the cardinal ligaments superiorly, may be needed to restore tension (and therefore sructural support) to the side walls of the vagina

The Role of Proximal Cervical Ring Fascia in Preventing Peripheral Neurologically Derived Symptoms

Symptoms of urge, frequency, nocturia and pelvic pain are attributed to failure of connective tissue to support the bladder base stretch receptors, and unmyelinated nerve endings of the uterosacral ligaments.

These are peripheral neurologically derived symptoms, so it is highly likely that they may be triggered by fairly minor degrees of connective tissue laxity. The cure rate for these symptoms with the posterior sling operation is in the region of 80%, (Petros 1997, Farnsworth 2002). Anecdotal evidence is emerging with use of the TFS (Chapter 4), that tightening the proximal parts of the pubocervical and rectovaginal fascia with a TFS tape may be important in better restoring function as regards these neurologically derived symptoms.

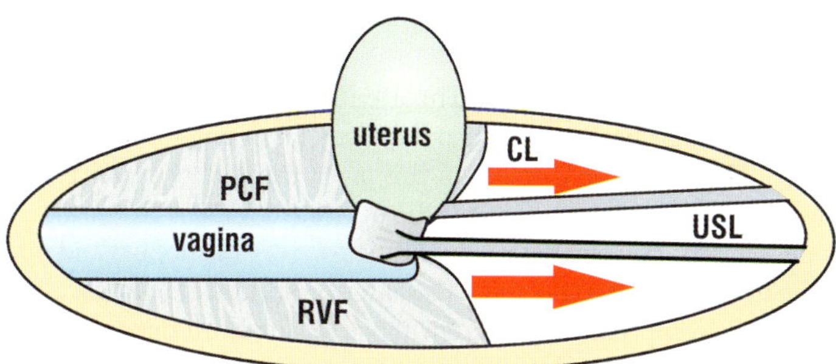

Fig. 2-10 Fascial re-inforcement of the upper walls of the vagina. The pubocervical fascia 'PCF' and rectovaginal fascia 'RVF' form a critical mass to support the upper part of the vagina, thus preventing its intussusception. CL = cardinal ligament; USL = uterosacral ligament.

2.1.5 The Muscles of the Pelvic Floor

In broad terms, the pelvic muscles form three layers: upper, middle and lower (fig 1-03) (Petros & Ulmsten, 1997). The upper layer consists of the anterior part of pubococcygeus muscle (PCM) anteriorly, and levator plate (LP) posteriorly. The middle layer consists of the longitudinal muscle of the anus (LMA), a short striated muscle not attached to the rectum which connects the upper and lower muscle layers. The lower layer consists of the muscles sited on the perineal membrane (PM), external anal sphincter (EAS) and postanal plate (PAP).

It is important to note that the three muscle layers do not necessarily correspond to the three levels of connective tissue structures. This is explained further below.

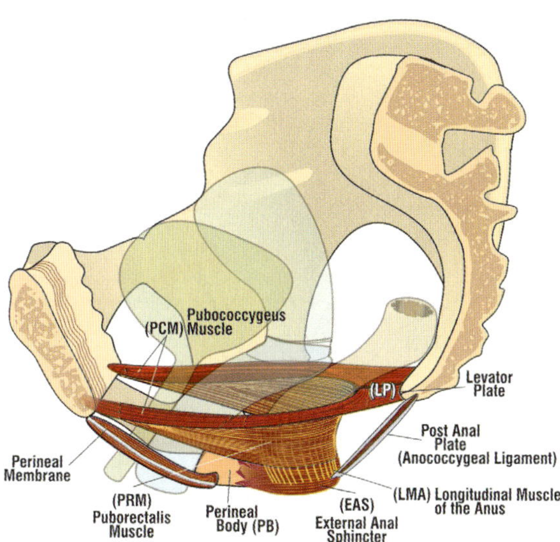

Fig. 1-03 The striated pelvic muscles and organs of the pelvic floor. This is a schematic 3D sagittal view of the pelvis, organs and their principal muscular relationships.

The Upper Layer of Muscles

The upper layer of muscles is horizontal in orientation. This layer of muscles stretches the organs forwards or backwards. Its pubococcygeus component (PCM) creates a forward force. The posterior segment of this layer, the levator plate (LP) attaches to the posterior wall of rectum and creates the backward force.

The upper layer of muscles have a dual function; organ support and opening and closure of the urethra, vagina and anus. The anterior portion of pubococcygeus muscle (PCM) has its origin approximately 1.5 cm above the lower border of pubic symphysis, and its insertion into the lateral wall of the distal vagina (fig 2-11) (Zacharin 1963). The lateral parts of pubococcygeus sweep behind the rectum to join with each other and fibres from coccygeus and iliococcygeus to form the levator plate (LP). The levator plate inserts into the posterior wall of the rectum, and so plays a major role in the backward movement of this organ.

The arrows (fig 2-11) indicate the direction of muscle forces. The anterior portion of pubococcygeus muscle, attached to the lateral walls of vagina constitutes the forward force. The levator plate, attached to the posterior wall of the rectum, constitutes the posterior force.

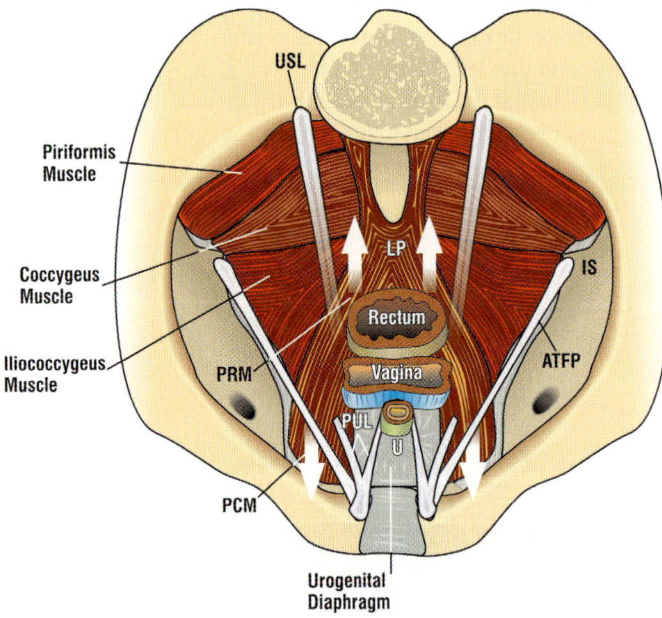

Fig. 2-11 Upper layer of muscles of the pelvic floor floor (after Netter 1989).

The Middle (Connecting) Layer of Muscles

The longitudinal muscle of the anus (LMA) (Courtney 1950) is a striated muscle which constitutes the middle layer (fig 2-12). The LMA is a vertically oriented muscle which creates the downward force for bladder neck closure during effort, and stretches open the outflow tract during micturition. It takes fibres superiorly from the levator plate (LP), lateral part of the pubococcygeus muscle and puborectalis. Inferiorly it inserts into the deep and superficial external anal sphincter (EAS). It appears to partly surround the rectum (R) posteriorly but does not insert into it, as indicated by the scissors tips (fig 2-12). It needs to be distinguished from the longitudinal muscle of the rectum, a smooth muscle which forms part of the rectal wall.

It follows from the anatomy that if LMA is well anchored by EAS, then LP will be pulled downwards. As LP inserts into the posterior wall of rectum (R), then the rectum will also be angulated downwards by LMA contraction.

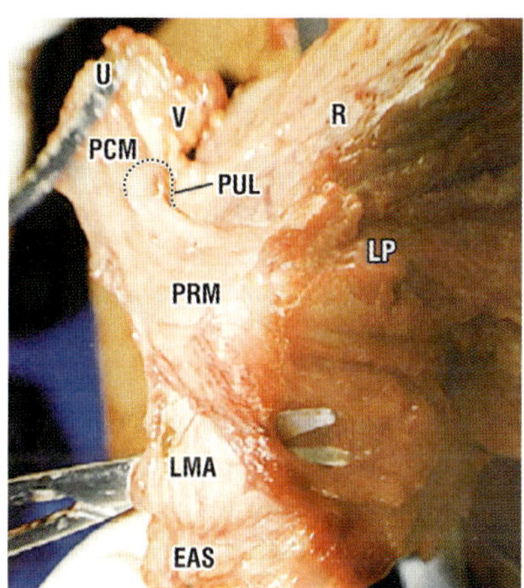

Fig. 2-12 Longitudinal muscle of the anus (LMA) – origins and insertions. This is an anatomical specimen from a female cadaver, cut away from its bony insertions. Bladder and vagina have been excised at the level of bladder neck.
U = urethra; V = vagina. PCM = anterior and lateral portion of the pubococcygeus muscle. These sweep behind the rectum (R) and merge with the contralateral side to form part of the levator plate (LP). PRM = puborectalis muscle; PUL = insertion of pubourethral ligament into PCM; EAS = external anal sphincter.

The Lower Layer of Muscles

The lower layer of muscles is the anchoring layer. It is composed of the perineal membrane and its component muscles: bulbocavernosus, ischiocavernosus and the deep and superficial transverse perinei muscles (fig 2-13).

The lower layer contracts to stabilize the distal parts of the urethra, vagina and anus. It also helps to contain the abdominal contents, but they (the muscles) also appear to exert a downward force on the distal parts of the urethra, vagina and (probably) the anus as well (see the x-rays in Chapter 5, Pelvic Floor Rehabilitation).

The perineal body is the key anchoring point for contraction of bulbocavernosus and the external anal sphincter (EAS) (Petros 2002). The deep transverse perinei anchors the upper part of the perineal body to the ischial tuberosity. It is a strong muscle and it stabilizes the perineal body laterally. EAS acts as the tensor of the perineal body and it is the principal insertion point of the longitudinal muscle of the anus. The bulbocavernosus stretches and anchors the distal part of the urethra.

The ischiocavernosus helps stabilize the perineal membrane and may act to stretch the external urethral meatus laterally *via* its effect on the bulbocavernosus. Between EAS and the coccyx is the postanal plate, a tendinous structure which also contains striated muscle inserting into EAS.

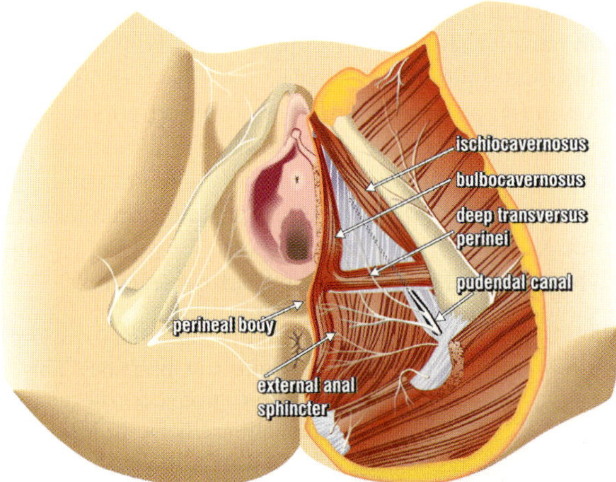

Fig. 2-13 Lower layer muscles of the pelvic floor anchor the organs distally (after Netter 1989).

The Special Case of the Puborectalis Muscle

The puborectalis muscle (PRM) (fig. 2-14) originates just medially to PCM and traverses all three muscle layers. It is included in the upper layer of muscles, even though it extends down to the middle layer. It is oriented vertically and runs forward medially below PCM. It is closely applied to the lateral walls of the rectum and inserts

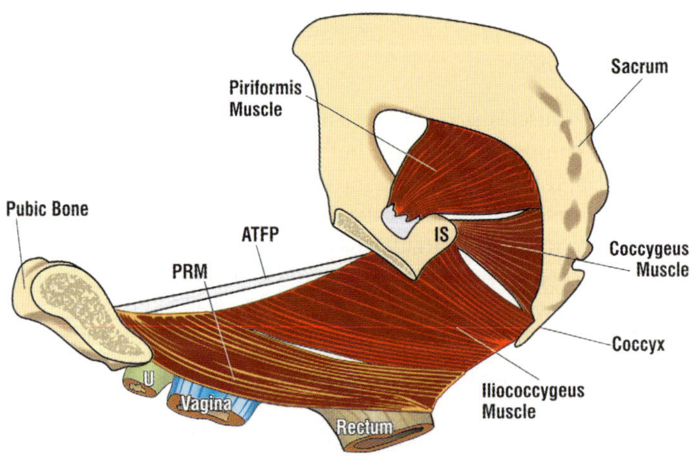

Fig. 2-14 Puborectalis muscle (PRM) (after Netter 1989)

into its posterior wall. Whereas PCM is a flat, horizontally placed muscle, PRM is more vertical and runs medial to, and partly below, PCM. As well as its pivotal role in anorectal closure, the puborectalis muscle is the voluntary muscle activated during 'squeezing' when it elevates the whole levator plate (LP) (See the section on pelvic floor rehabilitation later in this book). 'Squeezing' refers to the action that occurs when a patient crosses her legs and contracts the pelvic muscles upwards.

2.2   The Dynamics of Pelvic Floor Function

2.2.1   The Dynamics of the Striated Pelvic Floor Muscles

The pelvic floor muscles contain mainly slow-twitch fibres essential for their roles of containing the intra-abdominal contents and maintenance of pelvic organ shape, structure and closure. The pelvic floor muscles work in a co-ordinated manner to stretch and angulate the pelvic organs backwards and downwards (arrows, fig 2-15) so that they are compressed by intra-abdominal pressure. This helps prevent prolapse. The same muscle actions assist closure of the urethra and anus.

The lower two thirds of the urethra is densely adherent to the anterior vaginal wall. The distal part of posterior vaginal wall is densely adherent to the perineal body and the anterior wall of rectum. The upper parts of the urethra (U), vagina (V) and rectum (R) are not attached to each other. This freedom of movement allows the stretching of the organ which is so essential for opening and closure.

The Dynamics of Urethral Opening and Closure – Urethral Perspective

Urethral closure or opening is determined by contraction or relaxation of one muscle, the pubococcygeus.

A urethra adequately anchored by PUL and the forward muscles PCM, allows the backward acting muscles LP and LMA to stretch and close the proximal urethral cavity to 'C' (fig 2-16). Relaxation of PCM allows LP and LMA to stretch open the urethral cavity to 'O' during micturition.

Figure 2-16 is a schematic 3D view of the vagina (broken lines), urethra and bladder. The shared longitudinal smooth muscle of bladder and urethra is represented by thin black lines. Extension of this smooth muscle by the pelvic muscles is a prerequisite to closure 'C' and opening 'O'. An adequately tight pubourethral ligament (PUL) is needed to anchor all three muscle forces (arrows). The pubococcygeus muscle (PCM) also requires an adequately tight hammock 'H' to effectively close the urethra. If PUL is lax, the urethra is pulled into the 'open' position 'O' by levator plate (LP) and the longitudinal muscle of the anus (LMA) during effort. Anything which provides a firm anchoring point at PUL (e.g. a haemostat or a surgically implanted tape) will enable the 3 directional forces to close urethra from 'O' to 'C' during effort. This is the basis of the 'simulated operation' which involves anchoring the midurethra unilaterally (so as not to obstruct it) and asking the patient to cough (Petros & Von Konsky 1999).

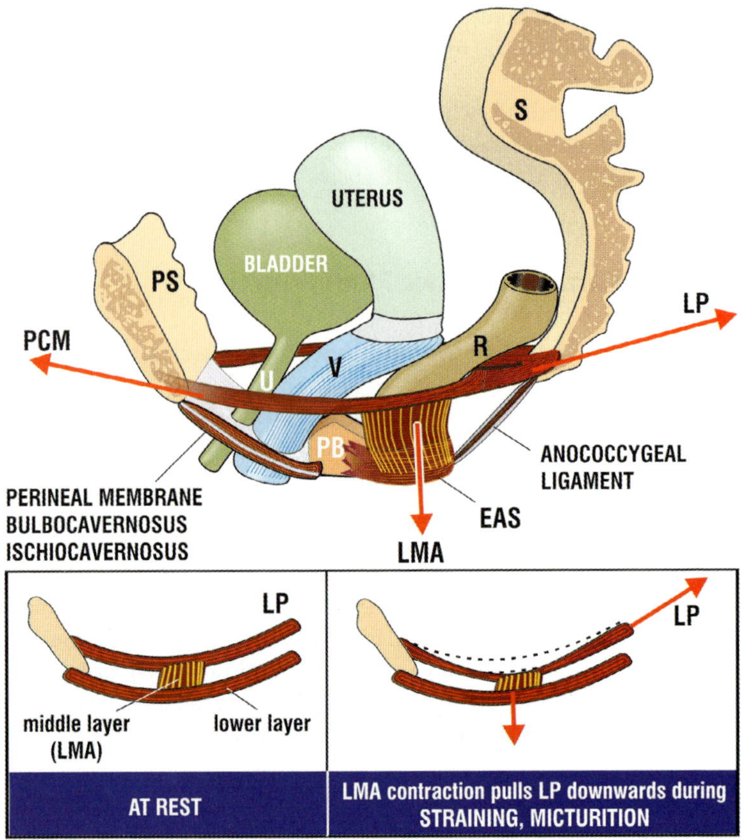

Fig. 2-15 Interaction of the upper and lower muscles of the pelvic floor.

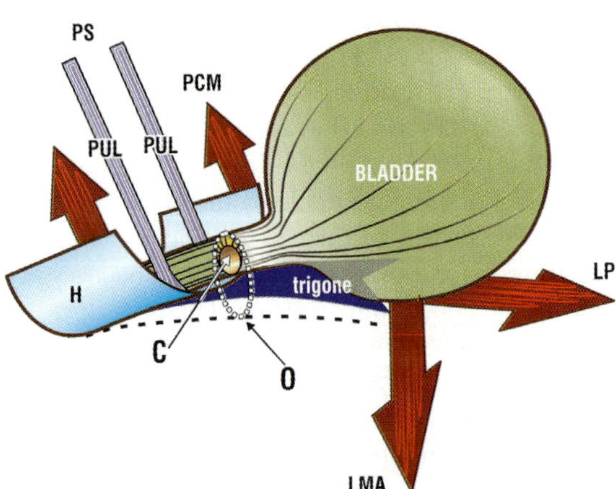

Fig. 2-16 Smooth muscle in the dynamics of urethral opening and closure

The Dynamics of Urethral Closure and Opening – Vaginal Perspective

Damage in the connective tissue of the ligaments or vagina may weaken muscle contraction, causing dysfunctional closure or opening of the outflow tract.

During effort (fig 2-17) the distal vagina is stretched forwards by PCM. The upper vagina and bladder base are stretched down and back by LP and LMA. PCM and LP contract against the pubourethral ligament (PUL). LMA contracts against the uterosacral ligaments (USL). The broken lines represent the resting position of the bladder.

During micturition (fig. 2-18), PCM relaxes.The stretch receptors activate the micturition reflex. The whole system is stretched down and back by LP and LMA, opening out the outflow tract. The detrusor contracts to expel urine. The broken lines represent the closed position of the bladder.

Note that, although the terms 'opening' and 'micturition' are used interchangeably, they are not exactly the same. 'Micturition' is driven by a neurological reflex whereas the 'open' state of the urethra may result from entirely mechanical factors, for example, 'genuine stress incontinence'.

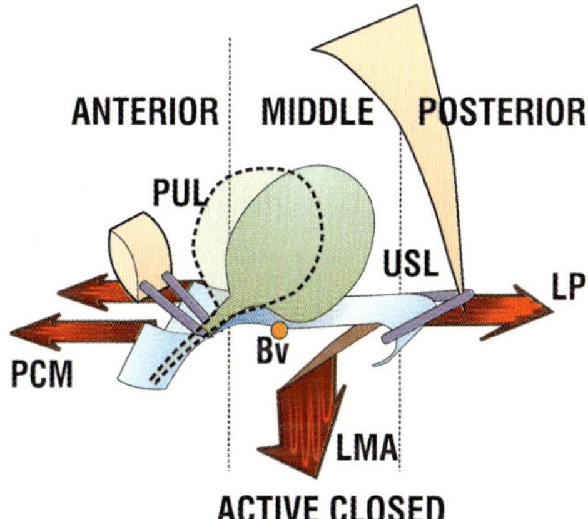

Fig. 2-17 Active Closure.
Bv = attachment of bladder base to vagina.

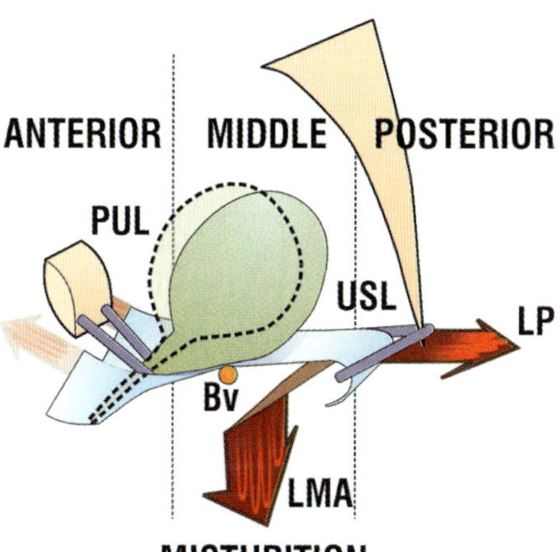

Fig. 2-18 Micturition

2.2.2 Pelvic Floor Dynamics - The 'Mechanical' Dimension

There are three normal states of the urethra: resting closed, closure during effort, and opening during micturition. Each state is a resultant of muscle forces acting mainly against anterior pubourethral ligament (PUL) or posterior uterosacral suspensory ligaments (USL). In this section, these states are demonstrated radiologically, using x-rays from the same patient in each of the three states.

Resting Closed

In the resting closed state (fig 2-19) the slow twitch fibres of the three directional muscles stretch the vagina (V) against the pubourethral ligament (PUL) anteriorly, and the uterosacral ligaments (USL) posteriorly. The white interrupted horizontal and vertical lines are drawn between fixed bony points. The backward angulation of the urethra and vagina at PUL clearly illustrates the effect of a backward force, the levator plate (LP).

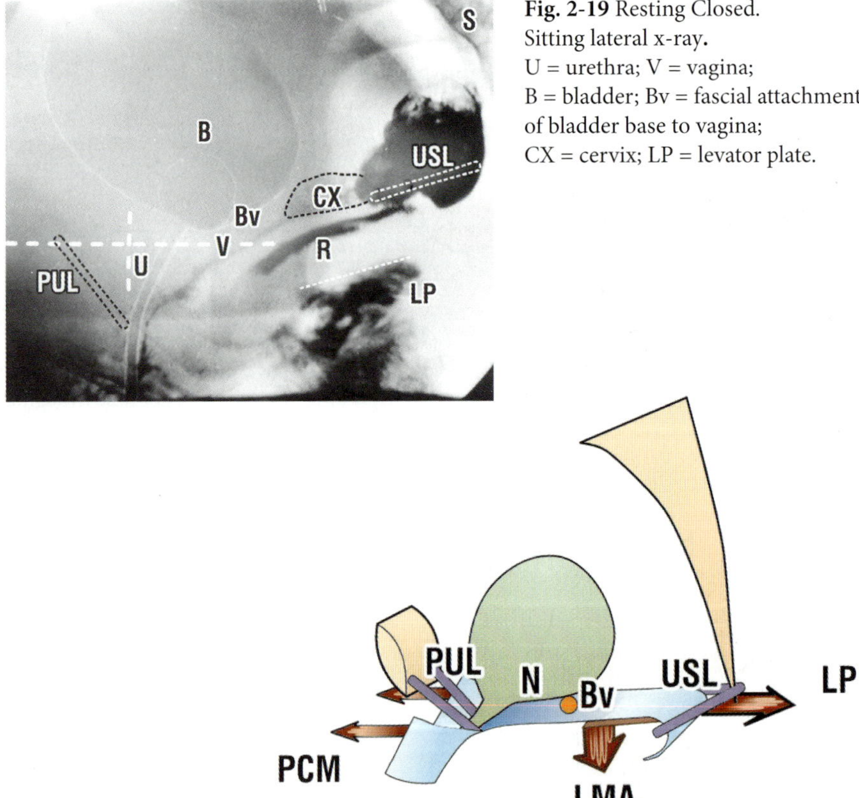

Fig. 2-19 Resting Closed.
Sitting lateral x-ray.
U = urethra; V = vagina;
B = bladder; Bv = fascial attachment
of bladder base to vagina;
CX = cervix; LP = levator plate.

Fig. 2-20 Schematic model of urethrovesical unit at rest, corresponding to the x-ray shown in figure 2-19. N = stretch receptors; Bv = attachment of bladder base to vagina.

Figure 2-20 schematically represents a 3D sagittal section of the bladder and urethra nestled in the anterior vaginal wall ('hammock'). It corresponds to figure 2-19. The distal part of vagina is tensioned by the anterior part of pubococcygeus muscle (PCM), and the proximal part by the levator plate (LP) and the longitudinal muscle of the anus (LMA). Inherent vaginal elasticity and slow-twitch muscle contraction maintains urethral closure.

Closure During Effort

Figure 2-21 shows urethral closure during effort. Compared to the 'resting closed' state shown in figure 2-19, three directional forces are evident. The bladder base, upper vagina and rectum appear to have been stretched backwards and downwards by contraction of LP and downward angulation of its anterior border. Furthermore, the distal vagina and urethra appear to have been pulled forwards (anterior arrow). The downward (LMA) force (downward arrow) acts directly against USL. The forward (PCM) and backward (LP) forces both act against PUL. The small downward arrows below 'V' indicate presumed contraction of the superficial and deep perineal muscles. The small arrows above 'R' (fig 2-21) signify the vector of the backward and downward forces.

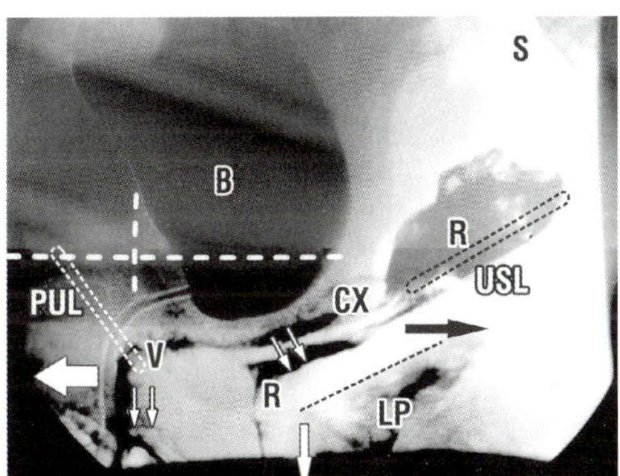

Fig. 2-21 Urethral closure during effort (coughing or straining). Same labelling as in figure 2-15. The upper vagina and urethra are stretched and angulated in a plane around PUL.

Note how the urethra has been stretched forward of the vertical line and the bladder base stretched below the horizontal line.

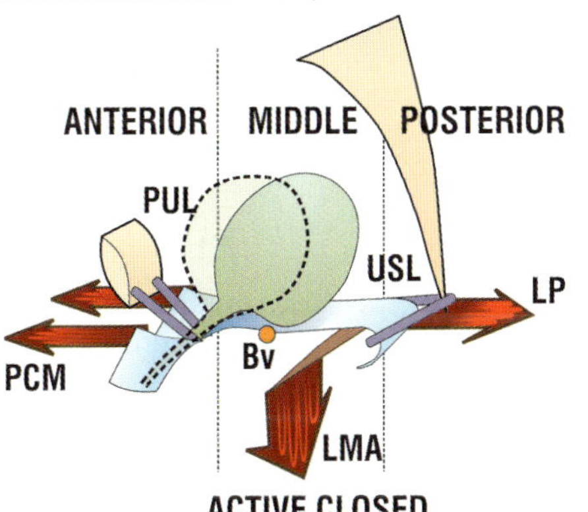

Fig. 2-22 The vagina transmits muscle forces to close urethra and bladder neck. This figure relates to figure 2-21. In comparison to figure 2-20 (resting state), the fast-twitch fibres of the three directional muscle forces PCM, LP and LMA stretch and rotate the vagina and bladder base in a plane around PUL to 'kink' the bladder neck, PCM closes the urethra along its length. The resting closed position is outlined with dotted lines.

Urethral Opening by External Striated Muscle Forces During Micturition

In comparison to figure 2-19, figure 2-23 shows that the urethra and bladder neck appear to have been opened out by the downward angulation of levator plate (LP) causing downward stretching of the vagina (V) and rectum (R). The directional stretchings of upper vagina, bladder, rectum, and levator plate appear identical to those in the 'closure during effort' position (fig 2-21). Note how the urethra is now well behind the vertical white line, consistent with PCM relaxation.

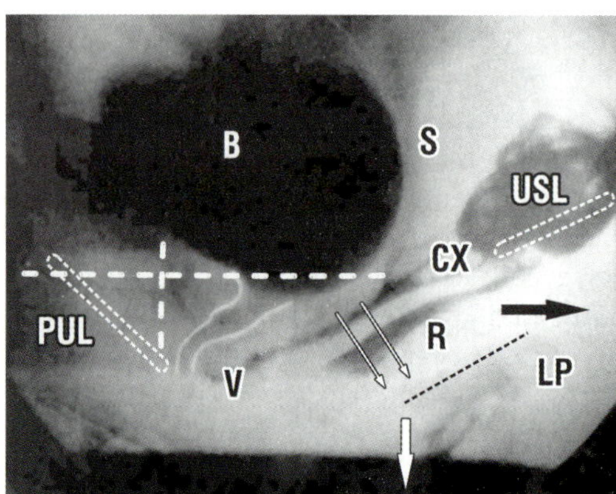

Fig. 2-23 Urethral opening during micturition. Same labelling as in figure 2-19.

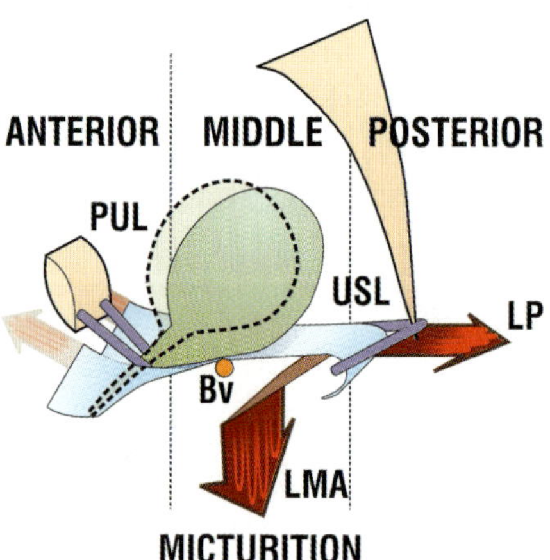

Fig. 2-24 Micturition (Schematic) This figure corresponds with the situation shown in figure 2-23.

In figure 2-24, relaxation of the forward force allows the backward and downward forces to open out the outflow tract. As the urethral resistance is inversely proportional to the 4th power of the radius (Poisseuille's Law, see 'Urethral resistance and the pressure-flow relationship' in Chapter 6), this action vastly decreases the detrusor pressure required to expel urine. The dotted lines (fig 2-24) indicate the resting position of the bladder.

2.2.3 Pelvic floor dynamics - the neurological dimension

Urethral Closure

In simple terms, the central nervous system co-ordinates and controls all the structures involved in opening and closure of the urethra and anus. The presence of nerve endings in ligaments and fascia indicates that they too are co-ordinated. The mechanical aspects of opening and closure of the urethra require that a critical tension is maintained in the vaginal membrane (fig 2-19) so that any force applied can pull open or close the urethra. Discovery of a muscle spindle (fig 2-25, Petros PE, Kakulas B and Swash MM - unpublished data) indicates the presence of a complex, balanced, finely-tuned control system.

Muscle spindles (fig 2-25) found in the anterior portion of pubococcygeus muscle suggest that a precise feedback system controls the tension in the vaginal membrane. Adequate tension of the tissues is essential if the woman is to maintain continence at rest.

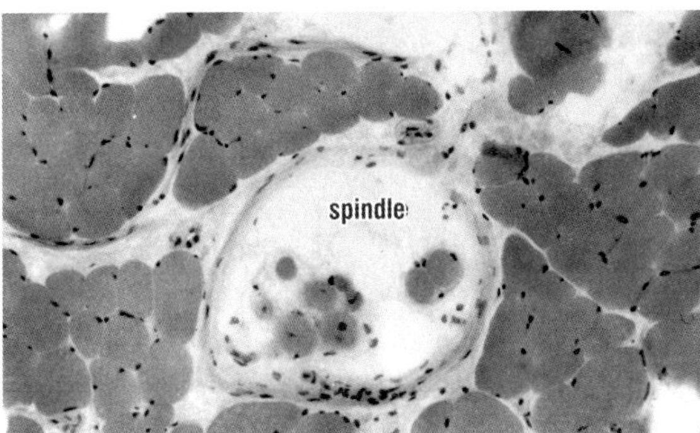

Fig. 2-25 Vaginal tension is controlled by muscle spindles. Muscle spindle found in the anterior portion of the pubo-coccygeus muscle.

Urethral Opening (Micturition)

Normal micturition may be defined as the controlled emptying of the bladder on demand and rapid restoration of the closed state on completion.

The micturition reflex is activated by both stretch and volume receptors at the bladder base. These vary in sensitivity from patient to patient. The control of the micturition reflex is essentially by a neurological feedback system which operates *via* these receptors. The normal micturition reflex is co-ordinated by the central nervous system and has four main components (fig 2-26):

1. The hydrostatic pressure of a full bladder activates the stretch receptors (N) which send afferent signals to the cortex.
2. The anterior striated muscles relax.
3. The posterior striated muscles (fast-twitch component) stretch open the outflow tract, greatly reducing urethral resistance, thereby allowing the expulsion of urine.
4. The detrusor contracts, creating a smooth muscle spasm to expel urine.

When the afferent stimulus ceases, the fast-twitch posterior muscle fibres relax. The stretched tissues 'rebound' to close the urethra. The anterior muscles contract. Because electrical transmission is from smooth muscle (Creed 1979) to smooth muscle, the detrusor 'spasms' to expel the urine. This can be seen on video x-ray studies.

It can be helpful to conceptualise the inhibitory centres as 'trapdoors' which can be opened or closed by cortical direction, thereby facilitating or blocking afferent impulses from the bladder base stretch receptors (fig 2-27).

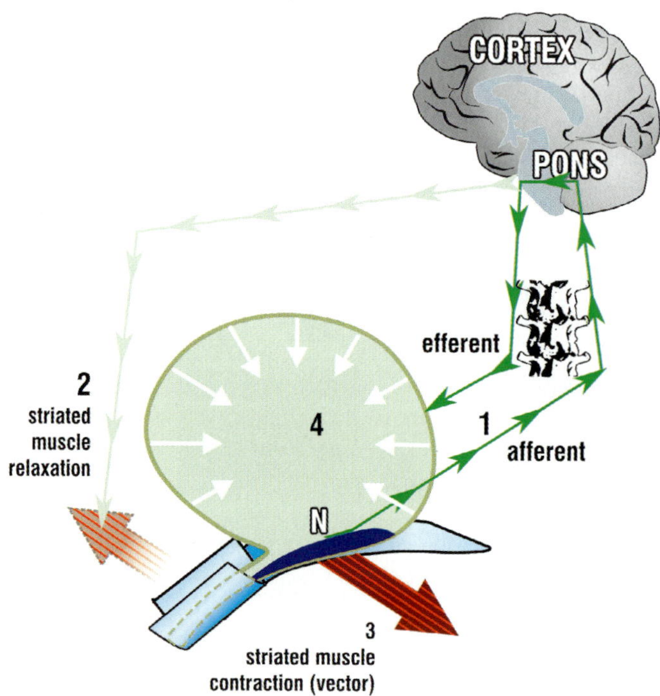

Fig. 2-26 The normal micturition reflex. The normal micturition reflex is activated by peripheral and volume receptors 'N' at bladder base.

The Role of Connective Tissue Tension in the Peripheral Neurological Control Mechanism for Micturition

In a functional sense, there are two neurological mechanisms for controlling inappropriate activation of the micturition reflex: central and peripheral. The central mechanism 'C' arises from the cortex and it acts through the micturition inhibitory centre (fig 2-27). The peripheral neurological control mechanism is a musculo-elastic complex which requires competent suspensory ligaments to work properly (fig 2-28 'trampoline analogy').

With reference to figure 2-27, spindle cells in the pelvic muscles (arrows) sense the tension of the membrane and the system is balanced by the cortex. As the bladder fills, the stretch receptors (N) send afferent impulses to the cortex. These are reflexly suppressed by activation of the central inhibitory centres (broken red lines). The central inhibitory centres have only a limited ability to suppress the micturition reflex, expecially if the vaginal membrane is too lax to support 'N'. As with a trampoline, even if one ligament (spring) is lax, the vaginal membrane cannot be stretched by the muscle forces. The hydrostatic pressure of the urine cannot be supported and 'N' may 'fire off' to initiate micturition at a lower volume. For the patient, these afferent impulses may be interpreted symptomatically as frequency, urgency and nocturia. Urodynamically, the patient may display a phasic pattern in the bladder or urethra ('detrusor' or 'urethral' instability) or a 'low bladder capacity'.

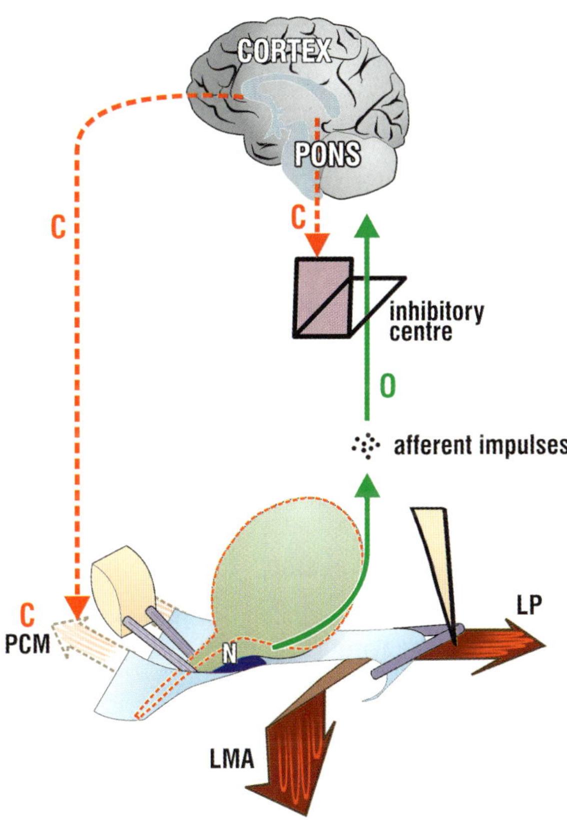

Fig. 2-27 Bladder control - the neurological dimension. Bladder in 'open' position. The closed phase 'C' is indicated by broken lines and the open phase 'O' by unbroken lines. Afferent impulses 'O' activate the cascade of events for micturition: relaxation of the PCM and de-activation of the inhibitory centre and closure reflex 'C'. 'C' activates the cascade of events for closure: activation of the inhibitory centres and contraction of PCM. Note the identical postion of LP and LMA in closure and micturition. N = stretch receptors, PCM = pubococcygeus muscle, LMA = longitudinal muscle of the anus, LP = levator plate.

2.3   The Role of Connective Tissue in Pelvic Floor Function and Dysfunction

A basic knowledge of the physical and biomechanical properties of connective tissue is a prerequisite for understanding function, dysfunction, the diagnostic process and the surgery of the pelvic floor. It is clear that a damaged muscle may modify the contractile strength of the muscles. However, high cure rates for a large range of symptoms following connective tissue repair indicates that muscle damage may be more of a modifying factor than a principal cause of urinary dysfunction.

Connective tissue is a living entity. Its structure changes with age and the influence of hormones. Connective tissue is a complex structure. Glycosaminoglycans (proteoglycans) constitute the ground substance and elastin fibres store energy. Collagen provides structural rigidity.

The ligaments attach the vagina to the bony pelvis. The three directional muscles act against these suspensory ligaments. Laxity in any of these ligaments may inactivate the muscle forces, causing dysfunction in opening or closure (c.f. the 'trampoline analogy' (fig 2-28) or the 'sail analogy' (fig 2-30)).

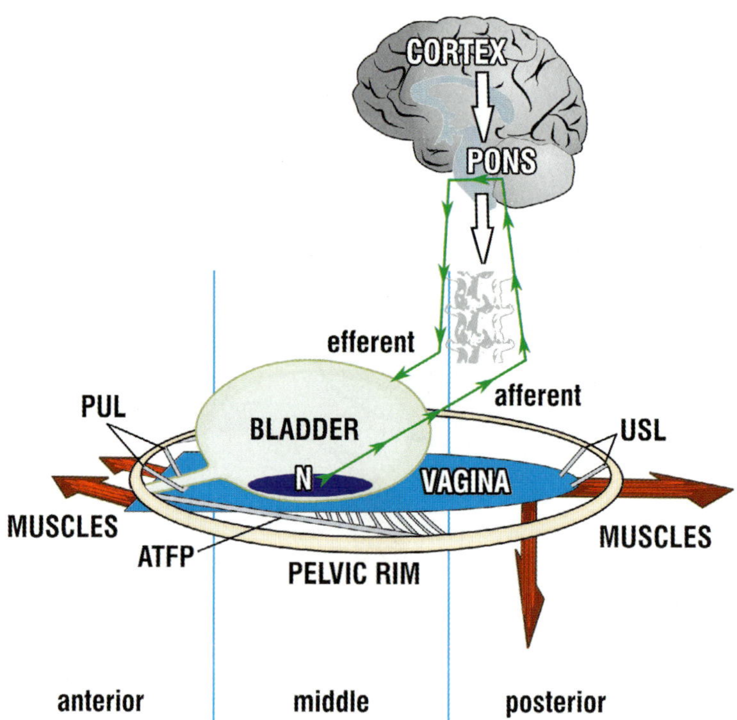

Fig. 2-28 Controlling the tension of connective tissue - the 'trampoline analogy'. White arrows = central inhibitory mechanism. Lax ligaments may not allow the muscles to tension the vaginal membrane, so 'N' 'fires off' prematurely: bladder instability.

Generally, pelvic floor surgery only addresses damaged connective tissue. Understanding how connective tissue weakens and alters the closure forces that act on the organs of the pelvic floor is, therefore, of vital importance when choosing a particular surgical technique. Biomechanics is the application of principles of physics and engineering to body function. It is used to mathematically analyse all the components that contribute to function, e.g. tissue quality, strength and direction of muscle force.

Structurally, collagen has an 'S' shaped fibril (fig 2-29). Once the curves are straightened out by distension, collagen acts as a rigid rod, preventing further distension. At this point, any force applied is transmitted directly. Thus the distensibility of a tissue depends entirely on the configuration of these collagen fibrils. In a tendon, there is no extensibility, as all fibrils are parallel. A ligament has limited distension, but skin and the vaginal membrane have much more.

The pelvic ligaments suspend the organs from the bony pelvis. They are strong, active structures and are only minimally distensile.

The muscle forces are transmitted to the bony pelvis by means of ligaments (estimated breaking strain approximately 300 mg/mm^2 (Yamada 1970). If the ligament is excessively weak, it cannot be repaired, and needs to be reinforced by a tape. This stimulates the deposition of collagen which forms an artificial neoligament.

Fig. 2-29

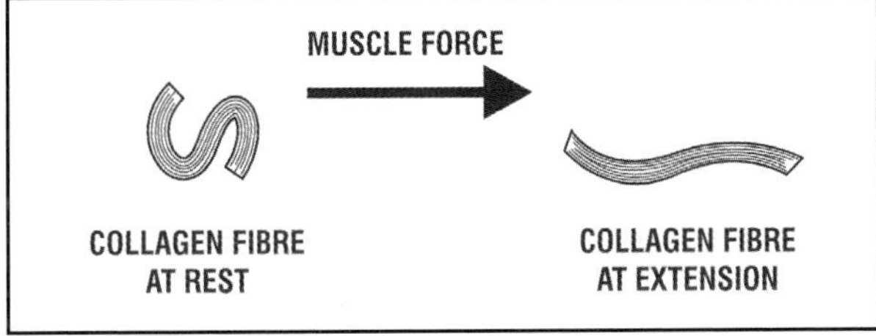

2.3.1 The Biomechanics of the Vagina

The vagina has an estimated breaking strain of approximately 60 mg/mm^2 (Yamada 1970). It is essentially an elastic membrane. Inherent elasticity provides a low energy urethral closure force applied from behind. The vaginal membrane has little inherent strength. It derives strength from its fascial layer, and, in a normal patient this is strongest in the area of ligamentous insertions, for example, the apex. The vagina stretches to transmit muscle forces for urethral opening and closure. This stretching counteracts the hydrostatic pressure at the bladder base and so prevents displacement of the stretch receptors which initiate the micturition reflex. The vagina is an organ which cannot regenerate once it is excised. Surgical excision, stretching and tightening of the cut edges of the vagina only serve to further weaken what is essentially a weak elastic membrane. Conceptually, vaginal prolapse is much like an intussusception of a visceral organ. During repair, there is a critical length along the side walls which may need to be reinforced in order to prevent further prolapse.

The Effect of Pregnancy Hormones on Connective Tissue

Connective tissue in the area of the urogenital organs is sensitive to hormones. During pregnancy, collagen is depolymerized by placental hormones, and the ratios of the glycosaminoglycans change. (The term 'proteoglycans' is used here interchangeably with 'glycosaminoglycans'.) The vaginal membrane becomes more distensile, allowing dilatation of the birth canal during delivery. There is a concomitant loss of structural strength in the suspensory ligaments. This explains the uterovaginal prolapse so often seen during pregnancy. Laxity in the hammock may remove the elastic closure force, causing urine loss on effort. This condition is described as stress incontinence. Loss of membranous support may cause gravity to stimulate the nerve endings (N) at the bladder base, so causing premature activation of the micturition reflex, expressed as symptoms of 'bladder instability'. This condition is perceived by the pregnant patient as frequency, urgency and nocturia. Laxity may also cause pelvic pain, due to loss of structural support for the unmyelinated nerve fibres contained in the posterior ligaments. The action of gravity on these nerves causes a 'dragging' pain. Removal of the placenta restores connective tissue integrity and the symptoms rapidly disappear in a large percentage of patients.

The Effect of Age on Connective Tissue

In younger patients, the 'S' shaped collagen (fig 2-29) easily extends. In older patients, the increased inter and intramolecular cross-bonding of the collagen stiffens the 'S' and so the tissue may shrink. Age related loss of elastin may cause tissues to 'droop' due to the effect of gravity realigning the collagen fibrils.

Though the individual collagen fibrils strengthen up to 400% with age, the total tensile strength of the urogenital tissues decreases to about 60% (Yamada, 1970). Excision and stretching of vaginal tissue during surgery may weaken it further. Therefore it is advisable to avoid excision of vaginal tissue during surgery where possible.

Loss of elasticity may take away the low energy elastic component of urethral closure. This explains the slow insensible urine leak often seen in patients with low urethral pressure ('intrinsic sphincter defect'). The patient must rely on the slow twitch component of the anterior closure force to close the urethra in a low effort situation, hence the frequent complaint of leakage after 20 minutes walking in patients with no demonstrable stress incontinence. The slow twitch closure muscles simply tire and urine leaks out. Oestrogen may prevent collagen loss and so is recommended as a preventative measure postmenopausally, at least as vaginal pessaries.

The Role of Connective Tissue in Transmitting Muscle Forces – The Sail Analogy

The muscle forces needed to close the urethra require adequately tightened connective tissues for proper functioning. The sail analogy (fig 2-30) is a simplistic illustration of this point: unless the sail and its holding ropes are firm, the force of the wind is not transmitted to drive the boat forward. The analogy drawn is that if the holding ropes (ligaments) are loose, the sail (vagina) flaps in the breeze. Just as a boat without

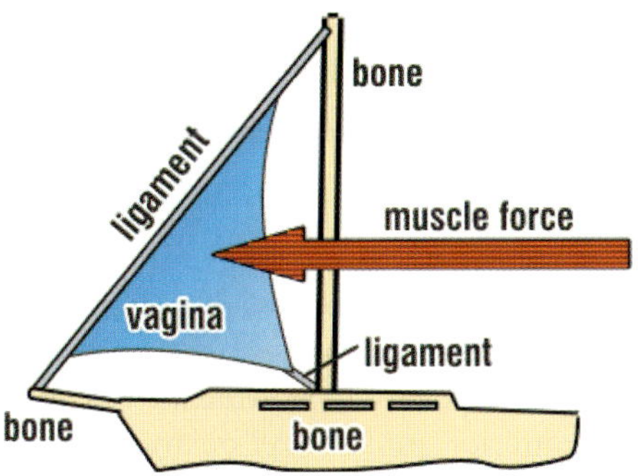

Fig. 2-30 The' sail analogy '– a loose vagina cannot be tensioned sufficiently to close off the urethra.

a taut sail cannot be driven forwards, so an untensioned vagina cannot be stretched forward to close off the urethra, or support the stretch receptors.

The Positive Effect of Uterine Conservation in Preserving Ligament Integrity

Patients undergoing hysterectomy are much more likely to suffer from urinary dysfunction later in life, and the incontinence is likely to be more severe (Brown 2000).

It follows that the uterus should be conserved where possible in vaginal surgery. The uterus occupies a central structural role in the pelvis, much like the keystone of an arch. The cervix is non-distensile and is a pure collagen structure with an estimated breaking strain of approximately 1500 mg/mm^2 (Yamada 1970). Because it is connected directly and indirectly with almost every pelvic ligament, any intra-abdominal force impacting on the cervix is distributed to these ligaments as a trophic force. Hysterectomy potentially removes this dispersion of forces, and results in the force being imposed on a weak vaginal membrane to cause herniation. Cervical conservation (subtotal hysterectomy) may be helpful, especially if the descending branch of the uterine artery, the main blood supply for the uterosacral ligament (USL), is conserved. Where cervical removal is essential, intrafascial hysterectomy, using a purse string suture pulls in the cardinal and uterosacral ligaments, and creates a fibrous plug in the centre.

2.3.2 The Role of Connective Tissue in the Maintenance of Form (Structure) and Function

'Function follows form, and dysfunction follows loss of form'.

A normal structure has form, function and balance. Dysfunction may be defined as abnormal symptoms consequent on damaged (unbalanced) structures. Damaged or unbalanced structures lose form and hence normal, healthy function.

Dysfunction is different from biomechanics because not all patients with damaged structures have symptoms. Dysfunction is different to anatomical prolapse in that symptoms may occur as a consequence of minor, barely detectable, anatomical abnormalities. Jeffcoate, in 1962, observed that some patients with gross degrees of prolapse had no symptoms at all. Others with minor degrees of prolapse complained bitterly of symptoms such as pelvic pain. The aim of this section is to demonstrate how connective tissue damage to key anatomical structures may cause abnormal symptoms.

The Causes of Damaged Connective Tissue

Childbirth is accepted as a major cause of uterovaginal prolapse, bladder and bowel dysfunction. Age and congenital collagen defects are also causal factors. Figure 2-31 schematically demonstrates how childbirth may damage specific connective tissue structures. Damage can be categorised as being of the anterior, middle and posterior zone.

Structural Effects of Damaged Connective Tissue

The circles (fig 2-31) represent the baby's head descending down the vagina damaging connective tissue (CT) thereby causing laxity. This, in turn, may cause urogenital prolapse, and urinary or bowel dysfunction. The numbers 1 through 4 in figure 2-31 represent connective tissue damage to the following structures:
1. Hammock, pubourethral ligament and external ligament laxity
2. Cystocoele and arcus tendineus fasciae pelvis defect
3. Uterine prolapse, enterocoele
4. Rectocoele, anal mucosal prolapse, perineal body and external anal sphincter damage.

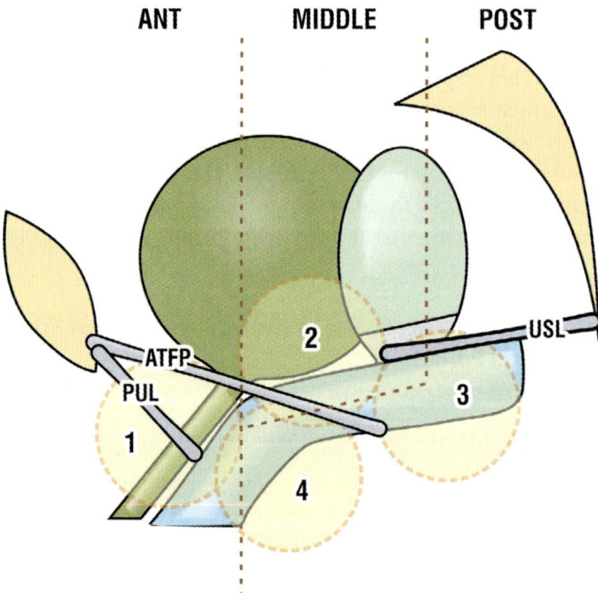

Fig. 2-31 Schematic representation of zones and structures of connective tissue damage at childbirth. PUL = pubourethral ligament; ATFP = arcus tendineus fascia pelvis; USL = uterosacral ligament

Lax Connective Tissue and Diminution of the Force of Muscle Contraction

Even at rest, sufficient tension is required in the vaginal membrane to close the urethra and support the stretch receptors (N) (fig 2-32) to prevent their 'firing off' prematurely. Vaginal tension is maintained by tissue elasticity and slow-twitch pelvic muscle contraction.

Connective tissue laxity 'L' (lower part, fig 2-32) may cause dysfunction. As the 'trampoline analogy' shows, laxity in the ligaments (springs) or vagina (trampoline membrane) will not permit tensioning of the vagina (trampoline membrane) by the muscles.

The muscle forces (arrows) can only be transmitted to open or close the urethra when point 'SE' has been reached on the stress-extension curve (upper part, fig 2-32). With damaged connective tissue, the muscle forces (arrows) must first 'take up the slack' (L) before sufficient tensioning of the vaginal membrane can be reached at SE_L. As a muscle can only contract over a finite length (E), SE_L cannot be reached, the muscle forces cannot close the urethra, and stress incontinence occurs. A lax vaginal membrane cannot support the stretch receptors (N), so these may prematurely activate the micturition reflex: 'detrusor instability'.

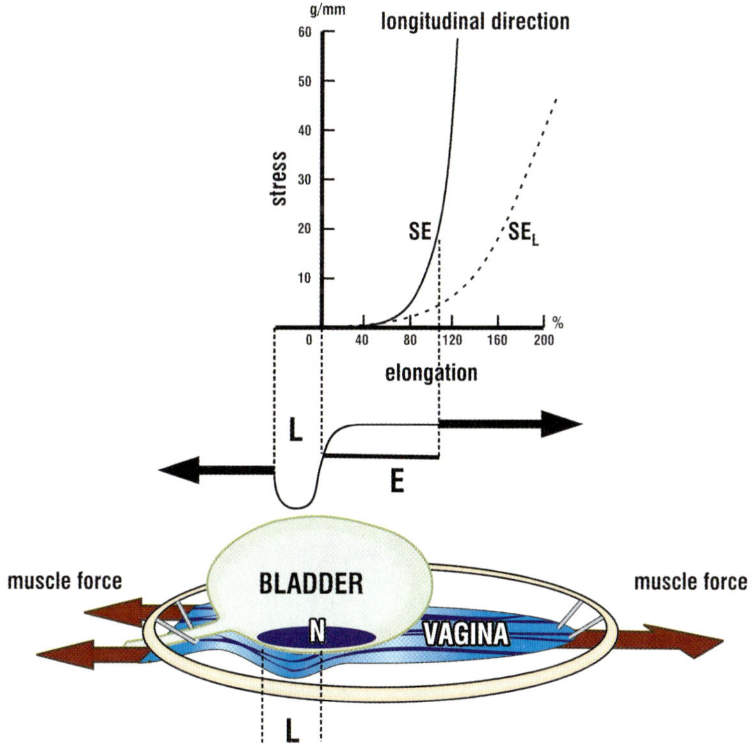

Fig. 2-32 Vaginal or ligamentous laxity may inactivate a muscle contraction. SE_L = stress-extension curve for lax tissues; SE = stress extension curve for normal tissues. (After Yamada 1970)

2.3.3 The Role of Connective Tissue in Balance and Imbalance of Pelvic Muscle Forces – Effects on Micturition and Closure

'Balance is a sign of health, imbalance, a harbinger of disease.' Hippocrates

Competent connective tissue is required for normal opening and closure of the bladder. Normal function is only achieved through a balance of the three directional muscle forces, PCM, LP and LMA (fig 2-33). Weakness in any muscle force may unbalance the system, causing dysfunctions of opening (micturition) or closure (continence). A series of diagrams is presented in this section, each illustrating a situation of balance or imbalance between the muscle forces within the three zones of the pelvic floor.

Closure at Rest and Effort

Closure at rest results from inherent elasticity and slow-twitch muscle contraction (fig 2-33). The bladder neck area of vagina must be elastic to allow the anterior and posterior muscle forces to function separately. This is called the 'zone of critical elasticity' (ZCE). The ZCE extends between midurethra and bladder base, and is stretched during effort and micturition. During effort, the fast-twitch muscle fibres of all three muscles are recruited to close the system further.

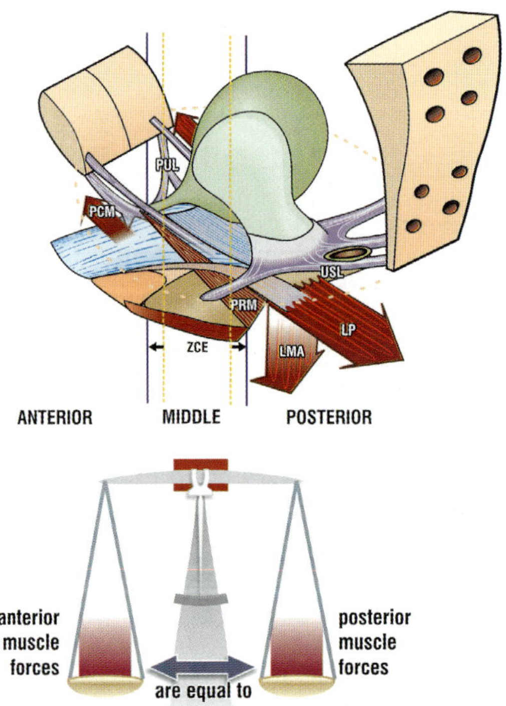

Fig. 2-33 Closure at rest - a balanced system

Normal Micturition – A Controlled Temporary Unbalancing of the Closure System

Competent connective tissue is also required for the normal micturition process (fig 2-34). Relaxation of the forward muscle pubococcygeus (PCM) causes the posterior muscles (levator plate (LP) and longitudinal muscle of the anus (LMA) to stretch the system backwards to the limit of tissue elasticity, expanding the outflow tract backwards, thereby decreasing intraurethral resistance to flow. At the end of micturition, the tissues recoil to close the urethra.

Fig. 2-34 (right) Micturition – a controlled temporary unbalancing of the closure system

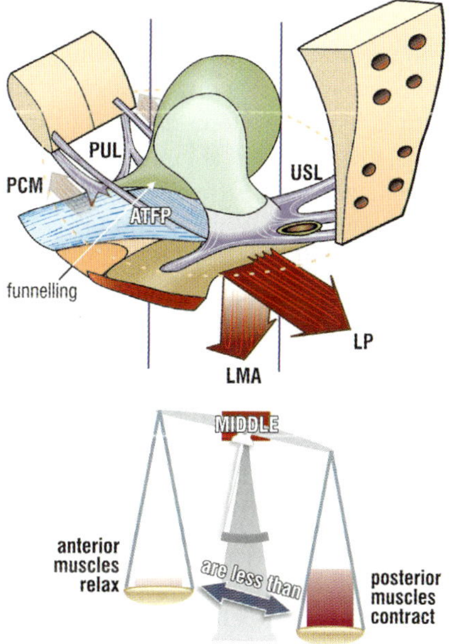

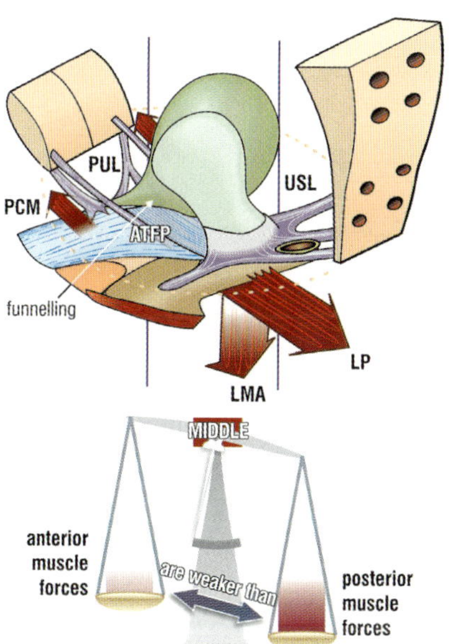

Fig. 2-35 (left) Stress incontinence – lax PUL fails to anchor the urethra and weakens the force of PCM contraction, so LP and LMA pull open the urethra during effort.

The Role of Damaged Connective Tissue in Incontinence Causation

'Mechanical' Imbalance

Stress Incontinence – A 'Mechanical' Imbalance

The cause of stress incontinence is mechanical failure of the connective tissue structures (fig 2-35). A lax pubourethral ligament (PUL) may unbalance the system by allowing LP to stretch open the outflow tract on effort, similar to that which happens during micturition.

The Role of Damaged Connective Tissue in the Pathogeneses of Intrinsic Sphincter Defect

Intraurethral pressure, as measured in one segment of the urethra, is equal to all the forces impacting on that segment divided by the area over which the forces are exerted (Pressure = force/area). The three directional muscle forces stretch the trigone to narrow the urethral lumen 'a', and cut off the venous return so that the vascular plexus swells into 'a' (fig 2-36). The horseshoe muscle contracts to seal the lumen 'a'. These components insert into the connective tissue of the vagina or pubourethral ligament (PUL).

Childbirth stretches connective tissue and ageing causes atrophy. Elastin begins to diminish in a female from her mid-twenties. This weakens the connective tissue of PUL, vagina, the urethral wall, and vascular plexus. The lumen 'a' loses its passive closure forces and dilates. The pubococcygeus (PCM) and the horseshoe muscles insert into connective tissue. As the connective tissue of the vagina and PUL atrophies, these muscles lose their contractile strength and may even atrophy to the extreme found by Huisman (1983). The combination of the diminished closure forces and the dilated lumen lower the intraurethral pressure: 'intrinsic sphincter defect'.

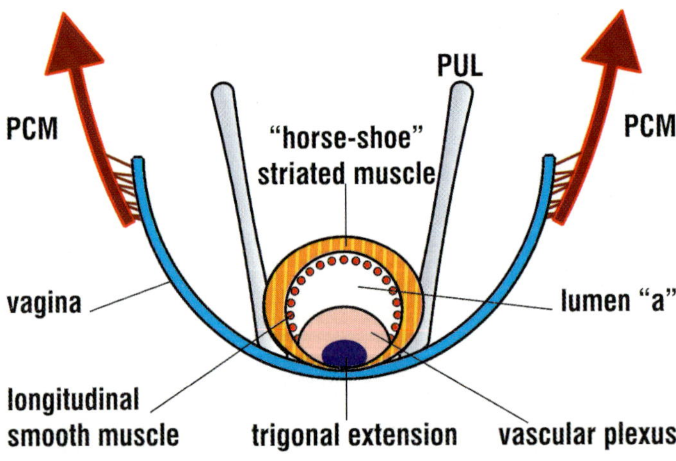

Fig. 2-36 The components of urethral closure. Perspective: vagina at midurethra

The Role of Connective Tissue in Peripheral Neurological Imbalance – Bladder Instability'

Connective tissue laxity in the suspensory ligaments or vaginal membrane (fig 2-37), may unbalance the peripheral neurological control mechanism, so that the stretch receptors (N) 'fire off' prematurely, causing manifestations of bladder (detrusor) instability.

The bladder lies on top of the vagina (cf. trampoline membrane), which is suspended from the pelvic girdle by the anterior (PUL), superolateral (ATFP) and posterior (USL) ligaments (cf. trampoline springs). As the bladder fills, the pelvic muscles reflexly stretch the vaginal membrane. This supports the hydrostatic pressure exerted by the urine column on the stretch receptors (N). It also explains the rise in urethral pressure observed during filling.

Laxity in the ligaments (cf. trampoline springs) or in the vagina (cf. trampoline membrane) (fig 2-37) may not transmit the forces applied and so the vagina cannot be adequately stretched. The stretch receptors may 'fire off' at a lower hydrostatic pressure (smaller bladder volume) and the cortex interprets this as urgency. The patient empties the bladder more frequently during the day (frequency). At night, there is nocturia. The sensitivity of the stretch receptors is clearly an important variable. Because a loose hammock may diminish the contribution of the forward forces to vaginal tensioning, hammock tightening is advised for patients undergoing anterior sling surgery for mixed incontinence.

This musculoelastic mechanism cannot counter bladder instability caused by damage to the cortical inhibitory circuits (white arrows, fig 2-37) say by multiple sclerosis, or excessive stimulation of 'N' by tumour or inflammation.

This process is further illustrated in the series of figures 6-15 to 6-18 in Chapter 6. Figure 6-18 shows how contraction of the puborectalis muscle (yellow arrow) can stretch the vagina forwards to support N and thereby restore balance in the system. This action can control an activated micturition reflex (fig 6-17).

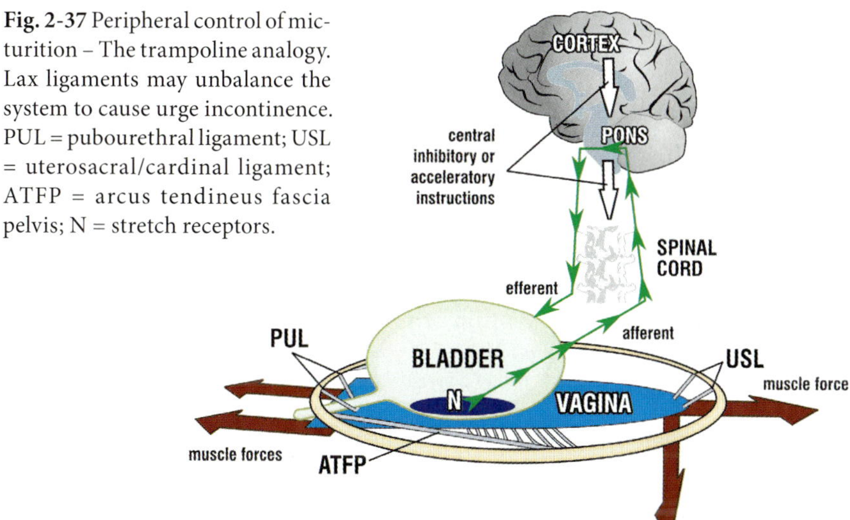

Fig. 2-37 Peripheral control of micturition – The trampoline analogy. Lax ligaments may unbalance the system to cause urge incontinence. PUL = pubourethral ligament; USL = uterosacral/cardinal ligament; ATFP = arcus tendineus fascia pelvis; N = stretch receptors.

The Role of Connective Tissue Damage in the Causation of Abnormal Bladder Emptying – A Mechanical Imbalance

Laxity in the ATFP, pubocervical fascia or uterosacral ligament (USL) may unbalance the external opening mechanism. Inability to stretch open ('funnel') the outflow tract may fail to lower the intra-urethral resistance to urine flow. As the urethral resistance varies with the 4th power of the diameter of the urethra, a high pressure may be needed to expel the urine. The clinical picture is one of obstructed micturition (Bush et al. 1997).

Symptoms for this condition are slow flow, 'stopping and starting', difficulty in initiating micturition, feeling of not having emptied, post-micturition dribble. A urodynamic demonstration of the consequences of inability of LMA and LP to open out the outflow tract, that is, a prolonged and slow micturition is shown in the series of figures 6-19, 6-20 and 6-21 in Chapter 6 of this book.

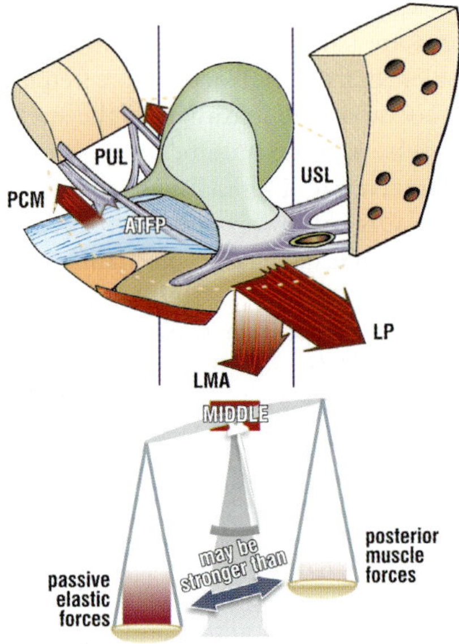

Fig. 2-38 Abnormal bladder emptying - inability to activate the external opening mechanism. A lax USL may inactivate the LMA contraction required to stretch open the outflow tract. A cystocoele may inactivate LP contraction.

Symptomatic Manifestations of Imbalance Caused by Damaged Connective Tissue

Proper functioning of the urethral tube requires firm connective tissue to be stretched open or closed by the pelvic muscles. Lax connective tissue therefore may result in a *mechanical* inability to open or close the urethra (cf. sail analogy). Failure of connective tissue to support bladder stretch receptors or pain fibres may result in *neurologically-based* dysfunctions, such as pelvic pain or premature activation of the micturition reflex (cf. trampoline analogy).

Mechanical Closure Defects

Symptoms of genuine stress incontinence, unconscious incontinence, continuous leakage and dribble incontinence (some types) are all consistent with a pathogenesis whereby lax anterior zone structures (PUL, hammock) may not permit urethral closure by the forward force, PCM.

Mechanical Opening Defects

Cystocoele or lax uterosacral ligaments may prevent the outflow tract being opened out by the backward muscle forces (LP and LMA). Inability to stretch open the urethra greatly increases the resistance to flow (to the 4th power) creating, in effect a functional obstruction. The patient perceives this as slow flow, feeling of not having emptied, post-micturition dribble, interrupted flow, dribble incontinence (some types), overflow incontinence, and difficulty in initiation of flow.

Peripheral Neurological Defects Caused by Connective Tissue Laxity

Lax connective tissue may cause the stretch receptors at bladder base to 'fire off' and activate the cascade of events which occur with micturition: sensory urgency, relaxation of PCM, opening out of the outflow tract, and detrusor contraction. Other causes of inappropriate activation of the micturition reflex are malignancy at bladder base, inflammation or even pressure on the stretch receptors by fibroids. The patient may present with symptoms of detrusor instability, low bladder capacity, sensory urgency, frequency, nocturia and motor urgency. All these symptoms are consistent with this pathogenesis. Poor sensitivity in the bladder base stretch receptors may prevent adequate activation of the micturition reflex. Hence the outflow tract has to be opened out by mechanical means only, that is by straining. This condition is described as 'detrusor acontractility' or 'under-activity'.

Pelvic Pain Caused by Connective Tissue Laxity

Pelvic pain related to laxity of the uterosacral ligaments (USL) is characterized by low dragging abdominal pain, (usually right-sided), deep dyspareunia, and often, low sacral backache (Petros 1996). It can vary in intensity. Sometimes it can be sufficiently severe for the patient to present as an emergency. It is often relieved on lying down, and usually exists as part of the 'posterior fornix syndrome' (posterior zone defect, fig 1-11) which may include urge, frequency, nocturia and abnormal emptying. The pain may occur with only minor degrees of prolapse. This pain can be reproduced ('simulated') by digital palpation of the USLs. It is hypothesized that the pain relief obtained after posterior IVS surgery is related to the physical support given to the S2-4 unmyelinated nerve fibres carried along the uterosacral ligaments. Ligamentous laxity may be causally linked to birth trauma in the multipara, or may arise in the nullipara soon after menarche.

2.3.4 The Role of Connective Tissue in Anorectal Opening, Closure and 'Idiopathic' Faecal Incontinence

This section is based on a series of clinical and experimental studies which indicate that idiopathic faecal incontinence, like urinary incontinence, may largely be caused by connective tissue damage. Thus it is related anatomically to the sections on urinary incontinence and prolapse. From the very first IVS prototype operations, patients with both stress (SI) and faecal incontinence (FI) volunteered that their FI had been cured by placement of a suburethral sling. Many reported cure of FI even when their

SI was not cured. Later, FI patients who did not have SI, but who had posterior zone defects also reported improvement of their FI (Petros 1999). These findings appeared to confirm Swash's observations that urinary and faecal incontinence may have a common origin. Using pudendal nerve conduction studies, Swash demonstrated that many (but not all) such patients had nerve damage. There were internal contradictions to this hypothesis. Many patients with FI had normal conduction times. In one study (Parks et al. 1977), 30% of FI patients referred for overlapping levator sphincter surgery had never been pregnant.

Existing Concepts for Anorectal Closure, Opening, and Faecal Incontinence

The mechanics of defaecation and faecal continence are not well understood. Existing valve-type theories for continence are not consistent with EMG and radiological data which suggest a striated muscle sphincteric mechanism, a concept supported by findings of neurological damage in patients with faecal incontinence (FI). Internal anal sphincter deficiency (Sultan et al. 1993) and motor endplate damage (Swash 1985) are considered to be important causes of faecal incontinence, but clinical studies (cf. Chapter 7) have demonstrated that these are not predictors for surgical success or failure using the anterior or posterior sling operations.

Anorectal Function According to the Integral Theory

In the Integral Theory, a similar mechanism to bladder neck closure is proposed, whereby directional muscle forces stretch the rectum backwards and downwards around an anus firmly anchored by the puborectalis muscle (PRM). Therefore, other than the puborectalis muscle, the ligaments and muscles involved in anorectal opening and closure are identical with those for bladder and urethra.

As the anus is a soft tissue structure with little inherent strength, it must be firmly anchored so that anorectal opening and closure may take place (fig 2-39). Dense fibromuscular tissue surrounds the lower 2-3 cm of urethra, vagina and anus. The perineal body (PB) is a key anchoring point for the distal vagina and anus. Contraction of the perineal membrane (PM) muscles and external anal sphincter (EAS) anchor the anus distally (Petros 2002). The deep transverse perineal muscles (fig 2-13) help anchor the upper part of PB to the descending ramus of the pubis.

The rectovaginal fascia (RVF) (fig 2-39) attaches to the perineal body (PB) below and levator plate (LP) above (Nichols 1989). It is stretched during anorectal closure and defaecation. Contraction of the levator plate (LP) stretches both walls of the rectum against an anus that has been immobilized by the puborectalis muscle (PRM) contraction. Contraction forwards of the anterior part of pubococcygeus (PCM) stretches the distal vagina and the anterior wall of the anus forwards creating, in effect, a semirigid tube for passage of faeces. LMA, on contraction, angulates the tip of LP downwards, creating the anorectal angle (figs 2-39 and 2-40).

PRM (fig 2-39) runs vertically below and medial to PCM, and inserts into the lower part of the pubic bone. It effectively compresses the sides of the anus and anchors its posterior wall. LP inserts directly into the posterior wall of rectum. On contraction,

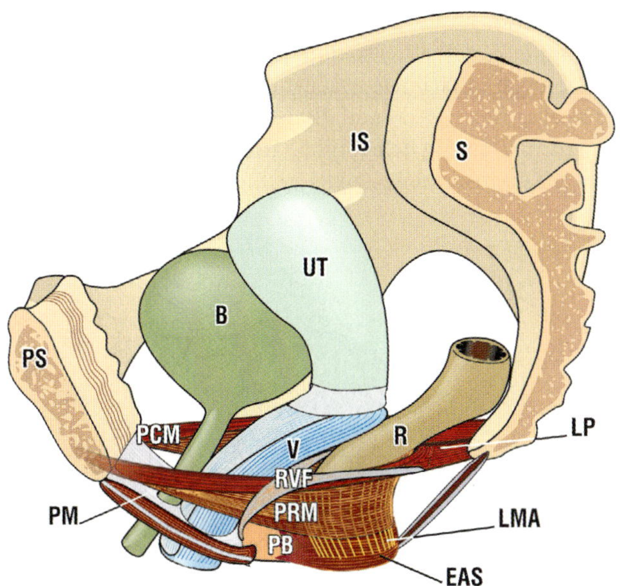

Fig 2-39 Anatomy of anorectal opening and closure. Schematic 3D view of the anus, rectum and relevant striated muscles.

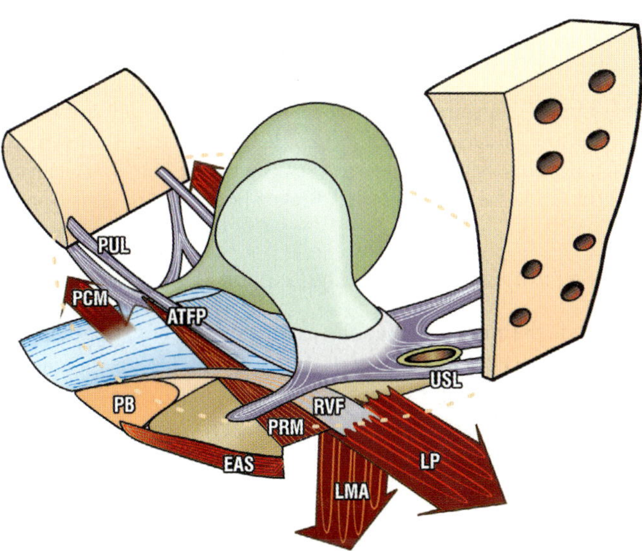

Fig. 2-40 Stable anorectal closure – Stable anorectal closure is similar to urethrovesical closure. LP and LMA contract to stretch the rectum and RVF backwards and downwards around a contracted PRM to create the anorectal angle. PCM tensions the perineal body and anterior wall of rectum. PRM acts directly against symphysis pubis.

it stretches the posterior wall of rectum backwards to create the anorectal angle. It is evident from figure 2-39 that relaxation of PRM will cause LP and LMA to open out the anorectal angle to facilitate evacuation of the rectum (fig 2-41). The deep transverse perineal muscles, PCM and PB, have an important role in anchoring the anterior wall of rectum during defaecation. The pubourethral ligaments anchor LP contraction and the uterosacral ligaments anchor LMA contraction (fig 2-41).

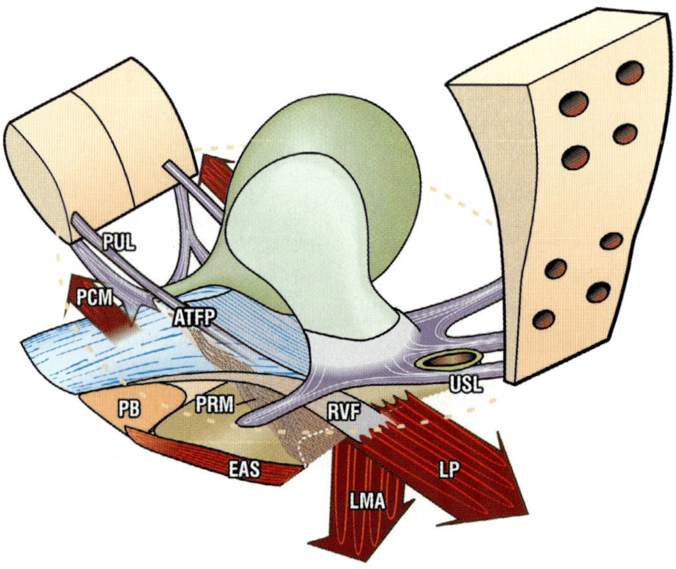

Fig. 2-41 Stable anorectal opening (defaecation). As PRM relaxes, LP and LMA stretch open the anorectal angle and posterior wall of rectum. RVF tensions the anterior rectal wall and PCM stretches it forwards, helping to create a semirigid tube (anus) to facilitate evacuation. The rectum contracts and faeces are expelled. Broken lines indicate 'closed' position.

Connective Tissue Laxity and Anorectal Dysfunction

Anal dysfunction is defined as the inability to evacuate ('constipation') or to contain the rectal contents ('incontinence'). Incontinence is graded (in increasing degrees of severity) as wind, liquid or solid incontinence.

Observational data collected from patients undergoing anterior and posterior IVS operations for FI suggest that anal sensation may work in a similar manner to the bladder: Anorectal stretch and volume receptors may initiate a defaecation reflex which can be controlled by puborectalis muscle (PRM) contraction.

Defaecation is different to anorectal opening. Like micturition, defaecation is driven by a neurological reflex which coordinates all the elements required to produce efficient evacuation.

Because LP and LMA also act during anorectal closure (fig 2-40) and defaecation (fig 2-41), if the ligaments against which these muscles act are damaged, dysfunctions of both closure and opening may occur. If the perineal body and rectovaginal fascia are damaged, the anterior wall of rectum cannot be stretched, and defaecation difficulties may occur simultaneously. This same laxity may also be an important cause of haemorrhoids. The inward collapse of the anterior rectal wall may inhibit the venous return, distending the veins and creating backward pressure which may cause pain and bleeding. It has often been observed that haemorrhoids disappear after a three level Posterior IVS repair.

If the insertion points of the levator plate (LP) (pubourethral ligament (PUL)) or LMA (uterosacral ligaments (USL)) are damaged, the backward and downward forces may not be able to create the necessary anorectal angle and faecal incontinence may occur.

The Role of Striated Muscle in Faecal Incontinence (FI)

A damaged external anal sphincter (EAS) is a major correctable cause of FI. It may contribute to FI in two ways. Firstly through its direct effect on distal closure of the anus and secondly, by its inactivation of LMA contraction. EAS is the insertion point of LMA. LMA is a key element in creation of the anorectal angle. The exact contribution of damaged pelvic muscle to FI is yet to be defined. Because the pelvic muscles effectively insert into the pelvic ligaments, a lax ligamentous anchoring point may cause that muscle to atrophy. The impact of damaged pelvic muscles on FI is likely to be minor, given the greater than 80% improvement rate following PUL or USL reinforcement with polypropylene tapes.

'Constipation'

During defaecation (fig 2-41), LP stretches the rectovaginal fascia (RVF) against the perineal body (PB) and RVF is then pulled downwards by LMA to open out the anorectal junction. Connective tissue laxity in USL, RVF or PB may weaken LP and unbalance this system, causing the puborectalis muscle to overcompensate and pull the anorectal junction forwards. Symptoms are 'straining at the stool' and 'constipation'.

Inability to splint the anterior wall of the anus explains difficulty in rectal evacuation ('constipation') in some patients, and why digital pressure on the perineum by the patient is often required to aid defaecation. Digital pressure anchors the perineal body. The anchoring effect of PB can often be demonstrated using synchronous perineal ultrasound. A lax PB may reduce the downward angulation of levator plate seen during straining to a mere flicker, while LP contracts exaggeratedly upwards and backwards. Anchoring PB can reduce this movement and restore the downward angulation of the anterior portion of levator plate (Petros 2002). As LP contracts against PUL and LMA against USL (fig 2-41), lax ligaments may weaken the backward force needed for anorectal opening, leading to 'constipation' (Petros, 1999). It is known that connective tissue weakens and loses elasticity with age, thus preventing the rectum being stretched to the semirigid tube required for evacuation. This may explain the increasing incidence of 'constipation' with age.

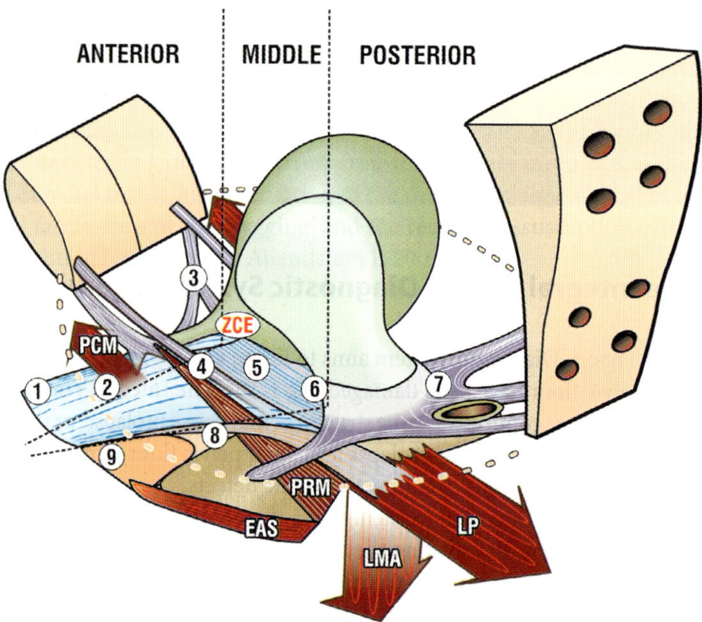

Fig 1-10 The three zone structure of the pelvic floor according to the Integral Theory showing the nine main structures and the special case 'ZCE' potentially needing surgical repair. A 3D view of the pelvis from above and behind. The dotted lines represent the pelvic brim. PCM = anterior portion of pubococcygeus muscle; LP = levator plate; LMA = longitudinal muscle of the anus; PRM = puborectalis muscle; EAS = external anal sphincter. 'ZCE' = 'Tethered vagina' - excessive tightness caused by previous surgery.

The Integral Theory Diagnostic System is an iterative process based on the perspectives of the pelvic floor anatomy and dynamics presented thus far in this book. There are two pathways: Clinical Assessment (fig 3-01) and the Structured Assessment (fig 3-02).

The Clinical Assessment pathway (fig 3-01) begins with the Pictorial Diagnostic Algorithm (fig 1-11), the starting point of the Integral Theory Diagnostic System. It provides a summary guide to diagnosis and management of pelvic floor dysfunction and is especially useful for generalist surgeons who do not have access to the facilities of a specialist clinic. When using the Pictorial Diagnostic Algorithm, the suggested 'zone(s)' of damage are checked by vaginal examination (fig 3-04) and confirmed by 'simulated operations' (fig 3-06). This is a relatively simple clinical technique which directly tests a connective tissue structure for stress or urge incontinence. A haemostat, finger, or ring forceps are used to anchor these structures in all three zones of the vagina with the patient providing feedback and response.

The Structured Assessment Pathway (fig 3-02) has been developed for use in a specialist referral clinic. The key elements and the 'decision tree' are summarized in figure 3-02. A questionnaire and urinary diary are completed by the patient. Pad

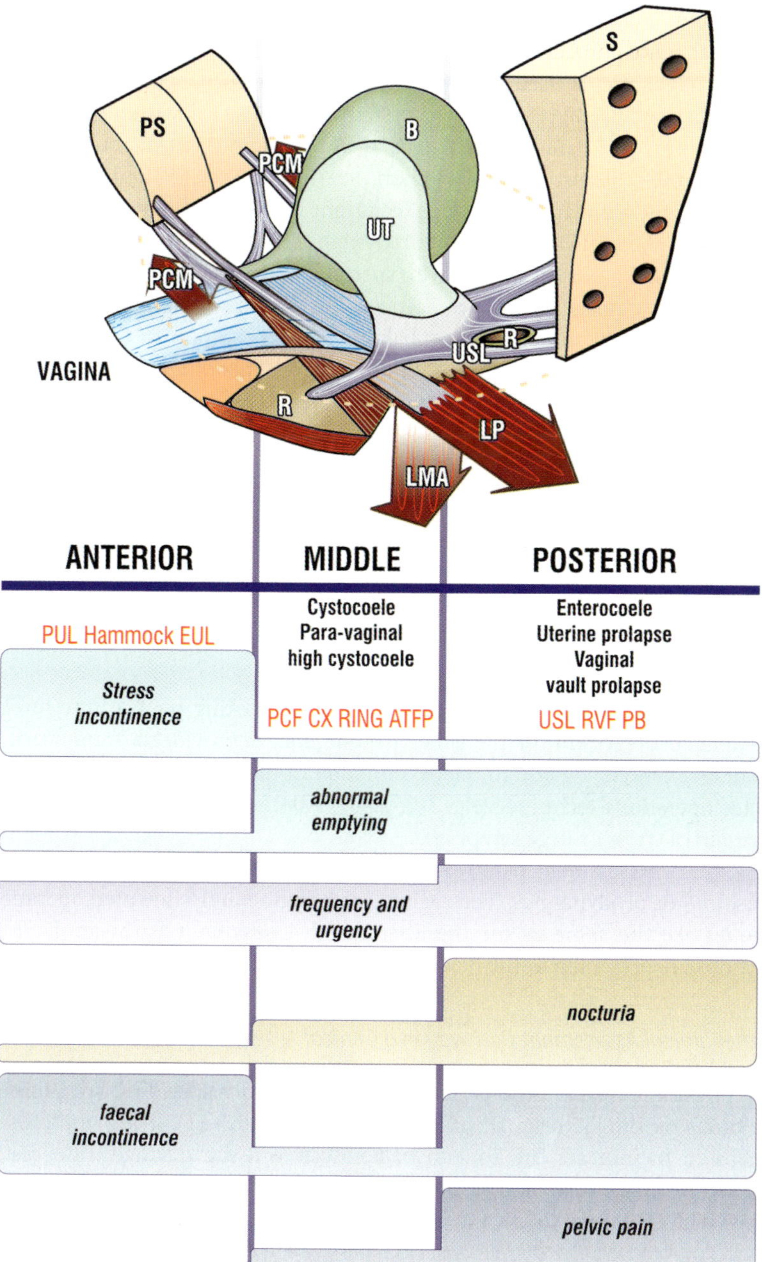

Fig. 1-11 The Pictorial Diagnostic Algorithm. This is a summary guide to causation and management of pelvic floor conditions. The area of the symptom rectangles indicates the estimated frequency of symptom causation occurring in each zone. The main connective tissue structures causing the symptoms are summarized in each zone, in order of importance. Note that there is no correlation between degree of prolapse and the severity of symptoms.

tests are used to quantify urine loss. There is a vaginal examination and, if available, transperineal ultrasound is used to assess the pelvic floor geometry. Similarly, if available, urodynamics is used to assess urethral competence, bladder stability and output. (The Structured Assessment is effective even if used without ultrasound or urodynamics). The data obtained from the Structured Assessment process are transcribed to the Diagnostic Summary Sheet (See fig 3-03, page 59) and the diagnosis tested by using the simulated operations technique (fig 3-07), if required.

The Integral Theory Diagnostic Support System (ITDS) consists of a data base and a computer based diagnostic system (with specially written software) to confirm the zone in which the damage has occurred. It uses the same decision making tree as the Structured Assessment and uses the probability of each component to diagnose the zone of damage. The ITDS component of the Integral Theory Diagnostic System is explained fully in Chapter 7, 'Current and Emerging Issues'.

3.2   The Integral Theory Diagnostic System

3.2.1   The Clinical Assessment Pathway

Introduction

The Pictorial Diagnostic Algorithm (fig 1-11) is the starting point of the Integral Theory diagnostic system for the generalist surgeon. It provides a framework for symptom assessment, a guide to the examination of the patient (fig 3-04), and the 'simulated operations' technique (figs 3-05, 3-07, 3-08, 3-09) for detailed localization of the origin of stress or urge symptoms.

The Clinical Assessment pathway does not require expensive equipment, such as ultrasound or urodynamics. The vaginal examination and 'simulated operations' techniques are the same as for the Structured Assessment Pathway. Detailed descriptions are presented in the next section.

Using the Clinical Assessment Pathway in a Clinical Assessment (fig 3-01)

1. The physician consults the patient and ticks the corresponding symptoms in the boxes on the Pictorial Diagnostic Algorithm (fig 1-11). The symptoms are organised to indicate the zone(s) of connective tissue damage. Information gleaned from the Patient Questionnaire (Appendix 1) helps the physician decide which questions to ask the patient. Responses from the patient allows the physician to assess the degree of seriousness of the condition.
2. The aim of the examination stage is to confirm the potential sites of damage. Using the Halfway Classification system (Fig 3-06), these sites are recorded as 1st, 2nd, 3rd or 4th degree prolapse on the Clinical Examination Sheet (Fig 3-04). The examination should always be done while the patient has a full bladder.

Experience has shown that accurate diagnosis of some anatomical defects (especially in the posterior zone) is not always possible in a clinical setting. Often the final diagnosis can only be made once the patient is actually in the Operating Room.

3. The 'Simulated Operations' technique involves providing mechanical support to specific connective tissue structures (either digitally or with forceps) to ascertain any change in urge and stress symptoms. Applying support may significantly relieve urge symptoms, which can give guidance as to causation. In the case of stress incontinence, anchoring each structure in turn may help determine and define the contribution of each of the three anterior zone structures (fig 3-08).

   If a patient does not have urge symptoms during the examination, they may need to drink water until urgency is felt. The 'Simulated Operations' technique can then be repeated. For patients with failed stress incontinence sling surgery, the cause may sometimes be laxity in the posterior ligaments (especially if the stress incontinence began after hysterectomy).

3.2.2 The Structured Assessment Pathway

Introduction

The Structured Assessment Pathway (fig 3-02) has been designed for use in clinics which specialise in pelvic floor disorders. It is essentially a clinically based process, although it uses ultrasound and urodynamics.

The Structured Assessment Pathway is an iterative process consisting of three stages: Collection and correlation of data, analysis of the data, and verification (or not) of provisional diagnosis.

Data is collected from the questionnaire, the urinary diary, the vaginal examination, pad tests, urodynamics and perineal ultrasound. (To remove bias, it is best if the questionnaire is completed by the patient.) Relevant data is transcribed on to the Diagnostic Summary Sheet (fig 3-03).

The Diagnostic Summary Sheet consists of four groupings which list the specific conditions which form the basis for diagnosing the zone(s) of damage. The groupings are:

- symptoms
- examination
- urodynamics
- ultrasound.

Each condition in these groupings is checked against the data collected. These entries on the Diagnostic Summary Sheet are then analysed by the physician and a provisional diagnosis of damaged structures is made.

This provisional diagnosis is then verified (or not) using the 'simulated operations' technique.

It is advisable for the physician to make a copy of figure 3-03 for each patient.

Note: The questionnaire, instructions on pad test usage and which data to use from ultrasound and urodynamic tests are detailed in Appendix 1.

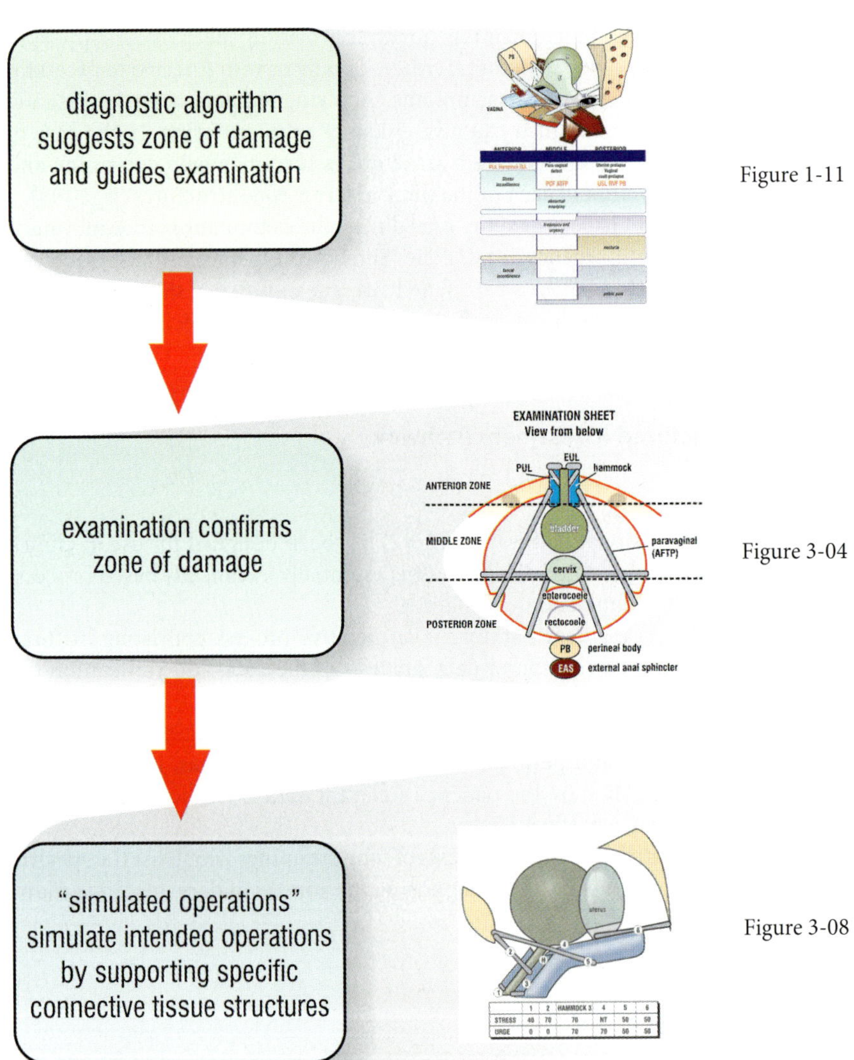

Fig 3-01 The Clinical Assessment Pathway. This figure shows the relationship between the Pictorial Diagnostic Algorithm, the Structured Assessment Diagram and the 'Simulated Operations' Validation Table.

Structured Assessment Path

Data Collection Stage

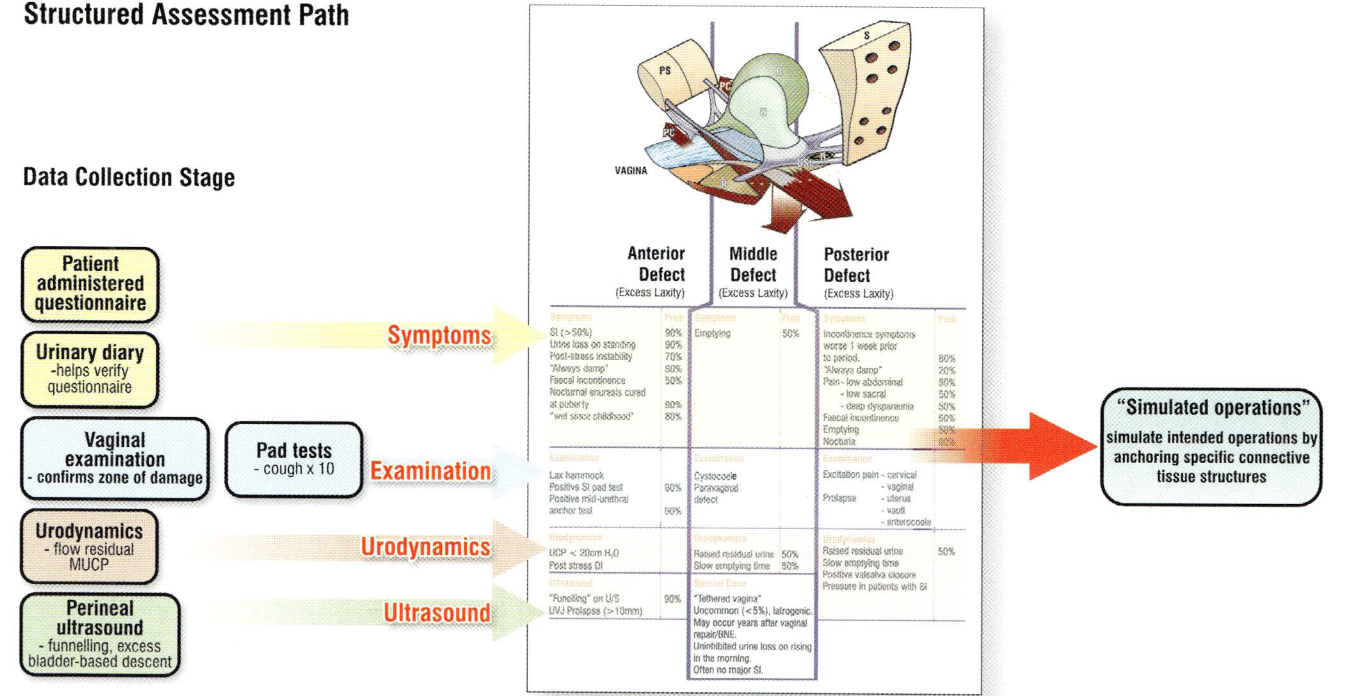

Diagnostic Summary Sheet (Fig. 3-03)

Fig 3-02 The Structured Assessment Pathway incorporates three stages: data collection, diagnostic summary and 'simulated operation'. The Diagnostic Summary Sheet lists the conditions specific for each zone of damage. The conditions are grouped under four headings: 'symptoms', 'examination', 'ultrasound' and 'urodynamics'. Each condition in each zone is checked against the data collected and 'ticked' if it correlates. The zone(s) of damage may then be identified according to the number of 'ticks' in each zone. Once the zone of damage is established it can be validated directly using 'simulated operations', that is, by anchoring specific structures and observing the percentage change in symptoms or urine loss.

Phase One: Data Collection and Correlation

The Patient Questionnaire (Appendix I, or visit www.integraltheory.org)

In the Integral Theory, symptoms are a useful guide to the site of damaged connective tissue. The patient questionnaire is used to provide comprehensive information about symptoms associated with the zone of damage.

Instructions for administering the questionnaire are included in Appendix 1. The patient places a 'tick' in a box next to a description of her symptoms. The physician collates the responses in the questionnaire into the Diagnostic Summary Sheet (fig 3-03) by ticking the symptoms listed in the columns where they appear on the sheet. Each column represents a zone of the vagina. If a symptom (for example, 'emptying') appears in two zones, it is ticked in both zones. After the symptom section has been completed, a reasonably accurate indication as to which zone may be damaged can usually be obtained. This helps guide the physician in the vaginal examination (fig 3-04). The data in the questionnaire help to improve the objectivity of the process and provides a valuable record for gauging improvement or otherwise post intervention.

The questions are grouped under specific headings: stress incontinence, urge incontinence, deficient emptying, bowel symptoms, pelvic pain and social inconvenience. Individual questions within these groupings may be linked to specific conditions and zone of damage. These questions are prefixed by the letters 'A', 'M' or 'P' to indicate likely connective tissue damage in the anterior, middle or posterior zone. The questions with a prefix 'A', 'M', or 'P' are so designated because affirmative answers indicate a high probability of being associated with a specific zone or damage. Urgency symptoms are a special case in that they are the only one which can be associated with all three zones.

The questions *without* the prefix have, as yet, no significant or clear probability link to a particular zone. Hence these questions are *not* included in the Diagnostic Summary Sheet (fig 3-03).

Some of the questions have a box for a third option that may be selected by the patient. The box is ticked by the patient if the symptom occurs more than 50% of the time. This response is an indication of severity of the symptom and is especially useful information to assess progress after an intervention when the questionnaire is used post-operatively.

A response in this box is also used as a 'filter' designed to give the physician an indication of patients that are likely to require surgery for stress incontinence (anterior zone damage), as against those that aren't. Only where there is more than 50% stress incontinence is the symptom ticked in the anterior zone of the Diagnostic Summary Sheet (see 'symptom variability', page 69).

For all other symptoms a tick in the 'sometimes' box is sufficient to warrant their inclusion in the Diagnostic Summary Sheet.

Some questions in the questionnaire are followed by a number in parenthesis. This is a numbered code that links with notes at the end of the patient questionnaire which explains and expands the information in the Diagnostic Summary Sheet.

The 24 Hour Urinary Diary

The information entered into the 24 hour urinary diary by the patient provides a check on the patient's historical accuracy. In particular, it excludes excessive fluid intake as a cause of frequency. The diary is not used directly in the diagnostic decision tree.

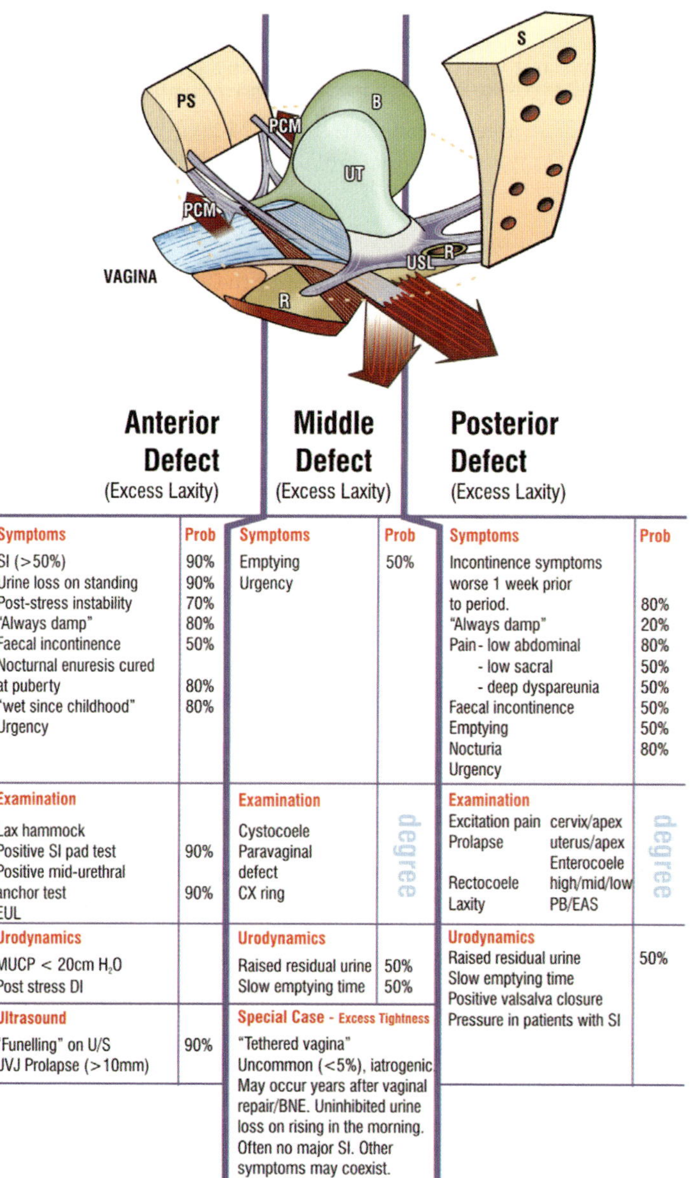

Fig. 3-03 The Diagnostic Summary Sheet as used in the Structured Assessment Pathway. It is designed to be copied by the physician and used as a record. Each condition is checked against the data gathered and ticked when appropriate. The more ticks in each column, the greater the confidence that the corresponding zone has been damaged. The probabilities listed against some symptoms indicate the likelihood that damage within that zone is causing that particular condition. The physician may record other relevant data onto the Diagnostic Summary Sheet, such as degree of prolapse, urge incontinence episodes per day, etc., as a record summary. An example of a completed Diagnostic Summary Sheet is included in Appendix 1, page 234.

Pad Tests

Pad tests are a simple and effective means for assessing severity of incontinence and the results of intervention. A rapid cough stress test (cough x 10) can confirm (or not) the likelihood of an anterior zone defect. The 24 hour pad test is performed in the same time period as the 24 hour diary. It is used to determine the severity of the incontinence problem.

The Vaginal Examination

The vaginal examination is always conducted while the patient has a full bladder. It is used to validate (or not) the zone of damage predicted by the clinician's interpretation of the data in the patient questionnaire. Damage to any of the 9 structures (fig 1-10) and degree of prolapse are noted on the Clinical Examination sheet (fig 3-04). The relevant parts are transcribed to the Diagnostic Summary Sheet (fig 3-03).

Direct confirmation of specific defects may be difficult in an Outpatient setting. The decision as to which structure to repair may need to be made in the operating room.

Testing for Vulvar Vestibulitis when Indicated

A cotton bud is gently applied at 0.5 cm intervals to the hymenal area of introitus in a circle. A hypersensitive reaction confirms a diagnosis of vulvar vestibulitis.

Anterior Zone Examination

Three structures are tested: the external urethral ligament (EUL), the pubourethral ligament (PUL) and the vaginal hammock. A 'pouting' (open) external urethral meatus generally signals laxity in the EULs, especially if associated with eversion of the urethral mucosa. The test for a damaged PUL involves two essential stages. The first is for the patient to demonstrate urine loss in the supine position on coughing (Petros & Von Konsky 1999). Then, a finger or a haemostat is placed at midurethra on one side and the cough is repeated. Control of urine loss signifies a weak PUL. The EUL can be similarly tested.

A lax hammock is evident on inspection, but it can also be tested by the 'pinch' test, taking a unilateral fold of the hammock with a haemostat (Petros & Ulmsten 1990). Diminution of urine loss during this test demonstrates the importance of an adequately tight hammock for urethral closure. These manoeuvres are an essential part of the vaginal examination. They also form part of the 'simulated operations' technique.

Middle Zone Examination

A pure midline defect (cystocoele) is shiny. A pure paravaginal defect has well marked vaginal rugae. A cystocoele can be differentiated from a paravaginal defect by placing ring forceps in the lateral sulci to support the ATFP and asking the patient to strain. Often, however, a patient has both midline and lateral defects. With a cervical ring defect (high cystocoele), there is a 'ballooning' of the vagina just anterior to the cervix or hysterectomy scar, often extending laterally along the cardinal ligament.

Excessive tightness in the bladder neck area of vagina (scarring, excessive bladder neck elevation) in patients who leak immediately on getting out of bed in the morning ('tethered vagina syndrome') should be noted on the Clinical Examination Sheet (fig 3-04). Observation of excessive tightness (or not) in the bladder neck area of the vagina ('ZCE') is more reliably made in the operating room.

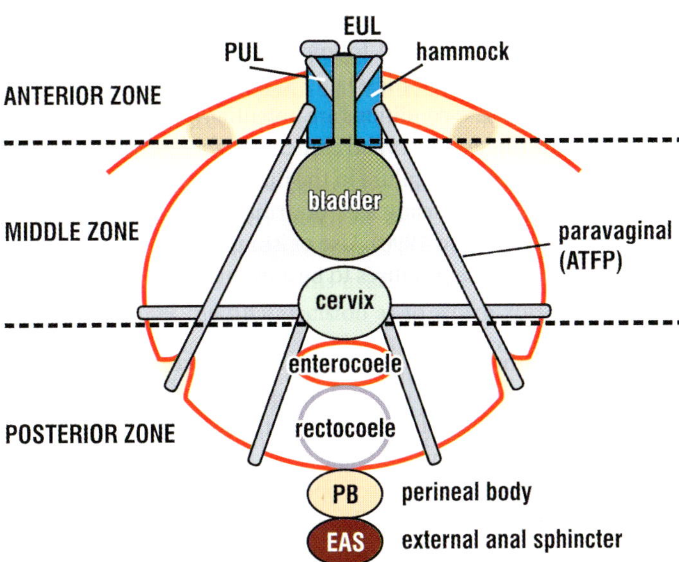

Fig. 3-04 The clinical examination sheet is designed to be copied and used by the clinician as a record. Each structure is assessed and notated, if possible as 1st, 2nd or 3rd degree prolapse, or for PUL and EUL, 'normal' or 'lax'. An example of a completed Examination Sheet is included in Appendix 1, page 235.

Posterior Zone Examination

Evidence of a bulge at the apex, vaginal wall or perineal body should be looked for during straining. Small degrees of prolapse in the apex of the vagina are easily missed. Therefore, always support the lateral sulci of the vagina with ring forceps and ask the patient to strain when examining the posterior zone. The posterior vaginal wall is tested for defects in the rectovaginal fascia (rectocoele) by asking the patient to strain, and also by digital rectal examination. The perineal body and external anal sphincter are tested by digital examination.

Physical Examination for Classification of Prolapse

The International Continence Society's POPQ classification system was designed to quantify prolapse. The Integral Theory system for examination is specifically oriented towards surgical correction of symptoms. Although the POPQ system is compatible with the Integral Theory approach, it plays no role in the Diagnostic Decision pathway. Furthermore, the POPQ diverts examination time away from the assessment of damage in the structures within the three zones (as described in the Integral Theory). As there is only a limited time available to reasonably examine a patient, a clinician may choose the simpler and more widely available Halfway Classification System (fig 3-06) to notate the Clinical Examination Sheet (fig 3-04).

In patients with lower abdominal or pelvic pain, palpation of the posterior fornix with ring forceps, or digitally, usually reproduces the pain complained of by the patient.

Patients with a cystocoele or enterocoele should always be examined with a full bladder and asked to cough before and after reduction of the prolapse so as to uncover 'latent' stress incontinence.

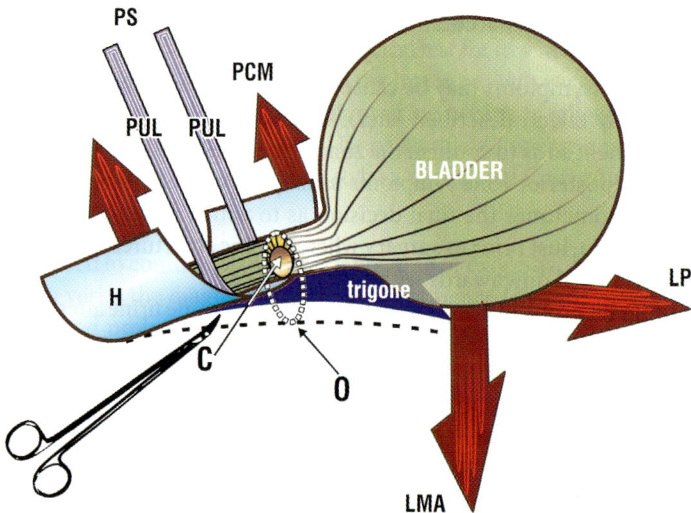

Fig. 3-05 Technique for diagnosing a damaged pubourethral ligament (L). Schematic 3D view of distal vagina (V), urethra and bladder. A haemostat applied unilaterally at midurethra mimics the effect of a midurethral sling. Midurethral anchoring restores the closure forces which narrow the urethra from 'O' (stress incontinence) to 'C' (continence) during coughing. Taking a fold of vagina 'H' ('pinch' test) may also decrease urine loss.

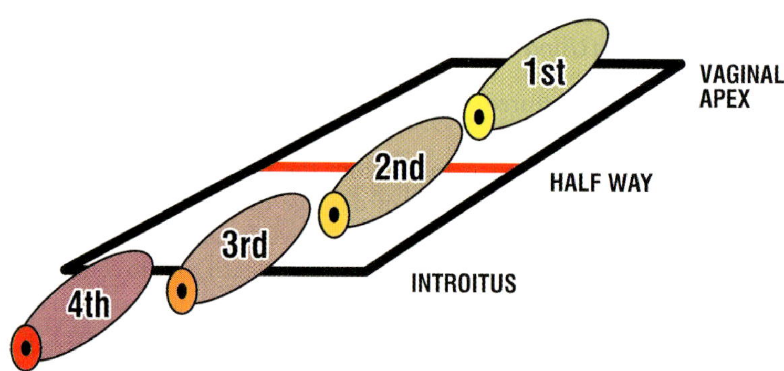

Fig. 3-06 Halfway Classification System. Perspective: schematic 3D sagittal view. The Halfway Classification System is used for prolapse from grades 1-4. Prolapse assessment is best performed under gentle traction, preferably in the operating room:

1st degree = prolapse to the halfway point;

2nd degree = prolapse between the halfway point and introitus, but not beyond;

3rd degree = prolapse beyond introitus;

4th degree = total eversion of either uterus or vaginal vault with traction.

Limitations of 'Simulated Operations'

Not all patients with a history of urge symptoms can reproduce their urge symptoms even with a full bladder when lying in the supine position. Occasionally the serial anchoring of specific structures listed in figure 3-08 makes no impact on the urge symptoms. In such patients, other causes such as bladder cancer should be rigorously excluded before proceeding.

In younger women, pelvic inflammatory disease or endometriosis needs to be excluded in patients with a positive pain response to palpation.

'Simulated Operation' Technique: Anterior Zone

The patient should always be tested with a full bladder. An artery forceps applied unilaterally at the pubourethral ligament (PUL) ('2' in fig 3-08) during coughing in a patient with stress incontinence may control urine loss in 80% of patients. This often relieves urge symptoms as well if the patient has mixed incontinence. The 'pinch test' (taking up a fold of vaginal epithelium unilaterally) '3' may control stress incontinence (SI) completely in up to 30% of patients and demonstrates the importance of an adequately tight hammock for continence (Petros 2003). In about 10% of patients, anchoring EUL may diminish urine loss or urge. Anchoring '2' and '3' (fig 3-08) together almost invariably controls urine loss with SI completely, demonstrating the importance of also tightening the hammock during midurethral sling surgery.

'Simulated Operation' Technique: Middle Zone

Gentle digital support at bladder base '4' (fig 3-07) usually improves urge symptoms. Alternatively, a fold of vaginal tissue can be taken below bladder base using Littlewood's forceps. Stretching the bladder base vigorously upwards towards the pubic symphysis almost invariably worsens urge symptoms. This explains why bladder neck elevation surgery may give rise to a new incidence of urgency and 'detrusor instability' (DI). Excess pressure with ring forceps in the sulci '5' may also worsen the urge. Gentle pressure may reduce urge. These manoeuvres demonstrate how extremely sensitive bladder base stretch receptors may be in some patients. Reduction of a cystocoele and asking the patient to cough may uncover latent SI. In such patients a suburethral sling should be inserted at the same time as cystocoele repair.

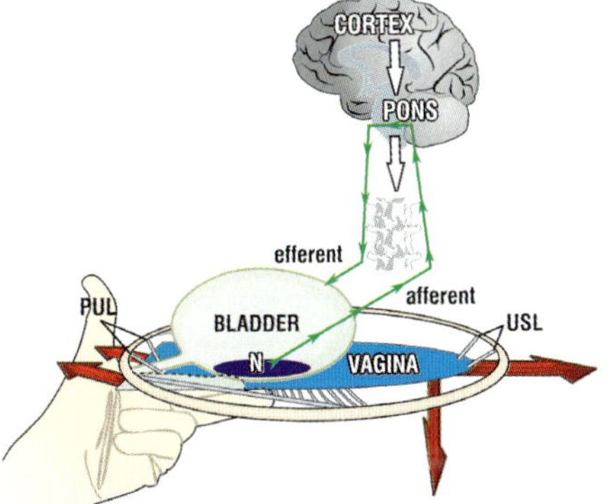

Fig 3-07 'Simulated Operation' Technique. The urine column is supported. The stretch receptors (N) do not 'fire off' prematurely. Afferents to do not reach the cortex. The sensation of urge diminishes.

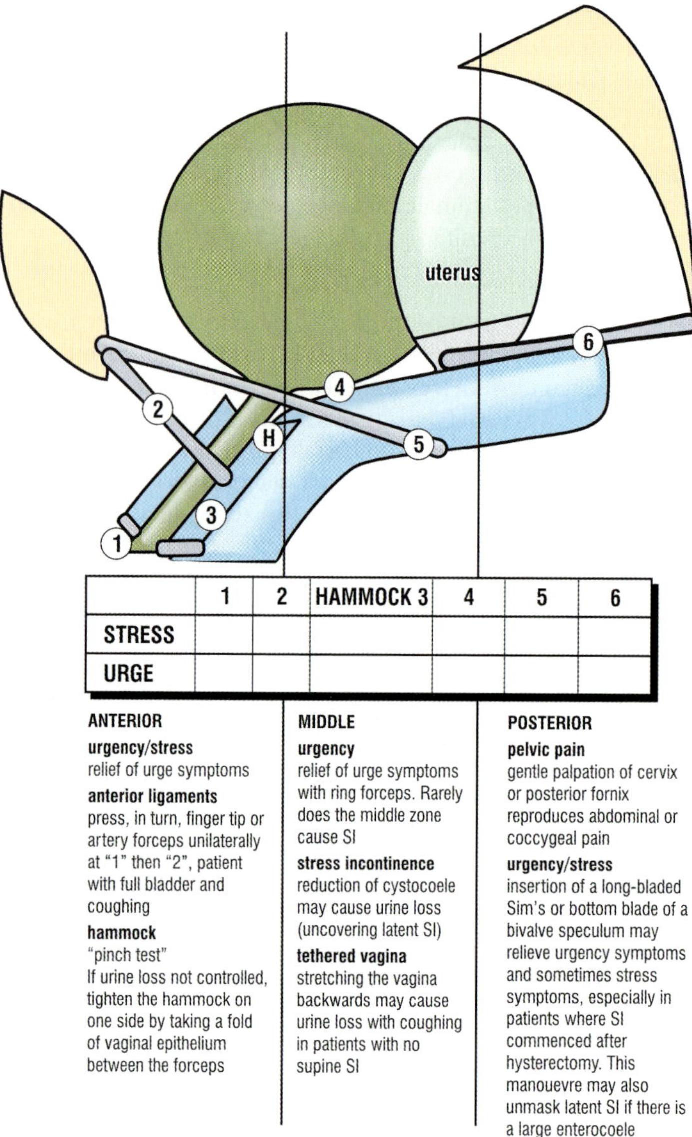

	1	2	HAMMOCK 3	4	5	6
STRESS						
URGE						

ANTERIOR

urgency/stress
relief of urge symptoms

anterior ligaments
press, in turn, finger tip or
artery forceps unilaterally
at "1" then "2", patient
with full bladder and
coughing

hammock
"pinch test"
If urine loss not controlled,
tighten the hammock on
one side by taking a fold
of vaginal epithelium
between the forceps

MIDDLE

urgency
relief of urge symptoms
with ring forceps. Rarely
does the middle zone
cause SI

stress incontinence
reduction of cystocoele
may cause urine loss
(uncovering latent SI)

tethered vagina
stretching the vagina
backwards may cause
urine loss with coughing
in patients with no
supine SI

POSTERIOR

pelvic pain
gentle palpation of cervix
or posterior fornix
reproduces abdominal or
coccygeal pain

urgency/stress
insertion of a long-bladed
Sim's or bottom blade of a
bivalve speculum may
relieve urgency symptoms
and sometimes stress
symptoms, especially in
patients where SI
commenced after
hysterectomy. This
manouevre may also
unmask latent SI if there is
a large enterocoele

Fig. 3-08 The 'Simulated Operations' Validation Table. The clinician uses this table to
record percentage decrease in urine loss with coughing (stress) or percentage decrease in
urge symptoms following digital support (anchoring) of the individual structures 1-6 in the
three zones. The patient should always attend with a full bladder, sufficient to cause urgency
symptoms when lying down.
1 = external urethral ligament (EUL); 2 = pubourethral ligament (PUL); 3 = hammock; 4 =
bladder base; 5 = ATFP (lateral sulcus); 6 = posterior fornix (USL).
Perspective: In a clinical setting, only structures 1, 2 and 3 are generally tested for *stress incontinence*. All the structures (1-6) need to be tested to locate the causes of *urge symptoms*.

'Simulated Operation' Technique: Posterior Zone

Gently stretching the posterior fornix '6' backwards digitally, with a Sim's type speculum or opened out ring forceps may relieve urge symptoms (see the 'trampoline analogy'). Excess stretching may worsen the urge, once again demonstrating the extreme sensitivity of the stretch receptors at bladder base in some patients. Digital or ring forceps stretching of the posterior fornix usually reproduces a patient's pelvic pain symptoms. In some patients reporting the onset of stress incontinence after hysterectomy, anchoring the posterior fornix may significantly diminish urine loss during coughing (Petros & Ulmsten 1990).

Deciding which Structural Defects to Repair Surgically in 'Difficult' Cases

It is emphasised that there is no correlation between quantum of prolapse and quantum of symptoms. Prolapse may exist without symptoms and no symptom is necessarily present in a particular zone.

There is no quantum of prolapse specified in figure 3-03 because the same operation is performed whether the prolapse is first or fourth degree.

Often, the final decision as to which structural defect(s) to repair can only be made in the Operating Room because confirmation in the outpatient setting may be difficult. For example, patients with posterior zone symptoms, (pelvic pain, urgency, nocturia and abnormal emptying) frequently have only minimal prolapse. In the author's experience, it is rare for such patients to not have at least first degree prolapse of the apex of vagina.

Another difficult diagnosis to make is the 'tethered vagina syndrome'. Older patients (>70 years) with previous surgery and classical symptoms of the 'tethered vagina syndrome' (losing urine immediately their foot hits the floor on getting up in the morning) may in fact be suffering from a weak pubourethral ligament. It is necessary to confirm tightness and/or scarring in the bladder neck area of vagina prior to surgically restoring elasticity in this area, and this may need to be done in the Operating Room.

3.3 Working with Symptoms in the Integral Theory Diagnostic System

3.3.1 The Reliability of Symptoms

Symptoms are the sentinels of the body and inform the cortex that something has gone wrong. The brain stores symptoms, orders them, and averages them out, and so presents the patient's collective experience over a period of time. From Hippocrates onwards, symptoms have been an essential element in a medical diagnosis. The symptoms displayed in figure 3-03 are essential for the diagnostic process with the Integral Theory. For example, a patient with symptoms of pelvic pain, nocturia, abnormal emptying and urgency ('posterior fornix syndrome', Petros & Ulmsten, 1993) has a greater than 80% probability of cure following reconstruction of the posterior zone with the posterior IVS operation.

Practical Application of the Structured Assessment

The structured assessment is best performed in two visits. The protocol outlined is that followed by the author. It can be altered according to the physician's or clinic's needs. It is advisable to perform Structured Assessment even in patients presenting with prolapse and few apparent symptoms. This process will generally reveal the presence of some accompanying dysfunction.

First Visit

The History

Prior to the first visit, the questionnaire is mailed to the patient to be completed by her at home. She then attends with a comfortably full bladder. The physician checks the questionnaire and completes the first part of Diagnostic Summary Sheet (fig 3-03). The information from the questionnaire guides the physician as to where to look during the examination.

The Examination

Using the Clinical Examination Sheet (fig 3-04) as a guide, the physician checks the three zones for evidence of connective tissue laxity. The findings are noted on the Clinical Examination Sheet. During the examination, patients with stress incontinence are asked to cough, and the midurethral anchor and 'pinch tests' are carried out to confirm PUL and hammock laxity. There is no other reliable way to test for these defects. If transperineal ultrasound is available, the patient may be tested for bladder neck descent and funnelling. All these findings are entered into the Diagnostic Summary Sheet (fig 3-03).

If the patient has urgency in the supine position, 'simulated operations' can be done whereby the six connective tissue structures are be anchored in turn to assess the contribution of each structure to the urge symptoms.

Prior to leaving the clinic, the patient is instructed by the nurse on how to do a 24 hour pad test and how to complete a 24 hour urinary diary which are done during the 24 hours preceding the second visit. Both are used to check for consistency in the questionnaire responses.

Second Visit

Ensure the patient attends with a comfortably full bladder.

24 Hour Pad Tests

The nurse weighs the used pads from the 24 hour pad test. Then the nurse administers the cough stress test and the 30 second hand-washing test. In the cough stress test, the patient is in the standing position and urine loss during 10 coughs is measured. If available, urodynamic testing is performed at this stage.

Review of Data, Diagnosis and Treatment Decisions

The physician reviews the patient along with all her data and then completes the Diagnostic Summary Sheet (fig 3-03) which is used to assess which zone(s) may have been damaged. The 'simulated operations' or the ultrasound may be repeated if clarification is required. On the basis of the quantum of urine lost, or the patient's needs, she may be referred for Pelvic Floor Rehabilitation or surgery.

3.3.2 The Variability of Symptoms in Patients with Similar Anatomical Defects

Specific symptoms do not always correlate exactly with the zones represented in the Pictorial Diagnostic Algorithm (fig 1-11). For instance, not all posterior zone symptoms are necessarily present in a given case of posterior zone prolapse, and these may vary from day to day. When symptoms vary from day to day, it means only that they may be the resultant of a complex series of events. The problem of symptom variability is overcome with the help of the patient's memory of a symptom, that is, referring to the 'sometimes' category from the questionnaire and applying it in the Diagnostic Summary Sheet (fig 3-03). The clinician can achieve a reasonably accurate clinical picture by checking the responses in the questionnaire against the urinary diary and the 24 hour pad test.

A urodynamic test for detrusor instability (DI) presents a 'snapshot' only at one point of time. Yet in answer to the question 'how many times do you get up at night to pass urine', a patient may unhesitatingly answer '3 or 4 times on average'. It is not surprising therefore that the correlation of the DI testing with the patient's history of urge, frequency and nocturia symptoms is rarely greater than 50%. From a scientific point of view, it can be argued that bladder instability symptoms (frequency, urgency and nocturia) are more reliable than urodynamically diagnosed DI because of 'logging' by the cortex. For DI testing to achieve the same 'accuracy' or level of probability as that obtained from a patient's 'logging' of urgency symptoms in her memory bank, the urodynamic test would have to be repeated hundreds of times, clearly not a feasible option.

3.3.3 Assessing Probability: The Impact of Different Structures on the Variability of Incontinence Symptoms

The pelvic floor functions optimally as a balanced system, with important contributions from muscles, nerves and connective tissues (CT). However, it is the connective tissues (CT) which are the most vulnerable part of the system. Each CT component of the overall structure - pubourethral ligament (PUL), hammock, arcus tendineus fascia pelvis (ATFP), uterosacral ligament (USL) and external urethral ligament (EUL) - contributes differently to the maintenance of continence. These contributions to stress incontinence can be represented in a normal probability curve (fig 3-09).

A damaged PUL is overwhelmingly the major cause of stress incontinence (SI). However, other structures – hammock, ATFP, USL and EUL – add variable contributions, depending on the patient. This difference in contribution explains the variable cure rate for SI that is obtained from the Kelly operation (hammock repair), the paravaginal repair (Richardson 1981), the EUL and PUL repair (Zacharin 1963, Petros & Ulmsten 1993), and the USL repair in some patients with post-hysterectomy incontinence (Petros 1997). From the viewpoint of restoration of function, it follows that restoration of damage to the whole system is desirable, if possible. As it requires only two more sutures to tighten the hammock and external urethral ligaments, both important components of the urethral closure mechanism, it is recommended these steps be added to reinforcement of PUL with a 'tension-free' tape or tissue fixation system (TFS) in surgery for cure of stress incontinence.

The concept of synergy also applies in patients with urge and abnormal emptying symptoms. The individual muscles, ligaments and stretch receptors contribute collectively to bladder closure and opening, but each structure has a different weight for each person.

Extreme examples are:

a) severe urgency in one patient may be caused by a cystocoele stretching very sensitive stretch receptors;

b) another patient with very insensitive stretch receptors and an equivalent cystocoele may have to empty by abdominal pressure because LP and LMA cannot gain sufficient 'traction' on the posterior urethral wall to open out the outflow tract;

c) in yet another patient, the cystocoele may stretch the hammock downwards sufficiently to tighten it during stress, creating the condition of 'latent stress incontinence' - appearing after surgical repair of the cystocoele.

Some insights into this concept of differential contribution to continence can be obtained by performing 'simulated operations', anchoring each supporting structure in turn and measuring the effect, e.g. diminution of urine loss on coughing, or diminution of urgency sensation in a patient with a full bladder, or reducing the cystocoele and asking the patient to cough. (See the section 'Simulated operations - case reports in the Diagnosis section.)

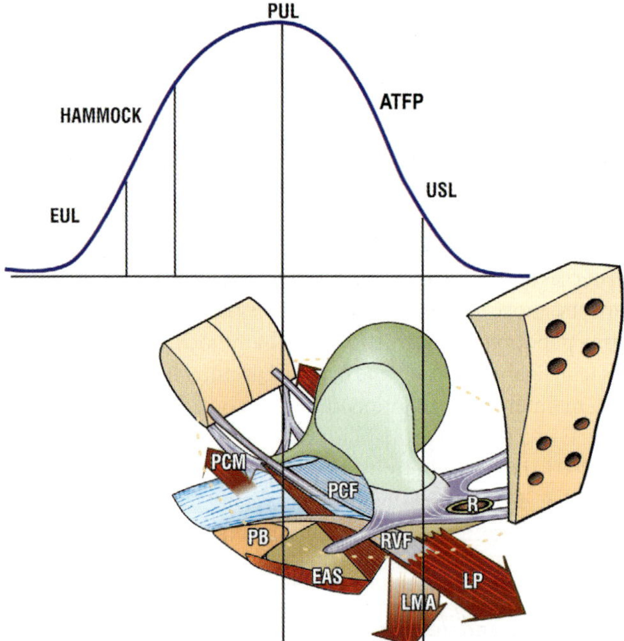

Fig. 3-09 Different structures impact synergistically to control stress incontinence in the individual patient. The impact of each structure *differs between patients*. The variance follows a normal distribution curve. This perspective is derived from application of the concepts of non-linearity to the dynamics of the pelvic floor (see fig 6-24, p 199 for a clinical example).

3.3.4 The Anatomical Basis for the Diagnostic Summary Sheet

The following section describes the components of the Diagnostic Summary Sheet (fig 3-03). The anatomical basis for these dysfunctions are presented according to the zone in which the dysfunction occurs.

Anterior Zone Defect Symptoms

Stress Incontinence (SI) > 50%

Symptomatic urine loss on coughing more than 50% of the time correlates highly with an anterior zone defect (Petros & Ulmsten, 1992).

Urine Loss on Standing

A weak PUL allows LP and LMA to pull open the outflow tract on standing up.

Post-Stress Instability

With a weak PUL, the bladder base is pulled backwards. Stimulation of the stretch receptors 'N' activates the micturition reflex, so that urine loss continues after coughing ceases.

'Always Damp'

In the absence of fistula, constant dampness may indicate Intrinsic Sphincter Defect (ISD), caused by inability of slow-twitch PCM to close the urethra because of possible damaged EUL, PUL and suburethral connective tissues.

Faecal Incontinence (Associated with SI)

These symptoms indicate a weak PUL preventing LP and LMA from stretching the rectum around a contracted puborectalis muscle to create anorectal closure.

Nocturnal Enuresis Cured at Puberty

Many patients who report nocturnal enuresis plus daily wetting up till puberty have a familial history of this, which also includes the male members. Improvement at puberty can reasonably be attributed to thickening of PUL under pubertal hormonal influence. Many patients only partly improve at puberty and these respond well to an anterior midurethral sling. This type of 'complicated' nocturnal enuresis is to be distinguished from the normal childhood wetting at night only.

Lax Hammock

Up to 20-30% of patients require unilateral tightening of the hammock ('pinch test') (fig 3-05) in addition to a midurethral anchoring to control urine loss on coughing when tested with 'simulated operations' (Petros & Von Konsky 1999). This demonstrates the synergy of these structures in urethral closure as well as the importance of tightening the hammock in addition to placement of a midurethral sling.

Positive Midurethral Anchor Test

This helps predict whether a midurethral sling may restore continence with stress. LP, LMA and PCM cannot close the urethra against a lax PUL (fig 3-05).

Lax EUL

In the absence of any significant stress incontinence, lax EUL may manifest as a light leakage 'like a bubble', or on sudden movement.

Funnelling on ultrasound and its reversal with a midurethral anchor

This indicates the importance of an adequately tight PUL for continence (see Ch 6).

Urethrovesical junction (UVJ) prolapse >10mm

This should be used only as a guide to look further. It is not possible to arbitrarily diagnose damaged PUL at 10.1 mm and intact PUL at 9.9 mm.

Urethral Closure Pressure (UCP) < 20cm H_2O

This confirms the diagnosis of intrinsic sphincter defect (ISD). ISD can usually be diagnosed without urodynamics using the 'slow leak speculum sign' (Petros & Ulmsten, Integral Theory, 1990), observation of a slow steady leak of urine on placing a Sims speculum into the vagina during examination. The speculum stretches the vaginal tissue downward to provide a counter force to the slow-twitch PCM-hammock closure mechanism, so that urine simply trickles out.

Middle zone defect symptoms

Emptying

During micturition the outflow tract is opened out by the posterior muscle forces "funnelled". The urethral resistance varies inversely with the length and diameter. Laxity in the middle zone due to cystocoele or paravaginal laxity may not allow LP to stretch open the outflow tract, so that the detrusor has to empty against greatly increased urethral resistance. The patient may experience symptoms such as 'stopping and starting', 'slow flow', 'difficulty in starting flow', 'feeling of not having emptied properly' and 'post-micturition dribble'.

'Tethered vagina' syndrome

Adequate elasticity at the 'zone of critical elasticity' is required for the anterior and posterior muscle forces (arrows) to function separately. Scar tissue at bladder neck may 'tether' these muscle forces. The more powerful posterior forces stretch open the outflow tract much like occurs at micturition, so that urine runs out uncontrollably, often without any accompanying urgency symptoms.

Posterior zone defect symptoms

Worse one week prior to periods

The cervix softens under the influence of hormones to allow egress of blood at period time. The posterior ligaments therefore loosen and produce worsening of posterior zone symptoms at period time.

'Always damp'

USL is the anchoring point for slow-twitch LMA muscles. It plays an important role in the bladder neck closure mechanism, stretching bladder base down and around PUL to achieve watertight closure in the proximal urethra (fig 2-17). If the hammock closure mechanism is insufficient, the patient may leak in a similar way to ISD. This mechanism explains the onset of urine loss after hysterectomy and the frequent improvement in SI symptoms after USL reinforcement with plastic tapes.

Pelvic Pain

Insufficient connective tissue support for the non-myelinated nerve endings which course along the uterosacral ligaments, may cause referred low abdominal pain or sacral backache (fig 3-10). Deep dyspareunia may cause pain by pressure on these nerves. The lower abdominal pain and sacral backache may be reproduced by gently touching the posterior fornix digitally, or with a ring forceps. This is described as 'cervical' or 'vaginal' 'excitation pain' in figure 3-03.

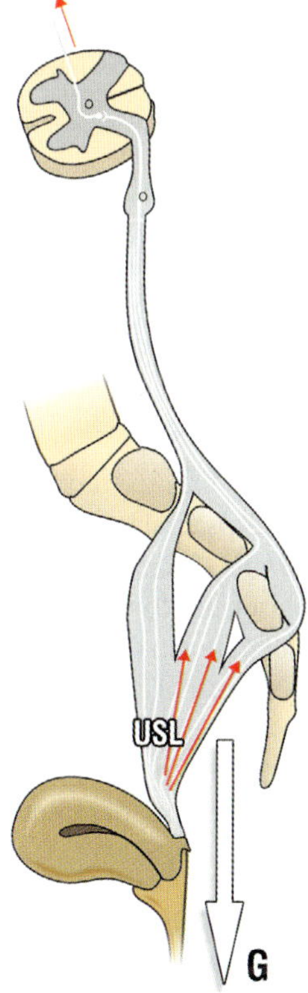

Fig. 3-10 The anatomy of uterosacral ligament (USL) referred pelvic pain. If the uteroscacral ligaments (red arrows) cannot provide adequate anatomical support for the unmyelinated afferent nerves (thin white lines) the force of gravity (G) may stretch them, causing referred abdominal and sacral pain. After Goeschen, by permission.

Nocturia

This is a symptom specific to posterior zone defects. Figure 3-11 shows the position of the organs when the patient is asleep. If weakened posterior ligaments cannot 'hold" the bladder base, the stretch receptors may be stimulated, and this is perceived as night urgency, nocturia.

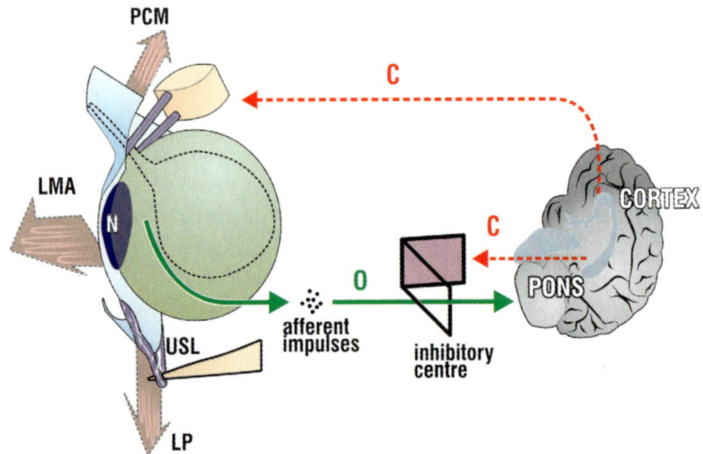

Fig. 3-11 Mechanical origin of nocturia- patient asleep. Pelvic muscles (arrows) are relaxed. As the bladder fills, it distends downwards. If the uterosacral ligamenst (USL) are weak it continues to descend until the stretch receptors 'N' are stimulated, activating the micturition reflex once the closure reflex 'C' has been overcome.

Emptying

Figure 3-12 demonstrates the physical origin of abnormal emptying symptoms, more fully explained in Chapter 6. The uterosacral ligament (USL) is the effective anchoring point of the downward force (LMA). USL laxity may not allow LMA to stretch open the outflow tract, so that the detrusor has to empty against greatly increased urethral resistance, producing symptoms of abnormal emptying, 'stopping and starting', 'slow flow', 'difficulty in starting flow', 'feeling of not having emptied properly' and 'post-micturition dribble'. Many patients presenting with indwelling catheters (inserted due to inability to empty their bladder), have been cured by the Posterior IVS operation (Petros, unpublished data, 2004, Richardson, pers. comm.).

Prolapse

The degree of prolapse has no relationship to posterior zone symptoms as minor degrees of prolapse may cause major symptoms.

Residual Urine

Given the non-linear nature of bladder emptying, arbitrary limits to residual urines, such as '30 ml' (the limit used by the author) have little meaning. Strictly speaking, any urine remaining after micturition is abnormal.

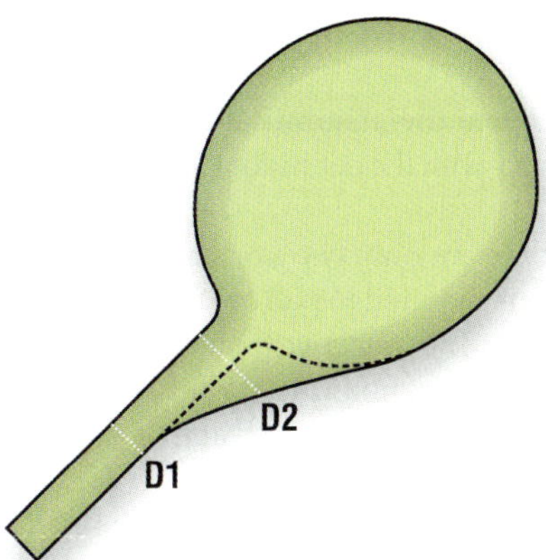

Fig. 3-12 Physical origin of abnormal emptying symptoms. Urethral resistance decreases by the fourth power of the diameter. D2 is twice the diameter at D1, therefore urethral resistance at D2 is 1/16th of the resistance at D1. ($2^4 = 16$)

Abnormal Emptying Time

A time limit of 60 seconds is generally used, but the same limitations as in the case of *residual urine* apply.

Diagnosing Causes of Symptom Recurrence after Surgery

Symptom recurrence after surgery may be due to:
1. Misdiagnosis as to which anatomical defect(s) may be causing dysfunction at the initial consultation.
2. Surgical error.
   a. Failure to adequately secure all elements of the system. For example, also tightening the hammock in stress incontinence (SI) surgery along with the mid-urethral sling should be routine with mid-urethral sling operations.
   b. Sutures tearing out.
3. Formation of another defect at a later date, with further onset of symptoms. Generally this occurs weeks or months after surgery, but it may occur within days.

For example, an enterocele which develops *de novo* after stress incontinence surgery may be associated with urge, nocturia, emptying problems and pelvic pain.

How to Address Symptom Recurrence

Have the patient repeat the questionnaire, then redo the Diagnostic Summary Sheet (fig 3-03). Always check meticulously to see if the patient's symptoms have altered. It must never be assumed that the cause is a failed operation. Creation of a strong repair in one zone will inevitably upset the balance of the three zones and divert the pelvic floor forces to the weakest point in the system. Beyond a critical limit, the 'new weak point' may give way, causing new symptoms to arise. The associated prolapse may be quite minor, especially in the posterior zone.

3.3.5 An Anatomical Basis For ICS Definitions and Descriptions

This section aims to correlate the anatomical explanations developed within the context of the Integral Theory with the definitions and descriptions of the International Continence Society.

In a normal patient, there are only two normal bladder states, stable closed and stable open. Muscle energy is required to pull open the outflow tract to the 'open' state and to close it. There are specific connective tissue structures in each zone which play a key role in these dynamics (ie opening and closure). In simple terms, the structures in the anterior zone are concerned with closure, and those in the middle and posterior zones are concerned with opening (fig 3-13).

The main connective tissue structures in each zone are printed in red (fig 3-13). These are listed in order of importance. The specific incontinence symptoms associated with damage to these structures, as defined by the ICS, are detailed in the columns representing each zone. The height of the rectangle in each zone represents an approximation of the probability of that symptom's occurrence in that zone.

These incontinence symptoms may be designated as dysfunctions of closure ('stress incontinence') or of opening ('abnormal emptying'). Dysfunctional closure occurs in the anterior zone, dysfunctional opening occurs in the middle and posterior zones. Bladder instability symptoms ('urgency', 'frequency', etc) may occur in all three zones.

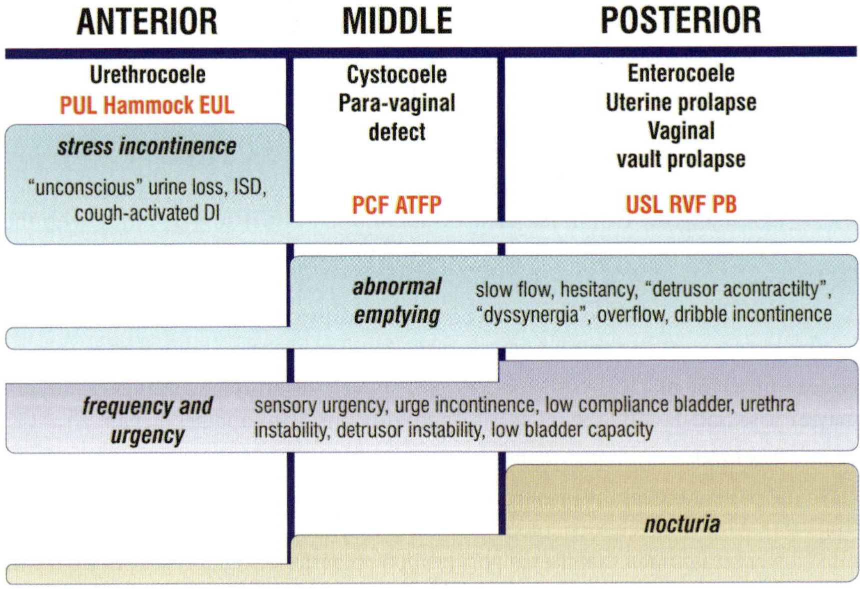

Fig. 3-13 ICS Symptom definitions allocated to the three anatomical zones, expressed as dysfunctions of closure or opening. Note the synergystic relationships between the middle and posterior zones.

The Role of the Peripheral Neurological Control Mechanism in the 'Unstable Open' State

In the normal patient, the peripheral neurological control mechanism consists of a musculo-elastic complex which controls afferent impulses from the stretch receptors 'N' (fig 3-14). This neuro-musculo-elastic complex is known as the 'micturition reflex'. This reflex acts as an 'engine' to accelerate opening out of the outflow tract.

The combination of damaged connective tissue and oversensitive nerve endings may lead to excessive afferent impulses from 'N' which may result in inappropriate activation of the micturition reflex at low bladder volume. This may be interpreted by the cortex as frequency, urgency and nocturia symptoms.

The afferent impulses activate the micturition reflex. Usually, the normal response to afferent impulses is the contraction of PCM, which pulls the hammock forward to stabilize the urethra and support 'N'. However, once activated sufficiently to override the inhibitory centres 'C' (fig 3-14), the micturition reflex drives the external musculo-elastic opening mechanism 'O' such that PCM relaxes, the urethra is opened out, the bladder contracts, and urine is expelled.

Conversely, a patient with insensitive nerve endings in the presence of connective tissue damage may present with bladder emptying problems or even urinary retention.

Fig. 3-14 The bladder is shown in the 'open' (micturition) phase. During micturition, the closure reflex 'C' (shown in red) is overcome by the opening reflex 'O', (shown in green). During closure, 'C' dominates. The inhibitory centre 'trapdoor' closes, PCM contracts to close the urethra and supporting 'N', thereby diminishing the number of afferent impulses.

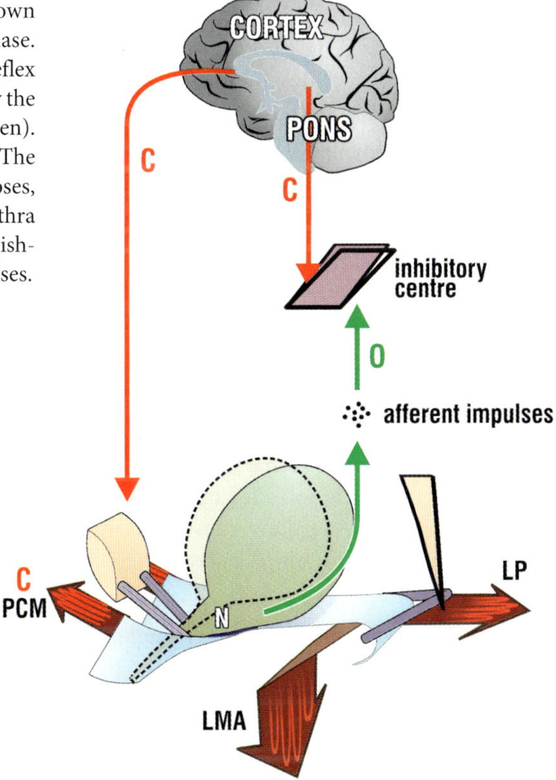

In the section below, the anatomical zones in which the symptoms originate are denoted in parentheses where relevant (Petros & Ulmsten, 1998, 1999). The terms used are as defined by the International Continence Society (ICS 1998).

'Detrusor instability' and 'bladder instability' are used interchangeably. In the Integral Theory framework they are both manifestations of a normal but prematurely activated micturition reflex.

Motor Urgency (Anterior, Middle & Posterior Zones)

According to the Integral Theory, motor urgency is mainly an uninhibited micturition. In patients with anterior ligamentous defect (PUL), the forward forces (PCM), (fig 3-14) cannot anchor the urethra. Instead, on being given the signal to close (e.g. when a patient stands up), the powerful backward forces (LP and LMA) open out the outflow tract much as occurs during micturition. This action further stimulates the stretch receptors 'N', already activated by urine in the bladder. The sheer quantity of afferent impulses may overcome the inhibitory centre. The micturition reflex is activated and massive urine loss ensues. These symptoms often commence after 70 years of age, and are presumably caused by PUL atrophy. In a patient with previous surgery, scar-based 'tethering' of the forward and backward forces may work in a similar way. The more powerful backward forces (fig 3-14) overcome the forward force to forcibly open out the outflow tract as adequate elasticity is required below bladder neck to allow the three directional forces to operate independently during urethral closure. Patients with these symptoms and previous surgery are unlikely to have the 'tethered vagina' syndrome if there is an absence of a fixed scarred bladder neck. A combination of sensitive stretch receptors and lax posterior ligaments may sometimes present a similar clinical picture.

Nocturia – Posterior Defect

The anatomical basis for nocturia is best understood by turning figure 3-14 clockwise through 90 degrees to represent the sleeping position (fig 3-11). As the bladder fills at night, the bladder fluid, assisted by the force of gravity, stretches the proximal vagina downward. If USL is strong, it will prevent excess stretching and will support the stretch receptors 'N'. If USL is weak, 'N' may 'fire off' at a low volume. This is interpreted as nocturia – that is, waking to pass urine. With very sensitive stretch receptors the micturition reflex may be activated and the patient may wet prior to arrival at the toilet. Alternatively, with insensitive stretch receptors and lax inelastic tissues, the urine may simply leak out so the patient wets her bed.

Sensory Urgency (Posterior, Middle, Anterior Zone Defects)

As the bladder fills, the afferent impulses from the stretch receptors 'N' reach the cortex and are interpreted as a full bladder, sensory urgency - the first warning of the activated micturition reflex. Central inhibition 'C' (fig 3-14) combined with vaginal stretching to support the stretch receptors usually prevents urine loss. If these are insufficient and the patient wets, the symptom is termed 'urge incontinence'. Intravesical lesions (cancer), chronic cystitis and extrinsic pressure (uterine fibroids) need to be excluded.

Unconscious Incontinence, Continuous Leakage (Anterior, Posterior Zone Defects)

Unconscious incontinence and continuous leakage is evidence of the inability of the urethral closure muscles PCM (fig 3-14) to stretch the vagina sufficiently for urine-tight urethral closure. Unconscious leakage may be mainly due to anterior zone laxity, but it may occasionally be due to inability of the slow-twitch backward and downward muscles to close off the bladder neck. Other cases, such as bladder fistula and multiple sclerosis need to be excluded.

Detrusor Instability (Posterior, Anterior, Middle Zone Defects)

Detrusor instability (DI), an abnormal phasic rise in pressure, is purely a urodynamic diagnosis and may be present in normal women. This contradiction disappears entirely if DI is considered as being part of an uninhibited, prematurely activated, but otherwise normal, micturition reflex (Integral Theory 1993). This perspective of a premature micturition reflex was supported by use of a provocative handwashing test. Handwashing may work by counteracting central inhibition (Mayer et al. 1991) of afferent impulses from the bladder base stretch receptors. The sequence of events observed in a group of 115 patients presenting with urge incontinence was, generally speaking, what one would find during normal micturition: a feeling of urgency within a few seconds of commencement of the test (108 patients), then, fall in urethral pressure (91 patients), rise in detrusor pressure (56 patients), and finally, loss of urine (52 patients) (Petros & Ulmsten 1993). The classical sinusoidal curve of DI can be explained as a 'battle' between two feedback systems: the micturition (opening) reflex 'O' (fig 3-14), and the closing reflex 'C'. In other words, the micturition reflex struggles to open the outflow tract, and the brain struggles to counteract this reflex by increasing central inhibitory impulses, and by contracting the pelvic floor, which, in turn, closes the urethra. If the detrusor is contracting at this point, detrusor pressure rises. If the outflow tract is being pulled open at this point, the detrusor pressure falls. The time delay in the transition between the 'open' and 'closed' is expressed urodynamically as a sinusoidal pressure curve indicating 'detrusor instability'.

Unstable Urethra (Posterior, Anterior, Middle Zone Damage)

The same explanation for the phasic contraction of the bladder applies for the urethra: both share the same smooth muscle and so both respond to the same feedback system. The fibre to fibre transmission of bladder smooth muscle (Creed 1979) not only precludes independent innervation of the bladder and urethra, but means that all the fibres contract 'as one' to expel the urine.

Inability to Micturate with Neurological Damage

This is explained by the spinal cord transection preventing working of the extrinsic opening mechanism. Therefore the detrusor contracts reflexly against an unopened outflow tract. As the urethral resistance varies inversely with the fourth power of the radius (r^4), a much higher detrusor pressure is required to expel the urine.

Change of Compliance (Posterior, Anterior, Middle Zone Defects)

'Low compliance' during cystometric filling is consistent with a micturition reflex activated by bladder filling, partly controlled by cortical inhibition 'C' (fig 3-14) and pelvic floor contraction. Pelvic floor contraction compresses the urethra thereby increasing the urethral resistance. This, in turn, increases the detrusor pressure. The latter is interpreted as 'low compliance'.

Bladder Sensation (Posterior, Anterior, Middle Zone Defects)

According to the ICS, bladder sensation is classified as 'normal', 'increased', 'decreased' and 'absent'. It was demonstrated, that the sensation of urgency, was the first and most constant manifestation of a micturition reflex prematurely activated by handwashing (Petros & Ulmsten 1993). Because of the complex feedback system, it is inevitable that these sensations will vary in intensity and frequency even within the same patient. Variable sensitivity of stretch receptors in patients with connective tissue damage may explain the ICS classification.

Bladder Capacity

The variables for bladder capacity are sensitivity of the stretch receptors 'N' (fig 3-14), competence of the central inhibitory mechanism, and competence of the musculo-elastic mechanism in stretching the vaginal membrane. How these merge is reflected as a particular bladder capacity on the day of testing.

Urethral Function During Storage (Anterior, Posterior Zone Defects)

In a normal patient, the urethral pressure rises during urodynamic bladder filling. Urine leakage in the absence of a detrusor contraction reflects the inability of the PCM/hammock (fig 3-14) complex to close off the urethra. A higher rate of cure for low urethral pressure incontinence, 'intrinsic sphincter defect' (ISD), or 'Type III' incontinence with the anterior midurethral sling procedure has been demonstrated when the hammock is also tightened. The importance of this mechanism has also been demonstrated when the hammock is surgically disconnected from the closure muscles. Urine may leak even in the presence of raised 'cough transmission ratio' (CTR) (Petros & Ulmsten, 1995).

Genuine Stress Incontinence (Anterior, Posterior Zone Defects)

According to the ICS definition (1988), genuine stress incontinence (GSI) is strictly demarcated from mixed incontinence, and implies that there is urine loss coincident with stress in the absence of a detrusor contraction. GSI is a confusing definition, as it attempts to separate conditions which, according to the Integral Theory's anatomical classification, derive from the same source, viz. laxity in the vagina or its ligaments. Indeed, the presence of DI was not a negative prognostic factor for the IVS operation (Petros 1997) or conventional bladder neck elevation surgery (Black 1997). Though testing for DI appears to be of little practical use in the Integral Theory decision path for surgery, dynamic urethral pressures, urine flow and residual urine determinations are of considerable assistance in improving the diagnostic accuracy of the basic pictorial algorithm.

Cough Activated Detrusor Instability

Although patients with symptoms of stress incontinence usually lose urine coincident with coughing, it is not always the case. Many previous investigators have observed that a cough may sometimes activate a detrusor contraction, so that leaking continues many seconds after the cough has ceased. This observation has been a key factor in the ICS labelling stress incontinence symptoms as unreliable.

However, an alternative explanation for this occurrence is as follows. A lax PUL (fig 3-14) may fail to anchor the urethra. The result of this is that LP and LMA stretch the bladder base backwards to stimulate the stretch receptors 'N' which activates the micturition reflex. This causes the bladder to contract, so that urine is lost after cessation of coughing. Urodynamic testing in this situation may show a phasic rise in pressure: detrusor instability. A midurethral sling usually cures this condition, but there has been at least one patient in the author's experience where a posterior sling was needed.

Although urgency and frequency may occur with damage in any zone, in the author's experience it is more likely to be caused by posterior zone defects, especially in older patients.

Reflex Incontinence

According to the ICS (1988), reflex incontinence describes urine leak in the absence of sensation. Neurological damage is equated with this condition. This concept is consistent with a neurological lesion such as multiple sclerosis which interferes with cortical or spinal cord inhibitory centres 'C' (fig 3-14). As the afferent impulses cannot be suppressed, they activate the cascade of events which form the micturition reflex 'O' (fig 3-14). However, patients with intrinsic sphincter defect and a very lax hammock can also leak urine without sensation. In this case the cause is purely mechanical.

may create a 'cascade' of *major* events (the 'butterfly effect'). The symptom-based emphasis of the Integral Theory stems from the fact that even minor degrees of ligamentous laxity (prolapse) may cause quite severe symptoms. For example, as explained earlier, in a patient with very sensitive nerve endings even minimal ligamentous laxity may cause the peripheral 'neurological' control mechanism to 'fire-off' at a low threshold.

The cascade of events which follow from this low threshold may be expressed as quite major symptoms such as urge incontinence, pelvic pain, cough-activated detrusor instability, etc. In surgery, some 'major events' (for example, thrombosis, haemorrhage and infection) are potentially fatal, yet their origins may be traced to apparently 'minor' events.

Accordingly, the Integral Theory system for surgery emphasizes a minimalist approach, with safety built-in to the techniques. For instance, wherever possible, conservation of the uterus and vaginal tissue is advised so as to avoid longer term complications for the patient. (These are explained later in this book). This approach is in keeping with the Chaos Theory perspective, as well as the historical concept that the consequences of surgery can not always be fully foreseen.

The Integral Theory surgical system introduces a specific methodology to the five elements which are characteristic of all surgery. These are:
1. Indications
2. Tissues
3. Structure
4. Methods
5. Tools.

By using the Integral Theory methodology in surgical practice, many conditions previously considered to be complex become treatable on a day-care basis.

The Indications: Major Prolapse, or Major Symptoms with Minor Prolapse

The diagnostic framework of the Integral Theory is summarised in the Pictorial Diagnostic Algorithm (fig 1-11). The Pictorial Diagnostic Algorithm brings together the key concepts at the core of this method:
- that restoration of structure will also restore function
- that even minor degrees of prolapse may cause dysfunction in the pelvic floor
- that the same minimally invasive surgical techniques can be applied regardless of the scale of damage to that structure.

This has meant, for instance, that patients with only minor degrees of damage and so-called 'incurable' symptoms such as frequency, urgency, nocturia, abnormal emptying and pelvic pain can now benefit from a posterior sling, even though its original indication was for utero-vaginal prolapse.

In the following sections, both structural and functional indications will be given for the surgical techniques described. Note that the same operations described for major degrees of prolapse may also be applied to improve symptoms associated with minimal anatomical defect.

The Tissues: Conservation and Reinforcement of Tissue

Conservation and reinforcement of tissue is the key to ambulatory surgery. Connective tissue loses strength with age. The vagina is an organ and cannot regenerate. To avoid vaginal shortening and dyspareunia, the Integral Theory approach recommends minimal and preferably no vaginal tissue be excised. Where required, damaged anterior (PUL) and posterior (USL) ligaments can be reinforced by using tapes, precisely inserted to create artificial collagenous neoligaments. Tissue conservation and a 'tension-free' technique while suturing will minimise post-operative pain. By avoiding surgery at the bladder neck area of the vagina 'zone of critical elasticity' (ZCE, fig 1-10), sufficient elasticity for funnelling during micturition is retained, thus minimising post-operative urinary retention.

The Structure: The Synergistic Interaction of Connective Tissue Components

There are nine main connective tissue structures which may contribute to pelvic floor dysfunction (fig 1-10). They are:

Anterior zone

1 = external urethral ligament (EUL)
2 = pubourethral ligament (PUL)
3 = suburethral vagina (hammock)

Middle zone

4 = arcus tendineus fascia pelvis (ATFP)
5 = pubocervical fascia (PCF)
6 = anterior cervical ring,
    ZCE = excess tightness, usually scar tissue below bladder neck ('tethered vagina')

Posterior zone

7 = uterosacral ligament (USL)
8 = rectovaginal fascia (RVF)
9 = perineal body (PB).

Three muscle forces stretch these structures (fig 1-10). As illustrated in the suspension bridge analogy, it is the 'tensioning' of the connective tissues that gives the pelvic floor system its structure and form.

Laxity in some or all of these connective tissue structures may affect position or function of the organs. Therefore the surgeon needs to address all damaged structures within each zone and across all three zones (fig 1-10).

The Methods: Avoidance of Post-Operative Pain and Urinary Retention

David Nichols (1989) stated that there may be multiple sites requiring repair, and therefore, it was important to address the reconstruction needs of each damaged site. Quoting Charles Mayo, he stated that there was no such thing as a 'standard operation' and that the operation must be tailored to the patient, not vice-versa. From the

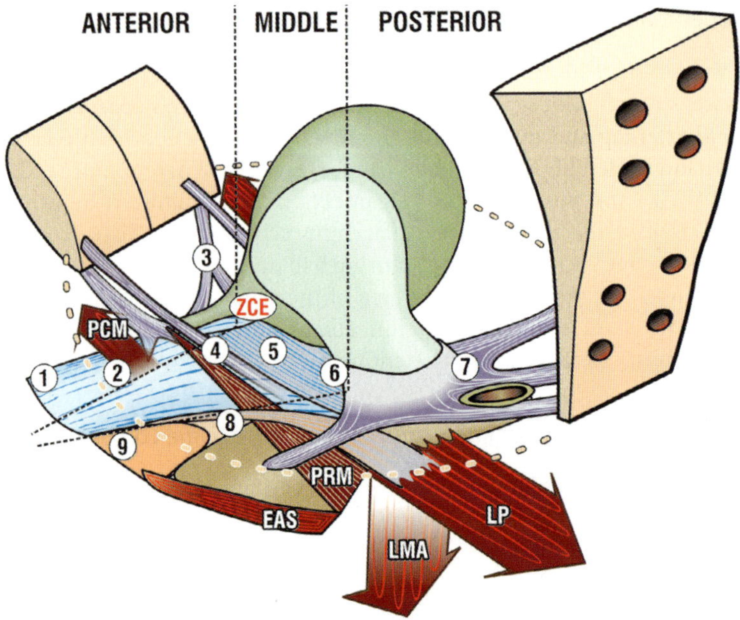

Fig. 1-10 The key connective tissue structures of the pelvic floor. Perspective: view from above and behind, level of pelvic brim. PCM = pubococcygeus muscle force; LP = levator plate muscle force; LMA = longitudinal muscle of the anus force; ZCE = Zone of Critical Elasticity.

perspective of this book, the final decision as to which structures need to be repaired can only be made in the operating room.

The surgeon particularly needs to be aware as to how the reconstruction *itself* may alter the dynamics of pelvic floor structure and function, leading to the development of a new set of abnormal symptoms soon after surgery, or even many years later. The best example is post-operative pain, urinary retention, neourgency and enterocoele formation after a Burch colposuspension. Other less common examples are possible sequelae from excision of vaginal tissue ('tethered vagina syndrome', hysterectomy (vault prolapse), and excessive tightness of tapes and sutures (pain and urinary retention).

The Tools: Reinforcement of Damaged Collagenous Tissues

The surgical operations based on the Integral Theory generally require special instruments to insert tapes in a minimally invasive way to reinforce damaged ligaments or fascia is fundamental to the Integral Theory System of surgery (Petros & Ulmsten 1993) (fig 4-01).

The initial aim of the anterior 'tension-free' sling operation was to create a day-care procedure by using a special instrument to insert a plastic tape in the position of the pubourethral ligament (fig 4-01) thereby reducing post-operative pain and urinary retention. Although this aim was largely achieved, other challenges have arisen, principally because the surgical procedure itself is 'blind'. There are reports of small bowel perforation (fig 4-02), major vessel perforations (external iliac, obturator), and major nerve (obturator) injury, all of which are directly attributable to the procedure being 'blind'. Lying just below and behind the pubic bone are venous sinuses, (fig 4-03) which, if perforated, have the potential to cause severe retropubic haematomas, given that tissue compression of the bleeding is not possible in the Space of Retzius. The transobturator approach 'TOT' (Delorme 2001) appears to be as effective clinically as the retropubic approach, and generally avoids the bladder, bowel, and external iliac complications which may occur with the retropubic approach. Nevertheless, bladder and urethral perforations have already been reported with the TOT. Damage to the obturator nerve and vessels always remains a possibility, especially with the

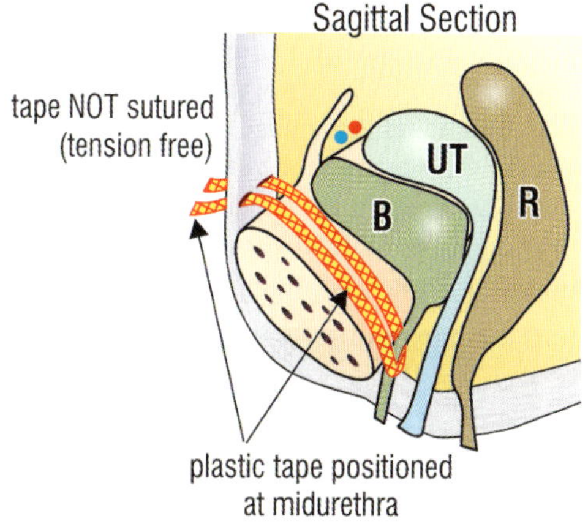

Fig. 4-01 The midurethral plastic mesh tape reinforces the pubourethral ligament.

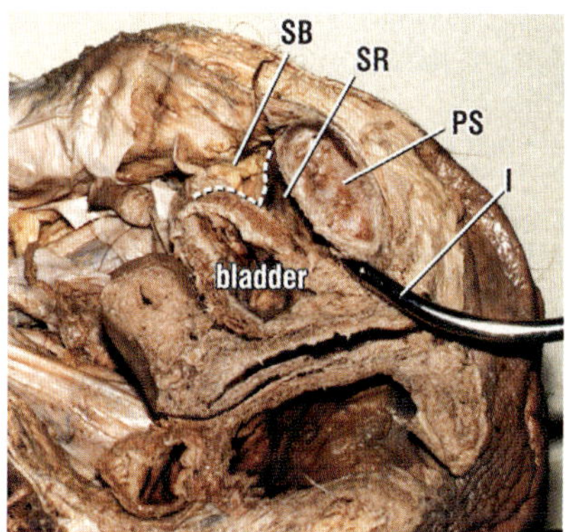

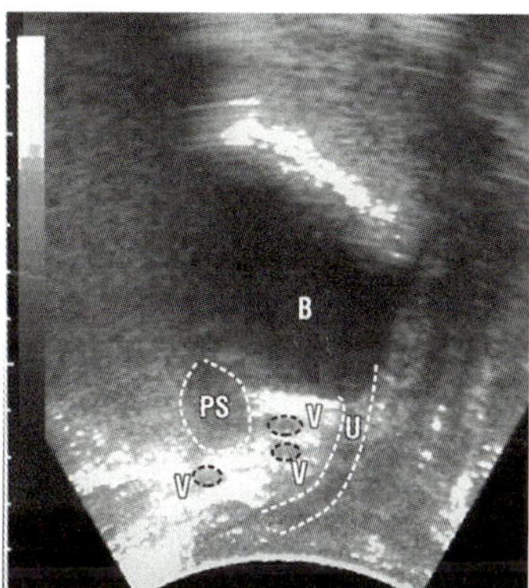

Fig. 4-02 Cadaver supine position shows how an instrument inserted blindly may damage bladder, small bowel (SB) and, if too lateral, the external iliac vessels. SR = Space of Retzius; PS = pubic symphsis; I = instrument.

Fig. 4-03 Venous sinuses. Ultrasound sagittal position, The venous sinuses 'V' are in the direct line of approach of a blindly inserted delivery instrument. PS = pubic symphysis; U = urethra; B = bladder.

blind vaginal approach. The posterior sling is inserted via the ischiorectal fossa and thus there is the danger that the rectum may be perforated and the distal branches of the haemorrhoidal or even pudendal vessels and nerves damaged inside the fossa. Special instruments have been devised to fix mesh with extended arms inserted via the transobturator or ischiorectal approach for repair of anterior or posterior vaginal wall prolapse. These, too, are 'blind' procedures.

Notwithstanding the success and efficiency of such 'tension-free' tape surgery, the complications that were reported created an impetus to develop a surgical method which could be performed largely under direct vision.

A Tissue Fixation System

A tissue fixation system (TFS) (fig 4-04), was developed to provide a less invasive means of inserting anterior and posterior slings, and to allow the surgery to occur largely under direct vision. The TFS system was also designed to avoid the 'slippage' which may occur when mesh tapes are applied 'tension free'.

The TFS uses a small, soft-tissue anchor to fix an 8 mm polypropylene tape into muscle or fascial tissue to reinforce the ligament or fascia. The sling is adjusted for tension using a one-way non-slip tightening mechanism at the base of the soft tissue anchor (fig 4-05).

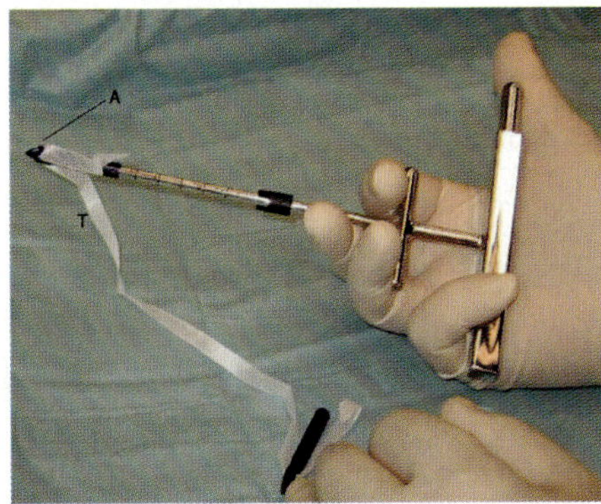

Fig. 4-04 TFS applicator. 'A' is the soft tissue anchor and 'T' is the polypropylene tape used to tighten lax ligaments or fascia.

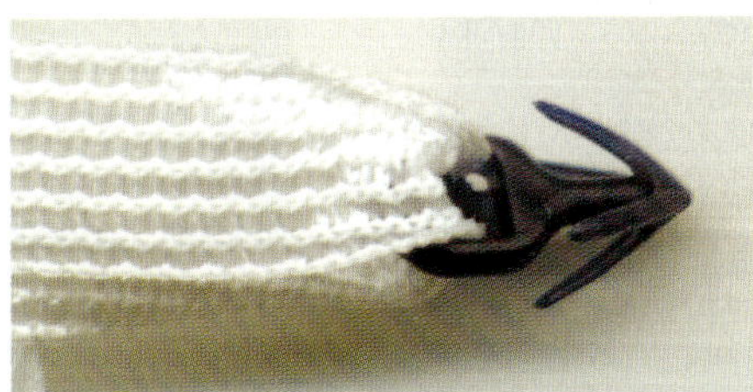

Fig. 4-05 TFS anchor. The polypropylene tape passes through the unidirectional 'trapdoor' at the base of the anchor.

The TFS can be applied to reinforce almost every ligament and fascial tissue in the pelvis. The polypropylene tape is inserted into the subpubic tissues anteriorly, the uterosacral remnants posteriorly, or ATFP laterally. The TFS can be applied transversely to reinforce damaged pubocervical or recto-vaginal fascia. Anteriorly, the tape is fixed to the muscle layer just below the pubic bone. Posteriorly, the tape is fixed to the uterosacral ligaments.

The multifilament tape was chosen for the first generation TFS operations because it does not stretch. Even with minimal tension the elastic nature of a monofilament tape may cause it to retract and constrict the urethra post operatively, as demonstrated by Rechberger (Rechberger et al. 2003). A multifilament tape is soft, has a greater surface area and so is less likely to damage the urethra.

To date, the TFS operations have had a remarkable lack of significant complications. They have a success rate equivalent to the older style anterior and posterior 'tension-free' tape slings, at least in the medium term (Petros & Richardson, 2005).

Tape slippage which leads to sagging of tissues is a possibility with any sling or mesh procedure. The TFS soft tissue anchor is especially designed to minimise slippage by 'gripping' firmly into the sub-pubic tissues. Clearly the efficacy of the 'gripping' is dependent on the quality of the tissue into which the anchor is inserted and the resilience of the anchor itself. Extremely weak tissues may, at least theoretically, make the anchoring mechanism of the TFS ineffective. There is no known way of determining the quality of tissues at the present time. However, experience to date has shown that, even in old and frail patients with poor quality tissues, the TFS appears to work as well as the 'tension-free' tape. Bench test research has shown that properly inserted anchors are capable of holding a weight of up to 2 kilograms. The Bio-engineering Department at the Royal Perth Hospital tested the anchor 'head' movement against the shaft to determine its resilience against fragmentation. The four prongs of the anchor head were still intact after 40,000 movements.

Notwithstanding the encouraging clinical results to date (Petros & Richardson, 2005), ongoing long term monitoring studies as well as comparative analysis with other surgical techniques will be required.

A Clarification: 'Tension-free' Tapes are Not 'Without Tension'

The term 'tension-free' tape surgery was first used in a 1994 (Ulmsten & Petros 1994). At the time, 'tension-free' was used to mean that the tape should not be applied under tension to the urethra. It is a term that, subsequently, has often been misinterpreted.

With 'tension-free' tape operations, the two ends of the tape are free. They 'grip' into the anterior abdominal wall muscles so that the sling provides a fixed anchoring point for the midurethra. This prevents the urethra being opened out during effort. Indeed, an essential element in the original descriptions of this technique (Petros & Ulmsten 1993, Ulmsten et al 1996, Petros 1996) was the insertion of 300 ml in the bladder, and pulling the tape upwards to tighten it sufficiently to prevent urine loss while the patient coughed.

4.2.2 The Surgical Principles of the Integral Theory

Introduction

> *'Restoration of function follows restoration of form (structure).'*

A central principle of the Integral Theory is that connective tissue damage in the fascia and ligaments of the three zones of the vagina may cause both prolapse and abnormal pelvic floor symptoms. Moreover, even minor connective tissue defects may cause abnormal symptoms.

Two major consequences follow from this: firstly, the same operation that is described for major prolapse surgery may be used for patients who, although exhibiting major symptoms, actually have only minor degrees of prolapse; secondly, symptoms become a major indicator for surgery, especially for patients with posterior zone symptoms. Hence the emphasis in the Integral Theory on the diagnostic system.

Before choosing a particular surgical technique however, the surgeon should try to assess the strength or weakness of a connective tissue structure, and contemplate the likely response of the functional anatomy to the intervention.

Guiding Principles for Day-Care Vaginal Surgery

To minimise pain

- Avoid tension when suturing the vagina
- Avoid vaginal excision
- Avoid surgery to the perineal skin

To avoid urinary retention

- Avoid tightness in bladder neck area of vagina
- Avoid indentation of the urethra with a midurethral sling.

The vagina is innervated by the parasympathetic nervous system, except for its introital portion, which is somatically innervated. Like the intestine, vaginal pain is elicited only by applying pressure, grasping or crushing.

Stretching and suturing the cut edges of vagina tightly potentially causes immediate, or longer-term pain by stimulating the parasympathetic nervous system. This explains the chronic post-operative pain experienced in up to 20% of patients after Burch Colposuspension. In particular, excess tightening of the cardinal and uterosacral ligaments during surgery is a potent source of post-operative pain, so one should be careful not to pull transvaginal holding sutures together very tightly. Avoidance of surgery to the perineal skin, and restricting vaginal incisions to within 1.0 cm of the introitus avoids post-operative somatic nerve pain.

The fibromuscular layer of the vaginal 'fascia' forms part of the vaginal wall. Therefore incisions need to be full thickness, avoiding surgical separation of the 'fascia' from the epithelium.

The midurethral sling must not indent (constrict) the urethra. Tightness at the bladder area of the vagina following vaginal repair may prevent the active stretching open of the outflow tract which occurs during micturition. This may result in diminished urine flow or even urinary retention.

Conservation and Reinforcement of Tissue: Implications for Surgery

The principles of conservation and reinforcement of tissue are fundamental to achieving connective tissue strength.

The vagina is essentially a tubular elastic membrane which derives strength from its fibromuscular layer. However, the elastic component of this layer is weak and susceptible to rupture. Once the elastin has been broken, (for example, through childbirth), the collagen fibres re-align along the lines of tension and may prolapse with gravity, resulting in herniation (rectocoele, enterocoele, cystocoele).

A high incidence of dyspareunia and apareunia has been reported (Jeffcoate 1962) following traditional vaginal repairs. These methods usually comprise excision of vaginal epithelium. It is important, therefore, to avoid excision of vagina where possible. As an organ, the vagina cannot regenerate. Stretching of urogenital tissue may weaken it by almost 30% (Yamada 1970). Thus it is best to avoid stretching of the vagina during surgery.

In patients with grossly redundant tissue, the surgeon can use a double layering technique such that the redundant tissue is used instead of mesh. This safely doubles the strength of the repair, while retaining elasticity.

In patients with poor tissues where surgery has failed, some form of polypropylene mesh or heterologous biological implant may be the best option available.

Collagen fibres within ligaments provide strong structural support. Unlike the vagina, ligaments have only limited stretching capacity (Yamada 1970). However, the breaking strength of these ligaments is far stronger than that of the vagina. The breaking strength of a pure collagen ligament (e.g. cervix) is approximately 1500 mg/mm^2 (Yamada 1970). In childbirth, just before delivery, the collagen of the cervix (and probably its associated ligaments) depolymerize, reducing their structural strength to a fraction of normal strength. Delivery may overstretch these tissues so that they 'reset' in an extended state. A stretched ligamentous anchoring point cannot adequately anchor the organ or the muscle force acting on it. Neither can it be shortened by suturing as it is already too weak. For these reasons, implanted polypropylene mesh tapes are used to create collagenous tissue to reinforce the ligament.

Post-operative Structural Adaption

A new group of symptoms occurring weeks, or even days after successful surgery is suggestive of another herniation. As shown in figure 1-10, *'Key connective tissue structures of the pelvic floor'*, all the components of the pelvic floor interact as part of a system for organ closure. It may be that strengthening one part of the system only diverts the muscle forces to another, weaker part of the system. This explains Shull's observations (1992) that herniations, usually in other parts of the vagina, occur in up to 38% of patients following vaginal surgery.

Adapting Surgical Technique for Wound Healing, Tissue Weakness and Scarring

Correct dissection technique can avoid much organ injury, especially in patients who have had previous surgery. The single most important dissection technique is to stretch the tissues to full extension prior to cutting. Once elastic tissue is cut under tension, it automatically retracts to reveal the dissection plane. With scarring from previous surgery, for example where vagina and rectum are fused by thick scar tissue, it is critical to precisely identify the organs and to cut the scar only while the organs (e.g. rectum and vagina) are being stretched in opposite directions by traction forceps. Stretching tensions the scar collagen, so that cutting it causes it to retract, revealing the plane between rectum and vagina, or bladder and vagina. Finger-tip dissection in patients with previous vaginal surgery should be avoided, as the organ often tears before the scar tissue separates.

In the early stages of setting, scar tissue has little strength (fig 4-06). The healing wound has very little structural strength during the first two weeks. During this time, the wound relies on the integrity of the suture in order to withstand the muscular forces pulling on the vagina. (The pressure needed to tear a suture out of the fascial layer of the vagina is approximately 8 lbs/sq inch (Van Winkle 1972).)

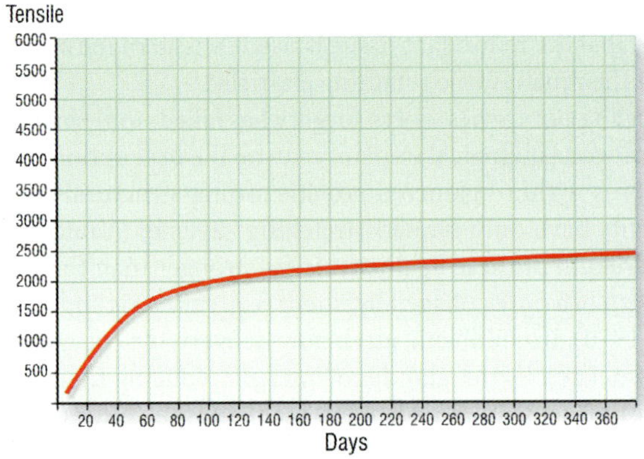

Fig. 4-06 Tensile Strength of healing fascia. (After Douglas)

As it is not possible to inhibit all natural reflex functions with bed rest, the surgical procedures themselves must contain the methodology to withstand such vaginal stretching.

Excessively tight sutures may compress the vagina and cause severe pain because of the sensitivity of visceral nerves to compression. Therefore, such sutures should be applied without excess tension.

Use of transvaginal 'holding sutures' help protect the healing wound for sufficient time until cross-bonding of the scar tissue collagen helps the wound to withstand herniation of the repaired tissue. The transvaginal holding suture derives its strength by penetrating the full thickness of the vagina. The new TFS soft tissue anchor system more strongly approximates laterally displaced tissues as the anchors have a 'tear out' resistance of up to 2 kg force.

Video observations show that some parts of the vagina may be stretched considerably during straining, micturition, and defaecation. In some instances, even a relatively low force may cause post operative tearing out of the retaining sutures, especially in a tight vaginal repair, where devascularization and restorative musculoelastic forces can combine to tear sutures out. Tearing out of sutures may cause wound dehiscence and recurrence of vaginal herniations.

For patients with previous surgery and poor tissues, mesh is often effective (when correctly used) in addressing patients with large herniations. However, it is technically difficult to restore the correct tissue tension using mesh, especially in patients with high cystocoele and high rectocoele. In such cases, restoration of correct tissue tension may be crucial if abnormal symptoms such as urge, frequency, nocturia,abnormal bladder emptying, even faecal incontinence are to be addressed (cf Chapters 2 & 3). The use of the TFS to approximate laterally displaced fascia is proving to be effective when used alone, in combination with 'bridge repairs' or even mesh.

Patient Care Issues Specific to Day-Care Pelvic Floor Surgery

With day-care surgery, special precautions need to be taken because the patient may be some distance from medical help if something was to go wrong. It is imperative that systems be in place to deal with any potential problems. These include ready accessibility to the surgeon, access to a hospital, as well as instructions such as immediately commencing a nil-by-mouth regime with acute emergencies such as post-operative haemorrhage.

Primary Haemorrhage

The vagina is a vascular organ, especially in the premenopausal female and the patient with previous surgery. Very small vessels may initially constrict only to bleed later. Suturing the vagina under tension may cause sutures to tear within 72 hours and this may result in considerable blood loss if there is delay in reaching a hospital. Therefore haemostasis must be meticulous, and sutures inserted without tension.

Cease aspirin and other analgesics which may alter blood clotting 10 days prior to surgery, and avoid pre-operative heparin if possible.

Adequate Fluid Replacement

Old or diabetic patients having their operation in the afternoon of a day admission list may already be 12 hours behind in their fluids. Dehydration may predispose to thrombosis and embolism. Arranging intravenous fluids on admission rather than during surgery may be useful.

Pre-operative Antibiotics

Where possible, all patients are given Tinidazole 2 gm pre-operatively, orally or 1gm Flagyl, rectally in the morning of the operation and a broad spectrum antibiotic such as a cephalosporin intravenously injected as a single dose at commencement of anaesthesia. Pre-operative vaginal swab cultures help to locate pathogenic bacteria such as staphylococci and beta haemolytic streptococci which should be treated before surgery.

Post-Operative Instructions

In general, the operations have been designed so that the patient can, within reason, return to fairly normal activities, such as household duties, driving a car, even

create a tight and inelastic vagina. It is clear that the rectum and posterior vaginal wall must be sufficiently elastic to move freely of each other, otherwise dyspareunia may occur. Similarly, the vagina and proximal urethra must be able to move independently of each other. Structurally, tapes positioned transversely between the ATFPs, or the lateral rectal ligaments, can potentially achieve the same effect as mesh by reinforcing weakened pubocervical (PCF) or rectovaginal fascia (RVF), much like ceiling joists hold up the plasterboard (vaginal epithelium).

The history of the Integral Theory surgical system has been an evolution towards safer and simpler surgical techniques to provide stronger, more effective repair to the connective tissues of the pelvic floor. The common theme has been the use of special precision instruments to insert mesh tapes to reinforce fascial and ligamentous defects in the three zones of the vagina (fig 1-12). In the next sections, options for surgical correction of connective tissue damage are explained, as well as the issues arising from these surgical correction techniques, particularly the use of mesh tapes, mesh, and the delivery instruments.

Repair of Damaged Ligaments through Creation of Artificial Neoligaments

A striated muscle requires a firm anchoring point to function optimally. It is the collagen component which gives a ligament strength. Once weakened or damaged, suspensory ligament such as PUL, ATFP or USL (fig 1-12) cannot be successfully repaired by suturing. Placement of a polypropylene tape in the position of these ligaments can strengthen them. The implanted tapes irritate the tissues causing a collagenous neoligament to form around the tapes. This linear deposition of collagen acts as an artificial neoligament (Petros et al (1990), Petros (1999), Doctor of Surgery thesis).

Principles and Research Underpinning the Strategy of Creation of Artificial Neoligaments

Very early in the development of the Integral Theory, it became clear that the characteristics and behaviour of the tapes to be used were critical to the practical success of surgery based on the Theory. A brief overview of the issues encountered is now provided, together with summaries of laboratory and other research undertaken to assess the characteristics of, and the histological reactions to the tapes used to create artificial neoligaments.

Eliciting a Useful 'Foreign Body' Tissue Reaction to Implanted Tapes

An early challenge was to determine if the foreign body tissue reaction elicited by the tape could be used in a positive way to reinforce the pubourethral ligament. Mersilene tapes were implanted between rectus abdominis and midurethra in 13 canines for periods of 6 to 12 weeks. Both tape ends were left lying free in the vaginal cavity (Petros, Ulmsten & Papadimitriou 1990). In all cases, a linear deposition of collagen was observed around the implanted tape, (fig 4-07), which persisted after the tape was removed (fig 4-08). Macrophages were observed in the tape interstices. There was no evident discomfort, pyrexia, change in appetite, or raised white cell count in the animals (Petros (1999), Doctor of Surgery thesis) or, subsequently, in the patients who had the prototype intravaginal sling procedures (Petros & Ulmsten, 1990, 1993).

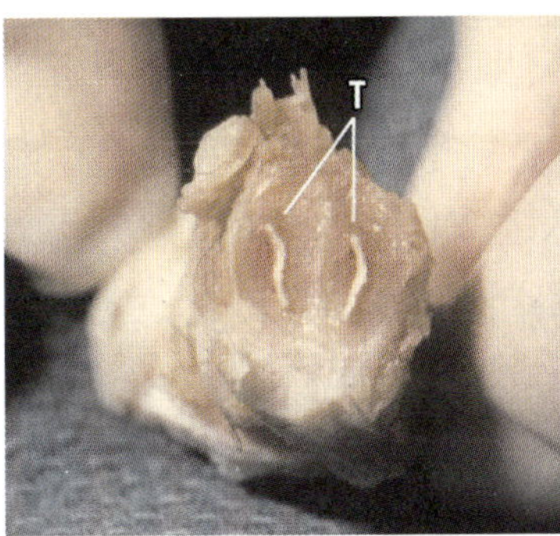
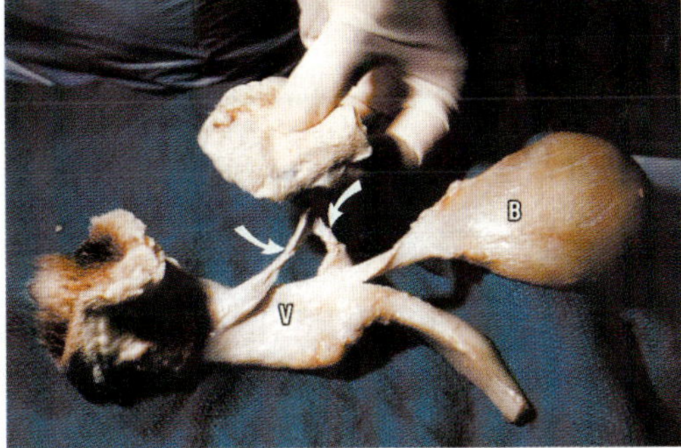

Fig. 4-07 (Above left) Tissue Reaction to implanted Mersilene tapes. Specimen from an experimental animal in which a tape had been implanted around urethra with ends free in the vagina for 12 weeks. The tape 'T' is surrounded by a layer of granulation tissue, then by a layer of collagen.

Fig 4-08 (Above right) Collagenous neoligaments 6 weeks after removal of the tape. Canine specimen. Arrows indicate the collagenous neoligament. V = vagina; B = bladder.

Assessing Different Tape Materials

Ulmsten et al. (1996) demonstrated that polypropylene mesh is better tolerated in human tissues than other materials (such as Mersilene, Teflon, PTFE). Polypropylene has low erosion rates and proven inertness, even in the presence of infection (Iglesia et al. 1997). It is the preferred material for reconstructive vaginal surgery.

Whatever the material, a mesh should not fray when trimmed because the frayed parts may exit through the vaginal epithelium to cause dyspareunia, or even perforate an organ to cause a fistula.

Mechanical Properties of Various Tapes

Both monofilament and multifilament tapes have been successfully used in incontinence surgery.

Monofilament mesh (fig 4-09) is very distensile, has thicker fibrils (100-150μ) than multifilament mesh, with relatively large diamond-shaped spaces between the fibrils. Monofilament mesh tape can be stretched under tension to a narrow string-like configuration. This stretching under tension greatly increases the pressure (force per unit area) that is applied, so that soft atrophic tissues such as the urethra may be easily transected (as reported by Koelbl et al (2001)). A distensile monofilament tape must always be set loosely under the urethra when used in stress incontinence surgery.

Multifilament mesh (fig 4-10) has more and smaller fibrils (20-30μ) and smaller spaces between the fibrils than monofilament tape. It is also softer and non-distensile. Multifilament mesh has a greater surface area to apply to the urethra, thereby vastly diminishing the pressure applied (force per unit area) and thus the possibility of perforation is reduced. When used in stress incontinence surgery, multifilament needs to just touch the urethra without indentation to be effective.

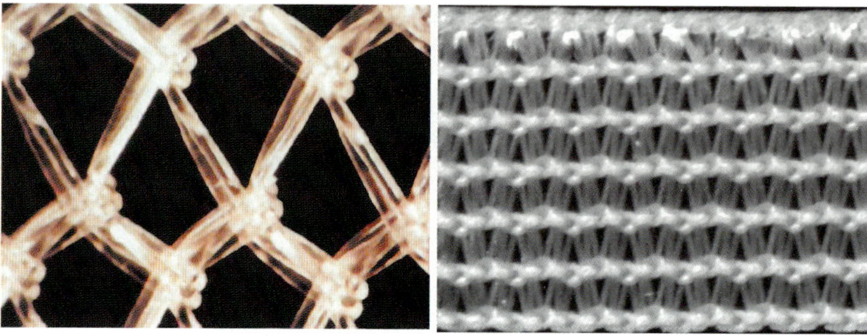

Fig 4-09 (Above left) Monofilament tape. The monofilaments are 100-150 microns thick. The spaces are relatively large. The diamond-shape allows the tape to be stretched into thin string which may transect the urethra.

Fig 4-10 (Above right) Multifilament tape. The tape is soft, non-elastic and non-distensile, and applies a smaller force per unit area to the urethra.The filaments are 20-30 microns thick. The spaces are 55 to 75 microns, significantly smaller than monofilament tape.

The Impact of Fibril Diameter on Tissue Reaction

The multifilament fibrils (20-30 microns) elicit much smaller individual tissue reactions and create a collagenous cylinder which surrounds the tape with fine, interconnecting collagen or glycasominoglycan fibrils. The thicker monofilament fibrils (100-150 microns) create a much denser collagen reaction around fibrils, a characteristic which may make surgical removal difficult. A multifilament tape is much easier to remove because it is encased in a collagen cylinder.

The Impact of Weave Density

Testing of monofilament and multifilament tapes at the School of Materials Engineering, University of Western Australia (unpublished data, 1999), showed that the multifilament tape was twice as dense per surface area as the monofilament tape, suggesting that a denser tissue reaction is more likely. This was confirmed histologically (Papadimitriou et al 2005).

In terms of the Integral Theory, the type of fibrotic reaction elicited by a multifilament tape is advantageous in ligament reconstruction because the ligaments are anchoring points for the three directional muscle forces that are the key to the structural integrity of the pelvic floor (fig 1-12).

A different type of scarring reaction is sufficient if relatively large sheets of mesh are used for repair of rectocoele or cystocoele. The pressures (forces per unit area) acting on fascia are far smaller than those acting on the suspensory ligaments, so only minimal monofilament fibrous tissue reaction is required.

Research into the Histological Reactions to Implanted Mesh

The second major theme of research was to investigate the histology of reactions to implanted mesh.

The Significance of the Size of the Interfibril Space

Without providing experimental evidence, Amid (1997) stated that a space between fibres of less than 10 microns is required for macrophages to penetrate mesh spaces, and that a space of 75 microns is required for a fibrovascular bundle. However, Papadimitriou et al (2005) have demonstrated experimentally that multifilament fibrils were surrounded by macrophages two weeks after implantation (fig 4-18) and fibrovascular bundles were penetrating between spaces often <5 microns (figs 4-13, 4-15). It is known from electron microscopic studies that macrophages can traverse interendothelial spaces which may have a diameter of less than 1 micron (fig 4-11) (Papadimitriou et al 1989). This capacity is achieved by shape distortion and development of thin 'lamellopodia'.

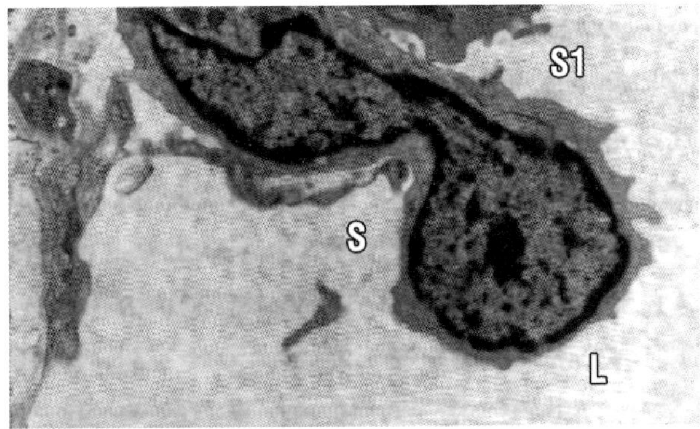

Fig 4-11 Electron microscopic image showing that macrophages can traverse interendothelial spaces, S-S1, which may have a diameter of less than 1 micron by development of thin 'lamellopedia' (L) (Papadimitriou et al 1989).

A randomised clinical trial (n = 100) by Rechberger (2003) between mono and multifilament tapes reported no erosions in either group, but a statistically greater incidence of post-operative urinary retention in the monofilament group. According to Rechberger, this is caused by pulling up of the plastic cover in the monofilament group (the only variable). Excessive tension applied to the tape may compress a soft and often atrophic urethra. Urethral erosion is more likely here with a monofilament tape because of its elasticity, wider spaces and thicker fibrils (100-150 microns). These apply a greater force per unit area to the urethra than a multifilament tape which is non-distensile, has more numerous and smaller fibrils (20-30 microns) and so it exerts a smaller force per unit area.

In 2005, a three way randomized trial by Lim et al (2005) reported vaginal erosion rates of 13.1% and 3.3% for two commercial brands of monofilament tape and 1.7% for a multifilament tape (n=180). In their analysis, they concluded that tape erosion was largely a matter of difference in technique, and was not related to the tape itself. This conclusion reinforces the views developed by the author over almost 20 years of experience.

Histological Patterns

The histological patterns formed around mesh is similar, regardless of the materials used in the mesh. In 1956 Harrison gave this description of foreign body tissue reaction following implantation:

> "In the acute stage, microscopically there is an early marked acute inflammatory reaction, characterised by an infiltration of polymorphonuclear leucocytes and macrophages. The acute reaction gradually subsides leaving a chronic inflammatory reaction, characterised by lymphocytes, plasma cells, macrophages and foreign body giant cells. This reaction diminishes over a period of six months, after which there can be found only an occasional macrophage or foreign body giant cell. Fibrosis is evident on the 7th day and the implant becomes completely encapsulated by proliferating fibrous tissue by 14 days."

Experimental work on animals with the Tissue Fixation System (TFS) (figs 4-12 & 4-13) and, previously, Petros & Ulmsten 1990) confirmed Harrison's descriptions. This work showed that fibrous tissue encapsulates the polypropylene anchors of the TFS system at 2 weeks and infiltrates the microfibrils of polypropylene multifilament mesh.

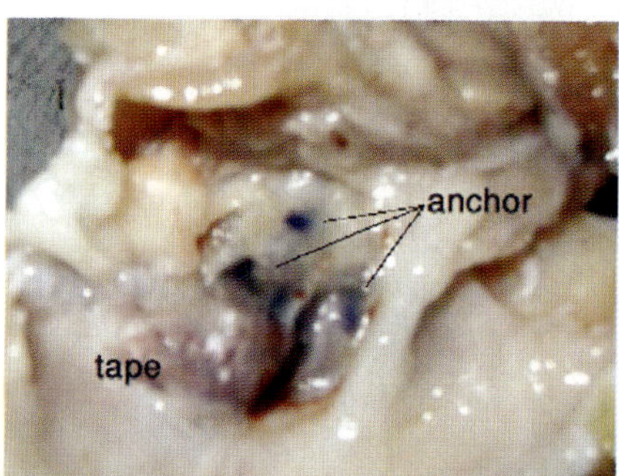

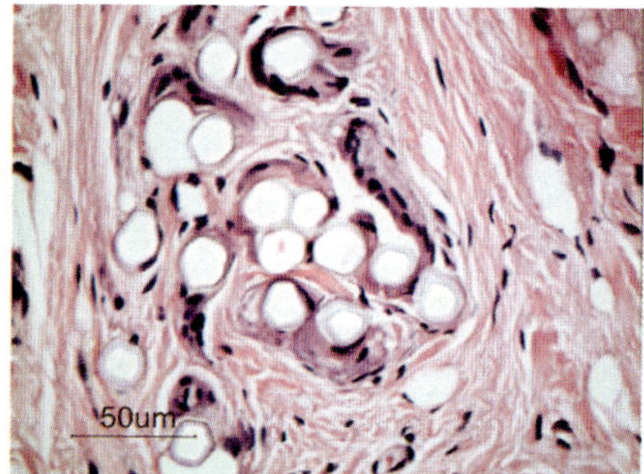

Fig. 4-12 Fibrous tissue at 2 weeks. This shows how tissue encapsulates the polypropylene anchors of the TFS system

Fig. 4-13 Fibrous tissue at 2 weeks. Shows how macrophages and fibrovascular tissue have infiltrated the microfibrils of a multifilament polypropylene mesh at 2 weeks

The Nature and Behaviour of Foreign Body Reactions

A foreign body inflammation is benign, irrespective of the amount of tissue reaction. A mature foreign body reaction is characterized by the presence of macrophages and multinucleate giant cells (figs 4-14 & 4-15). It was found that the intensity of tissue reaction varies according to the volume of the implant. It also varies markedly from patient to patient, from minimal to copious sterile pus (Petros PE, Doctor of Surgery thesis, 1999). A sterile tape abscess is rare and is an extreme foreign body inflammation, not dissimilar to a splinter abscess. The pain caused by tissue distension disappears on removal of the foreign body.

Figures 4-14 to 4-17 are derived from histological study of mono and multifilament meshes in the human by Papadimitriou at the University of Western Australia

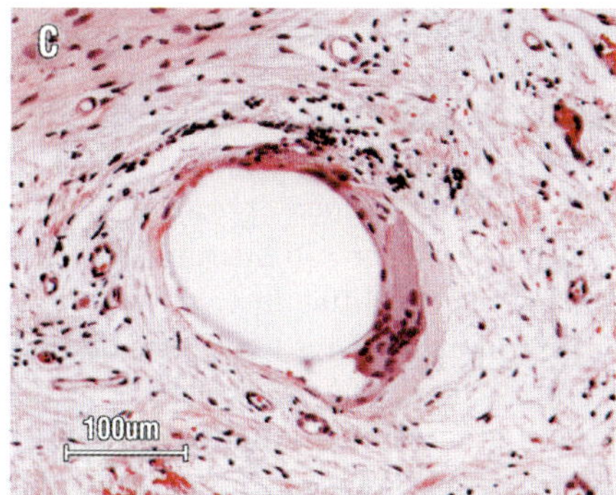

Fig. 4-14 Connective tissue in the vicinity of the monofilamentous mesh. Note the relatively small, poorly compacted collagen bundles, the large multinucleate giant cells apposed to the monofilamentous mesh and the presence of inflammatory cells in the adjacent connective tissue.

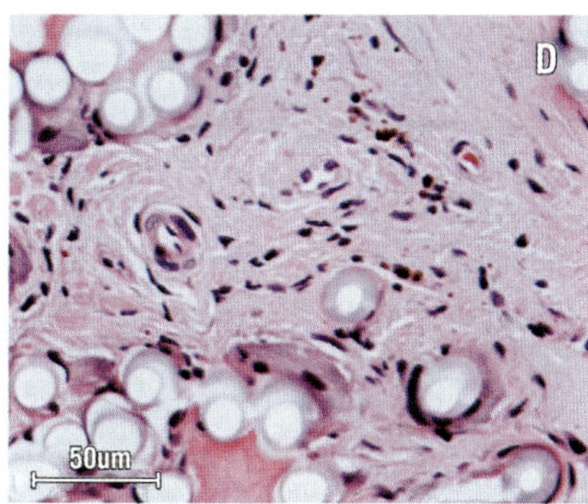

Fig. 4-15 Connective tissue in the vicinity of the multifilamentous mesh. Note the relatively thicker, more compacted collagen bundles. Small multinucleated cells are apposed to the components of the multifilamentous mesh. Amorphous pink coagulum (proteoglycan) can be seen in interstices. Only a few inflammatory cells are present in the adjacent connective tissue.

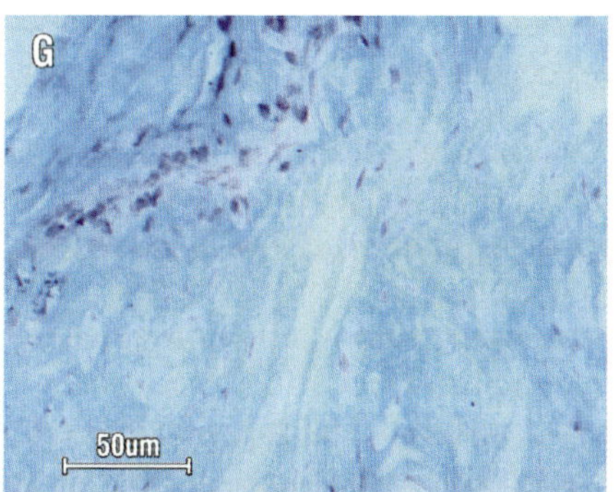

Fig. 4-16 Alcian blue stain showing the presence of proteoglycans in the connective tissue adjacent to the monofilamentous mesh.

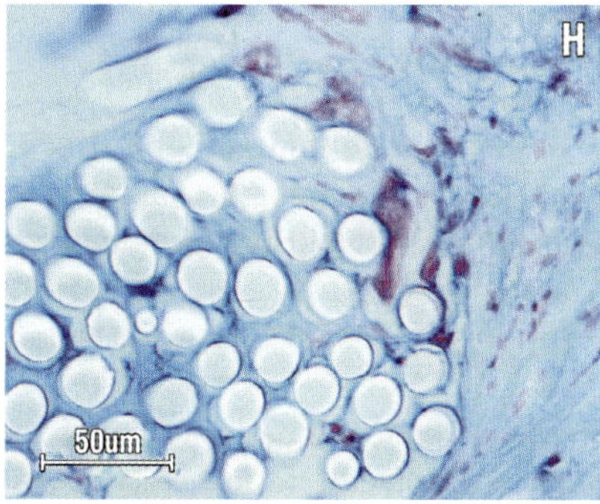

Fig. 4-17 Alcian blue stain showing the presence of proteoglycans between the interstices of the multifilamentous mesh as well as in the adjacent connective tissue.

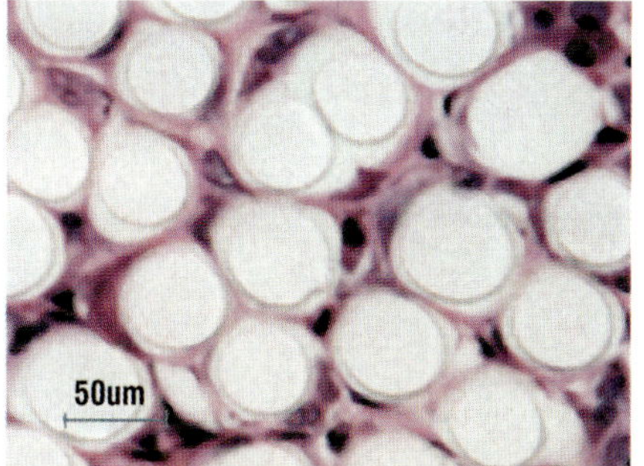

Fig. 4-18 (left) Macrophages surrounding multifilament fibrils. Rat specimen, 2 weeks after implantation. The microfibrils are surrounded by macrophages, proteoglycans and collagen III. (Papadimitriou J. and Petros, PE, (2005)).

(Papadimitriou et al. 2005). The slides were stained for collagens 1 and 3 and proteoglycans. The collagen 1 fibres were found to be somewhat thicker and more tightly compacted forming a cylinder around the multifilamentous mesh. This indicates that the quantum of collagen formation is directly proportional to the density of the mesh (ie more mesh = more collagen). The collagen cylinder greatly facilitates the tape removal. In contrast, the dense collagen around the 150 micron fibres of a multifilament tape may embed into the organ and may be difficulty to remove.

Proteoglycans, (fig 4-17), and even some argyrophyllic fibres (collagen 3 fibrils) were found between the multifilaments, proof that connective tissue is deposited between the multifilaments and macrophages (fig 4-18). It is known that Type 3 collagen is the collagen that is secreted by fibroblast early in the process of repair and is generally degraded by macrophages and fibroblasts as the wound ages. Its presence in a 2 year old implant may indicate a certain plasticity in the implant.

Repair of Damaged Fascia

There are two types of fascial damage, discrete tears in the rectovaginal and pubocervical fascial sheets, and homogenous overstretching thereof. It is not always possible to distinguish between the two types of damage. Whereas it is possible to directly repair a break in the fascia, direct repair to an overstretched sheet of fascia is not likely to be as successful.

The Critical Role of Optimally Tensioned Fascia to Restoration of Organ Function

A striated muscle contracts only over a fixed distance. Any laxity 'L' (fig 4-19) means that the vaginal membrane cannot be fully stretched, so that the function determined by those muscles will be suboptimal. So any of the symptoms detailed in the Pictorial Algorithm may persist, even though the implanted mesh may act as an effective barrier to further prolapse. For example, inability to stretch the vagina sufficiently to support 'N' (fig 4-19) may result in persistence of urge and frequency symptoms.

Because the vaginal fascia transmits the striated muscle forces which activate organ opening and closure, it is important to restore the original tension of the fascia, if organ function is to be restored. Figure 4-20 illustrates the prolapsed state of the fascia 'F'. In such a case, any mesh applied as a passive barrier will not restore function *unless* the natural tension of the fascia is also restored. This means that the laterally displaced fascia should be approximated towards the midline prior to placement and

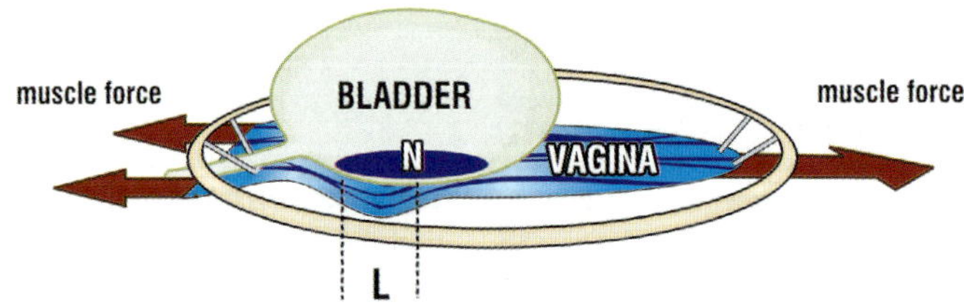

Fig. 4-19 A lax vaginal membrane will not permit adequate tensioning by the muscle forces. Lax fascia 'L' prevents the muscle forces (arrows) from fully tensioning the vaginal membrane. 'N'= stretch receptors.

attachment of the mesh. If the the fascial or mesh sutures do not tear out within 10 to 14 days the fibrogenesis induced by the mesh will strengthen the fascia, which will then 'set' in the restored tensioned position.

However, it is risky to rely on sutures to apply tension to mesh. It is extremely difficult technically and inaccurate (in terms of achieving the optimum tension).

More recent whole-mesh replacement techniques use a mesh that has four 'arms' attached to address the problem of anterior vaginal wall prolapse. The four 'arms' are threaded through the supero and infero-medial borders of the obturator fossa, and then pulled to apply tension to the mesh. This method has potential limitations because it is not a natural anatomical restoration.

A mesh attached to a posterior sling is used to address posterior vaginal wall prolapse. This method has limitations because of the inability to tension laterally displaced recto vaginal fascia.

The TFS system uses a soft-tissue anchor with a built in mechanism that allows the tension of the tape to be adjusted. This method can accurately restore fascial tension in any part of the anterior or posterior vaginal wall (fig 4-21).

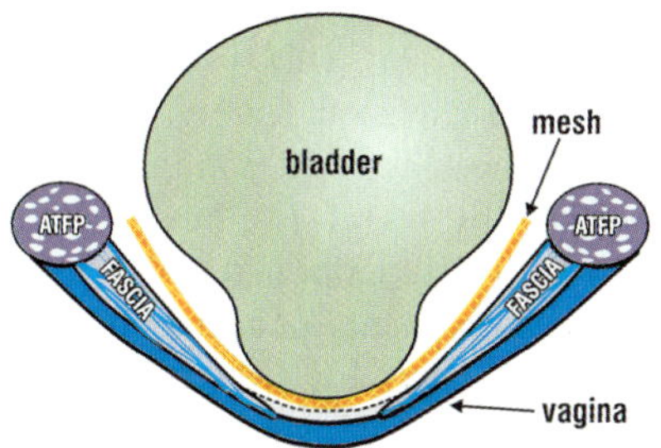

Fig. 4-20 Large mesh placed as a barrier. Note the prolapsed state of the fascia 'F'.

Fig. 4-21 A tensioned mesh also tensions the fascia. The tensioned mesh restores form and, therefore, function.

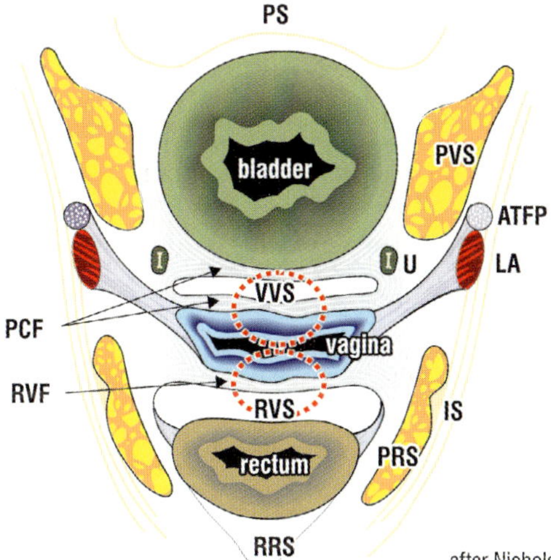

Fig. 4-22 The importance of preserving the spaces between the organs. The red circles indicate how the spaces between the organs may be obliterated when vaginal tissue is excised from the anterior or posterior walls of the vagina. U = ureter; PVS = pubovesical space; VVS = vesicovaginal space; RVS = rectovaginal space; RVF = rectovaginal fascia; RRS = rectorectal space; IS = ischial spine; ATFP = arcus tendineus fascia pelvis; LA = intermediate pubococcygeus muscle.

Direct repair of fascia

Preservation of spaces between the organs is important to allow their indepenent movement. Excision of excess tissue (red circles, fig 4-22) may only intensify mesh scarring, and cause organ adhesion. It is safer to excise no tissue at all, and to simply reposition any excess tissue.

Even with surgeons who favour mesh implantation, the first question which must be asked is, 'does this patient really need mesh reinforcement of the vaginal repair?' In the author's experience, in patients who have not had previous surgery, it is possible to repair most types of fascial damage without any mesh implantation and still achieve an 80% success rate.

Reinforcement of fascial tissue using homologous tissue, mesh sheets or heterologous tissue

Use of Homologous Tissue to Reinforce Fascia ('Bridge repair')

In a 'bridge repair' the excess tissue from a rectocoele is used to create a double layer of tissue over the central part of the herniation, its weakest part (fig 4-23a to fig 4-23c). This also brings together the laterally displaced fascia (F) (figs 4-24a & b). Allis forceps are placed on the right and left sides of the vaginal wall and brought to the centre so as to determine the width of the bridge incision. This is an important step because an overly wide bridge may lead to excessive tension, tearing, and post-operative herniation. Once the length and width has been assessed, a full thickness, leaf-shaped 'bridge repair' is cut into the vaginal wall (fig 4-23a). The 'bridge repair' surface is cauterized to destroy the surface epithelium. The superior part of the 'bridge repair' is attached to the fascia around the uterosacral ligaments, or anchored with a TFS or posterior sling tape. Inferiorly it is attached to the perineal body, and laterally it is attached to the underlying fascia with interrupted absorbable sutures (fig 4-23b). If required, a transvaginal 'holding suture' can be used to help retain the tissues in position while the scar tissue strengthens (fig 4-24b).

The 'bridge repair' is especially useful for the posterior vaginal wall, but it should only be used where there is excess vaginal tissue which would normally be excised. A 'bridge repair' can also be used in the anterior vaginal wall. However, if there is a paravaginal defect as well as a central defect, a post-operative recurrence involving the whole anterior wall may emerge weeks or months after surgery. Although there are few glands in the vagina, retention cysts may occur many months later in up to 5% of patients. This is treated by aspiration or excision of the cyst and repair of the vaginal wall.

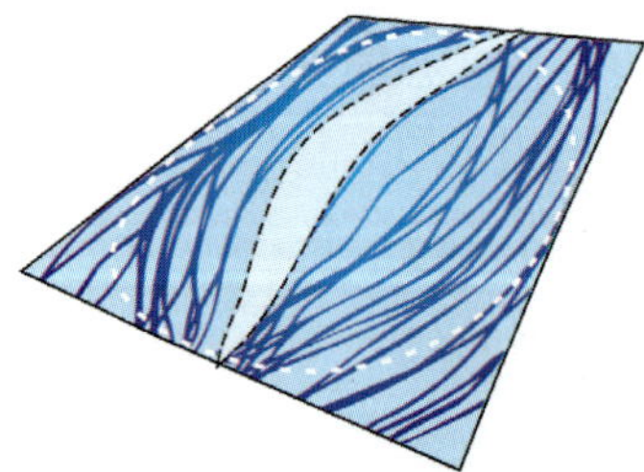

Fig. 4-23a 'Bridge' repair. A 'bridge' between 1 and 2cm wide is created by full thickness vaginal incisions.

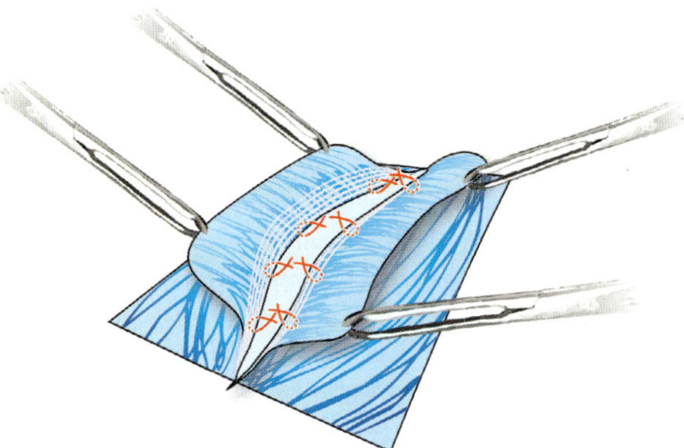

Fig. 4-23b 'Bridge' repair. A full thickness leaf-shaped ellipse is cut into the posterior vaginal wall. The lateral vaginal walls (V) are then sutured over the 'bridge'. The ellipse is sutured laterally to healthy fascia with interrupted sutures.

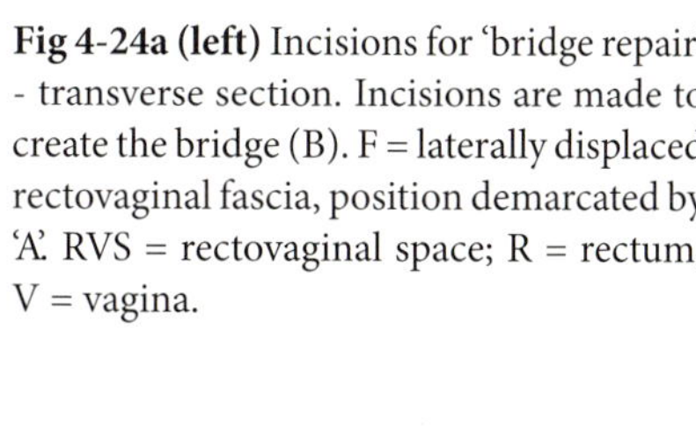

Fig. 4-23c The 'bridge' is covered by approximation of the vaginal edges.

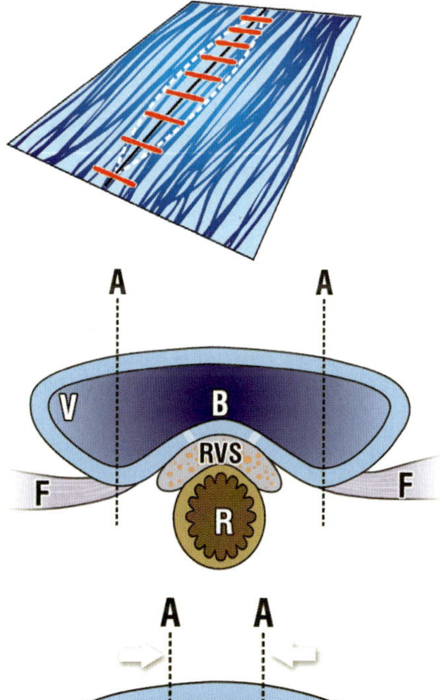

Fig 4-24a (left) Incisions for 'bridge repair' - transverse section. Incisions are made to create the bridge (B). F = laterally displaced rectovaginal fascia, position demarcated by 'A'. RVS = rectovaginal space; R = rectum; V = vagina.

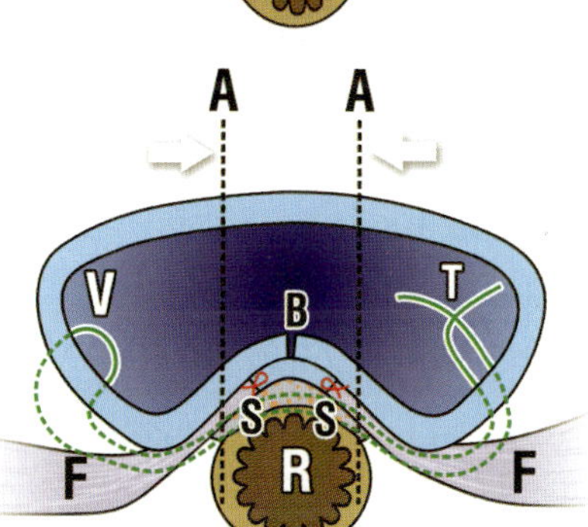

Fig 4-24b (left) 'Bridge repair' completed. The bridge (B) is attached laterally to fascia (F) by sutures (S). Note approximation of 'A' to 'A'. T = transvaginal holding suture.

Use of Mesh Sheets to Reinforce Fascia

Where the fascial layer has been weakened by age or previous surgery, there may be little option but for the surgeon to use mesh sheets or porcine dermis to reinforce the thinned out fascia.

It is probably best to use mesh sheet only where previous surgery has failed to repair the condition. In such cases, especially when the whole membrane is thinned out, there is often little musculofascial tissue available to create underlying support.

One technique is to cut the required size of mesh with two elongations placed below the pubic bone into the Space of Retzius, or to use various configurations which pass through the obturator membrane. The bottom end may be rounded to minimize erosion or viscus perforation. Many surgeons prefer to leave the mesh 'tension-free', and they advise a wide dissection to free the bladder or rectum from vaginal tissue laterally so that the mesh is held in place by tissue pressure. Others prefer to suture the mesh laterally and to the cervical ring posteriorly. In this case, the mesh must be sufficiently large to extend laterally towards the ATFP without stretching. The anterior border of the mesh should be 1cm behind the bladder neck so as to not interfere with the bladder neck closure mechanism (c.f. 'tethered vagina syndrome', this chapter).

The use of mesh is still controversial in some quarters. For instance, Milani et al (2004) advised against mesh implantation during vaginal surgery. They reported up to 13% vaginal erosion rates, a 63% increase in dyspareunia, and a 20% decrease in sexual activity following mesh implantation during vaginal repairs.

The histology of mesh implants is identical to that for tapes, as described earlier.

Use of Heterologous Tissue to Reinforce Fascia

Only acellular porcine tissue is addressed here: cadaveric fascial tissue cannot avoid the criticism of transmissible viral diseases, an issue which must impose an attitude of zero tolerance to its use.

When used to reinforce fascia, porcine skin or intestinal mucosa is treated so that all cellular tissue is removed. It is then manufactured into thin sheets which can be used as an alternative to polypropylene mesh. Porcine tissue is said to avoid many of the complications encountered with mesh, for example, surfacing, inflammation, infection, dysparuenia. Short and medium-term success rates from use of porcine tissue have been reported. However, there are complexities, as the efficacy of a heterologous tissue implant for a particular patient is species, donor, site and age dependent. Animal collagen may only be 85% homologous with human collagen (Peacock 1984). These are fundamental immunological issues and raise some concerns about the long-term viability of this material.

Repairing Damaged Fascia: Ongoing and post operative considerations

Possible Effects of Long-term Change in the Properties of Collagen

Collagen stiffens and contracts with age (Peacock 1984). The collagen of a 70 year old is 4 times stiffer than that of a 25 year old. A suburethral sling may contract with time and present many years later as urethral obstruction. The scar tissue around large mesh in the vagina may also contract years later to restrict the free movement between rectum and vagina. Therefore care needs to be taken with the selection and placement of mesh so as to avoid future long-term complications.

Fistula

The pelvic organs are constantly moving. So mesh may move or tear out even if sutured, resulting in surfacing, erosion, or fistula. If the mesh is too narrow, it is more likely to fold and penetrate a viscus, bladder or rectum. The fibrosis from such a perforation is intense, and repair requires a wide dissection so as to restore mobility to the bladder and vagina, a pre-requisite for operative success of the fistula.

Adherence of One Viscus to Another.

The organs are densely bound only at their distal 3 cm. Beyond that distance, they need to be able to slide on each other. Large sheets of mesh may cause dense fibrous adherence between rectum and vagina, or vagina and bladder base. This may lead to dyspareunia, or even abnormal function in the longer term given that collagen scarring stiffens and contracts with age.

Mesh Rejection

Mesh 'rejection' may be due to surfacing, foreign body reaction or sometimes, infection. Its incidence varies between 3% and 28% (Von Theobold P, and Salvatore, S., Pers. Comm.).

All implanted materials cause a foreign body reaction, which may vary widely in its intensity. A foreign body reaction and infection are both defined as inflammatory reactions. Historically, John Hunter differentiated between a foreign body reaction and infection. He defined the former as "adhesive inflammation", and the latter as "suppurative inflammation". Whereas a foreign body reaction is relatively benign, a tissue infection may not be. Before the diagnosis of infection can be made, a significant bacterial culture (>1,000,000 organisms/mg) is required, (Van Winkle and Salthouse, 1976). Tapes and mesh entirely rejected by a foreign body reaction or infection are surrounded by fluid, and usually pull out easily if totally rejected. Total rejection is more common with nylon or polyester (Mersiline) tapes. It is less common with polypropylene tapes.

Surfacing

In the first 48 hours after an operation, there is an efflux of fluid around the tape, similar to a wound reaction. In some patients, this may lead to 'slippage', usually minimal at this early stage. If the tape is close to the vaginal scar, the foreign body reaction to the tape may cause dissolution of the scar. This may lead to surfacing of the tape some weeks or months after surgery, especially in patients with weak or thin vaginal tissue. Sometimes there is no granuloma formation or vaginal discharge. Such 'surfacing' may become re-epithelialized spontaneously in time.

Tightening the overlying fascia of the hammock anteriorly and the uterosacral ligaments (USL)posteriorly will hold the tape in position and create a barrier between the tape and the vaginal scar. Restoring hammock tightness will also give an improved cure rate for SI and Intrinsic Sphincter defect (ISD) because of their contribution to the urethral closure mechanism. Uterosacral ligament tightening is likely to give a higher cure rate for 'posterior fornix syndrome' symptoms.

Granulomatous Erosion into the Vagina

Tape or mesh erosion in the vagina, where accompanied by granulation tissue, is almost always a foreign body reaction. It is a usually a minor problem which can be dealt with as an office procedure in most cases by trimming the extruded segment. Individual patient's immunological systems reacted very differently to an implanted Mersiline tape with its ends left free in the vagina (figs 4-25, 4-26) (Petros Doctor of Surgery Thesis 1999). In that study, it was found that, at six weeks, some patients had very little granulation tissue. Others had moderate amounts and a few had a sterile purulent reaction. Yet no patient had a raised temperature or white cell count. Swab and bacteriological culture of vaginally extruded tapes during anterior and posterior sling surgery rarely grew bacteria (Petros 1990, 1996, 1997, 2001), even when bacteria were detected on the tapes by gram staining, a not unexpected finding, given the abundance of bacteria in the vagina.

Van Winkle and Salthouse defined bacterial contamination in their 1976 monograph (Ethicon):

> "It is important to distinguish between contamination and infection. Contamination exists when bacteria are present, but their numbers are not so great that the body defences cannot dispose of them locally. Infection exists when the level of contamination reaches a point where local tissue defences cannot cope with the invading bacteria. It has been shown that the level at which contamination becomes infection for most organisms is about 1,000,000 bacteria per gram of tissue. Contaminated wounds can be converted to infected wounds when necrotic tissue, devascularised tissue, blood clots, etc., are present. Bacteria can multiply in such circumstances, safe from the cells that provide the local tissue defences."

It follows (from Van Winkle 1976) that the presence of a few bacteria on a tape implanted in healthy tissue are unlikely to be a factor in its rejection, whatever the configuration of the tape, as any bacteria will be 'mopped up' by macrophages on an ongoing basis. Findings of proteoglycans and macrophages between the fibrils of multifilament tapes (figs 4-17, 4-18) provide further evidence that macrophages and fibroblasts have penetrated between the fibrils and laid down connective tissue. This makes the 'concealment' of bacteria between fibrils (as asserted by Amid (1997), unlikely.

The erosion rate for polypropylene tape in patients undergoing stress incontinence surgery is approximately 1-3%. This complication very rarely causes major problems, such as abscess. Tape slippage and mechanical factors may be important factors in tape erosion. Thin vaginal tissue will more easily allow the tape to surface.

When a tape erodes or surfaces into the vagina, the first sign is usually a thick yellow painless discharge. The site of erosion can usually be identified by an area of granulation tissue which forms around the tape (figs 4-25, 4-26), although sometimes the tape surfaces without any erosion at all. The patient is almost invariably afebrile, with normal white cell count. It is rare to culture bacteria from the tape. Histology demonstrates granulation tissue around the tape. This consists mainly of macrophages, multi-nucleated giant cells, lymphocytes and neutrophils. The granulation tissue is surrounded by a layer of collagen (figs 4-25, 4-26). To remove the extruded tape segment, the tape is grasped with a haemostat and stretched. A totally rejected tape pulls out easily. Once resistance is encountered, cease pulling, trim the extruded segment by placing scissors around the tape, pressing down on the vaginal surface and cutting. Pulling forcibly against a firmly implanted tape may cause trauma and a small haematoma, a perfect culture medium for abscess formation. Extreme care needs to be taken if the mesh is monofilamentous and suburethral, as it is very easy to perforate the urethra during the removal process. Removing a multifilament tape is safer and easier as it is usually surrounded by a fibrous capsule and so can usually be removed from within the capsule.

Infection

In cases of significant clinical infection, the clinician would expect to find erythema, pyrexia, raised white cell count and microabscesses on histological examination, and bacterial growth of >1,000,000 organisms/mg.

A low grade infection may co-exist with the foreign body reaction. Even here the clinical course is usually benign. If there is any concern about infection (a rare occurrence in my experience), bacteriological investigation of the extruded segment is appropriate, and where relevant, appropriate antibiotics administered prior to removal. An abdominal skin sinus usually originates from a vaginal granulation. In this case, the tape should be removed vaginally only, by pulling on it, but only after investigation and treatment for pathogenic bacteria. Under appropriate antibiotic cover, an incision is made exactly at midurethra and the tape is removed simply grasping and pulling on it, as it will be surrounded by fluid all the way along its track. A perineal sinus consequent on a posterior sling is removed with a vertical incision in the posterior vaginal fornix. Any sinus usually seals within 48 hours of tape removal. At all times, excision of the sinus should be avoided, as this may spread any bacterial infection contained by the collagen cylinder into the surrounding tissues. Whether, or how much, infection contributes to tape erosion is a controversial issue. It is unlikely that infection occurs

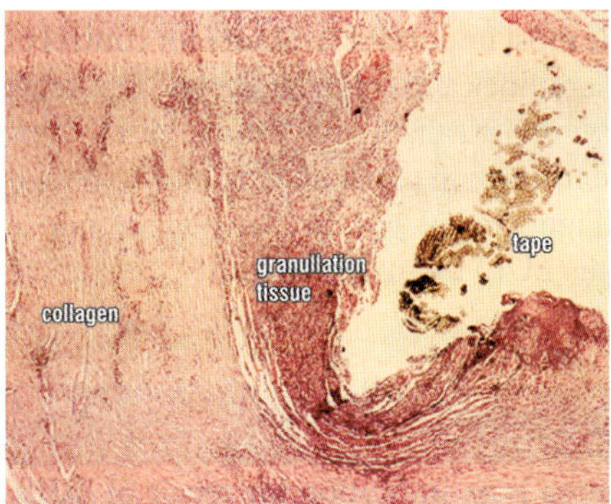

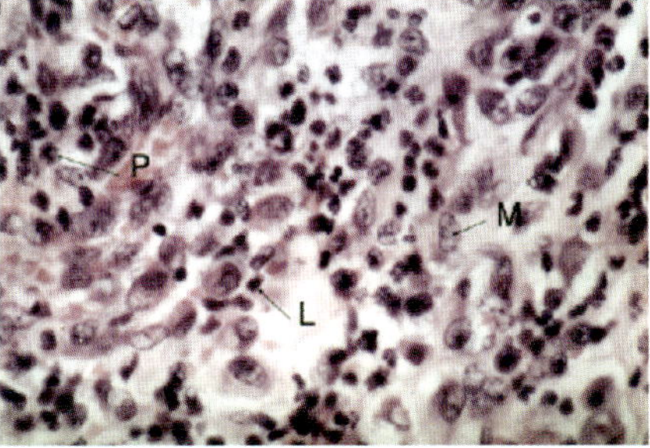

Fig. 4-25 Tape erosion in the vagina. The granulation tissue has surrounded the tape and the collagenous layer surrounds the granulation tissue.

Fig. 4-26 Tape erosion in the vagina - high powered microscopic view of the granulation tissue surrounding the tape in Fig 4-10a. Note the paucity of polymorphonuclear leucocytes 'P' and the preponderance of lymphocytes, 'L' and especially macrophages, 'M'.

The Methods: Strengthening a Weakened Pubourethral Ligament with a Tape

If the pubourethral ligament is weak, LP and LMA may stretch open the outflow tract from 'C' (closed) to 'O' (open during effort) (fig 4-30). The tape is used to reinforce the pubourethral ligament (figs 4-30). The levator plate muscle (LP) stretches the urethra backwards against the tape. This action tensions the trigone. The trigone extends to the external urethral meatus and acts as a 'splint' for the hammock during closure by PCM. Therefore the vaginal hammock needs to be adequately tight for adequate closure to take place.

If either the hammock or tape is excessively loose, the operation may fail, allowing the urethral diameter to be stretched open from 'C' (closed) to 'O' (open during effort) (fig 4-30). Conversely, excessive tightness of the sling may cause urethral constriction. Rotation of the trigonal plane around the tape is activated by LMA, which relies on an adequate uterosacral ligament for the downward force to work properly. This mechanism explains the improvement frequently seen in stress incontinence symptoms after the posterior sling operation.

The aims of anterior zone defect repair are to reinforce PUL by implanting a tape *without constricting* the midpart of urethra, to tighten the vaginal hammock (H) if loose, and to anchor the external meatus by shortening its anchoring ligaments (EUL) if they are also loose. A firm EUL is needed for bulbo and ischiocavernosus muscles to anchor the meatus, and for proper functioning of the hammock closure mechanism (fig 4-32).

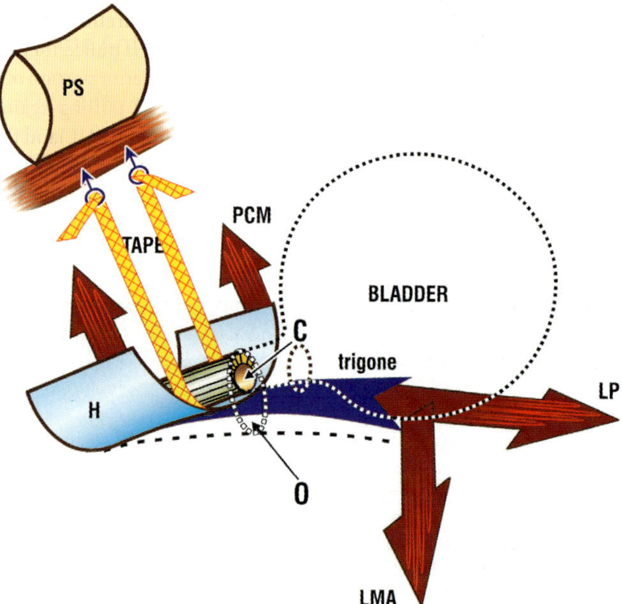

Fig. 4-30 Subpubic TFS – A polypropylene mesh tape sited at midurethra reinforces the pubourethral ligament (PUL) by providing a firm anchoring point for all muscle forces (arrows). If PUL is weak, the posterior muscle forces (arrows) may forcibly open the urethra from the closed position 'C' to the open position 'O'. H = vaginal hammock.

Rationale for Repairing External Urethral Ligament (EUL) and Hammock

Urethral closure occurs distally (fig 4-32). Usually one, but at most two extra sutures are required to tighten the hammock and EUL. If there is intrinsic sphincter defect (ISD) (maximal urethral pressure less than 20 cm H_2O), then also repairing both the hammock and the external urethral ligament (EUL) may be critical as success will undoubtedly be higher if a full restoration of anatomy is made. In a subgroup of 11 patients, a cure rate of more than 90% was obtained for patients with ISD, higher than the main group (cure rate 88%) (Petros 1997).

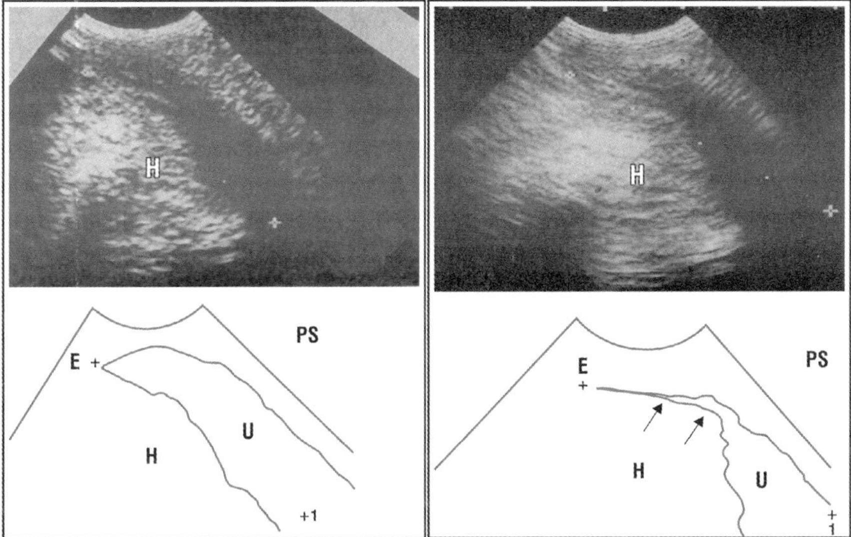

Fig. 4-31 At rest – This is an abdominal ultrasound in a continent woman.
E= insertion of external urethral meatus, (external urethral ligament).
U = urethra; PS = pubic symphysis; H = hammock.
(From Petros & Ulmsten, 1990))

Fig. 4-32 Straining – The arrows demonstrate how the urethral cavity (U) is closed by muscle forces acting on the attached vaginal wall from behind (arrows). 'E' denotes the attachment of the external urethral meatus to pubic symphysis (PS). Clearly, if 'E' is loose, then distal closure may be compromised.

Surgical Technique for Repair of the Anterior Zone Anatomy

'Tension-Free' Suburethral Sling

The main indication is for cure of stress incontinence. A polypropylene sling is inserted in a 'U' shape, below the mid-point of the urethra, to the level of the rectus sheath (fig 4-33) (Petros & Ulmsten 1993, Petros 1996, 1997, Ulmsten et al. 1996). The tape can be inserted via an abdominal or a vaginal approach using a number of commercially available delivery instruments. The hammock should be adequately tensioned. The difference between continence and incontinence may only be 2 mm. Accuracy is critical.

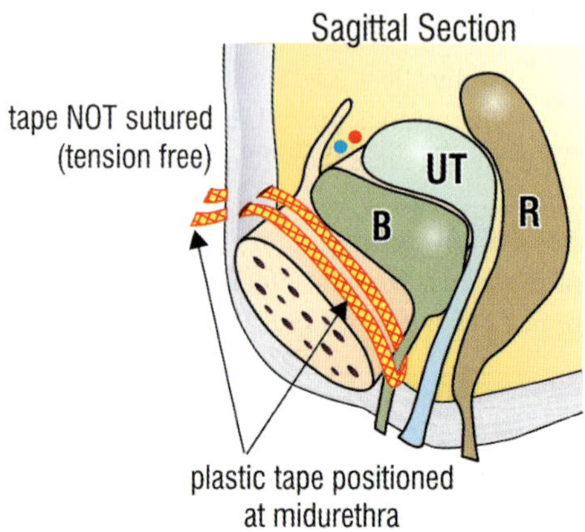

Fig. 4-33 'Tension-free' midurethral sling reinforces the pubourethral ligament (Petros and Ulmsten 1993).

Slippage of tape to the bladder neck is a cause of post-operative retention. If slippage is likely in a particular patient, suture the tape into the paraurethral tissues on one side with a 2-0 Dexon suture.

Four approaches to the 'tension-free' suburethral sling are presented below: the midline vaginal approach, the suprapubic approach, the paraurethral approach and the trans-obturator approach.

Midline Vaginal Approach

A catheter in the urethra is used as a splint to lessen the possibility of urethral perforation. Place the vaginal epithelium under stretch. Make a full thickness incision in the midline from meatus to midurethra (figs 4-34, 4-34a). Dissect between vagina and urethra laterally with scissors. Proceed with perforation of the diaphragm with scissors between the periosteum and subpubic ligaments, creating a space approximately 6mm in diameter, sufficient for entry of the delivery instrument. The description below applies to all vaginal delivery systems.

Making a hole in the perineal membrane is the most critical step, no matter which delivery instrument is used, because it confers built-in safety to what is, essentially, a blind procedure. The hole prevents excessive thrust and allows perfect control of the instrument at all times, helping avoid the major complications of this procedure, bladder and major vessel damage. Furthermore, if the subpubic venuous sinuses are breached, this can be identified because the bleeding flows out through the hole. The bleeding can be controlled by applying digital pressure for three minutes against the pubic bone from below.

Once the tip of the delivery instrument has entered the diaphragm, move the delta wing handle so it is horizontal. This is another critical step, as the external iliac vessels may be only 1.5-2 cm lateral to the exit point of the delivery instrument. The instrument can only move upwards if the delta wing is horizontal. No pressure is applied against the posterior part of symphysis pubis.

Use fingertip pressure only to gently roll the tip of the instrument over the posterior surface of the pubic bone. This vastly reduces the incidence of bladder perforations. A resistance is met at the level of the rectus sheath. At this point sufficient pressure is applied to 'pop through' the tip. The insert is left *in-situ*, and the procedure is repeated on the contralateral side.

With both inserts now *in situ*, the bladder is filled with 500 ml of saline and a cystoscopy is performed. A volume of 500 ml is required to distend the bladder sufficiently to ensure there are no folds obscuring any perforation. Care is taken to search especially around the air bubble at the 11 and 1 o'clock positions, the most common perforation sites.

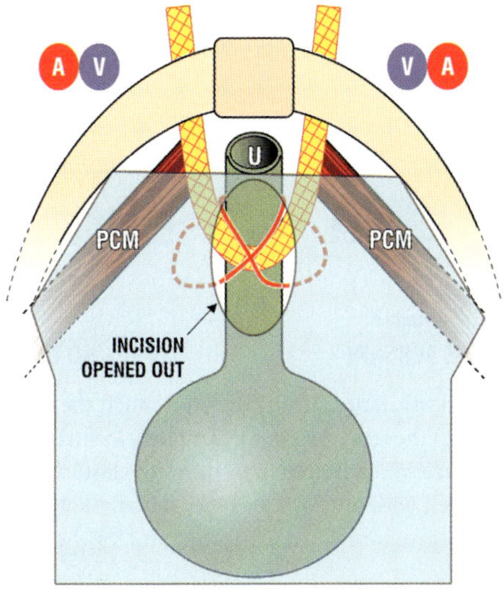

Fig. 4-34 Midline incision. Hammock tightening supports the tape from below. Perspective: Looking into anterior vaginal wall

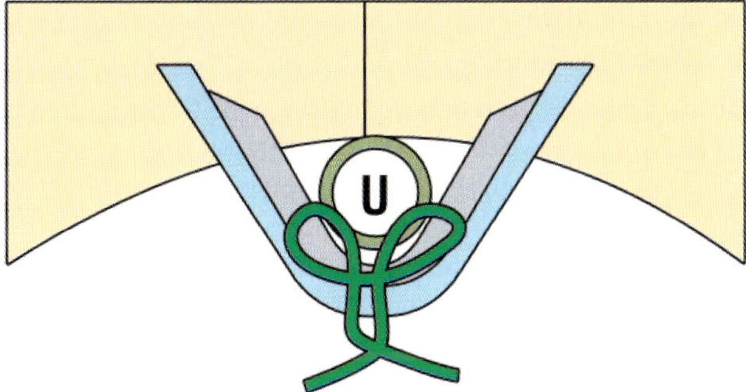

Fig. 4-34a Hammock suture. The vaginal fascia is tightened so the vagina functions as a buttress just below the urethra. Lax EUL is tightened by suturing the cut ends below the external urethral meatus. Note how the urethra is displaced upwards towards pubic ramus. Perspective: Coronal section level of external urethral mentus.

If a non-stretch tape is used, a No. 7 Hegar dilator is inserted to splint the urethra, and the tapes are pulled up one by one. Sufficient tension is exerted to ensure the tape has no folds. At all times during this step, the dilator is pushed downwards to minimize urethral constriction. At this point, the tape is directly inspected for excessive tightness. The tape should be touching the urethra without indenting it (fig 4-35). If there is indentation, loosen the tape. The tape is left 'tension-free', and is *not* sutured in any way to the abdominal muscles.

If an elastic monofilament tape is used, a 0.5mm space should be left between the tape and the urethra to allow for subsequent retraction of the tape.

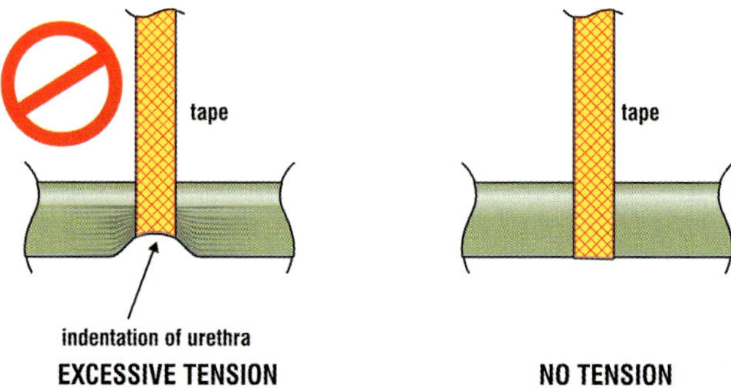

Fig. 4-35 Lateral view, non-elastic tape. The tape should touch the urethra. Touching increases the adhesive frictional force of the tape, making it less likely to surface. With an elastic tape, the surgeon has to "guess" the space which is needed to allow for elastic contraction post-operatively. Indentation is contraindicated with any type of tape, as it is likely to create obstruction. The closure mechanism works by providing an anchoring point for the 3 directional muscle forces, not by obstruction.

The Suprapubic Approach

Anatomically, the suprapubic approach is similar to the midline vaginal approach, except that entry of the application instrument is from above, downwards.

The Paraurethral Approach

The paraurethral approach was first used in the Goebell-Frangenheim-Stoeckel sling in the early 1900's. It allows a more anatomically accurate restoration in that the hammock can be re-attached to the closure muscles. It is especially indicated if the sulcus is shallow. Repair of EUL is more anatomical, as it cannot constrict the external urethral meatus. Its disadvantages are that it requires two incisions. Also a tunnel has to be made in the tissue between vaginal epithelium and urethra, something which is difficult to accomplish in patients with a deep paraurethral sulcus.

Two full-thickness longitudinal incisions are made in the lateral urethral sulcus, extending from just below the level of the external urethral meatus to the level of midurethra (fig 4-36). A Foley catheter identifies the bladder neck.

A suburethral tunnel (Tu) is created between vagina and urethra at the level of midurethra. The tape is inserted into the tunnel and brought through the anterior

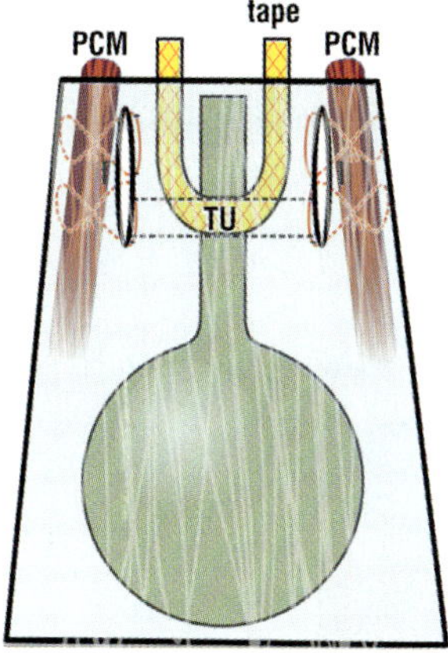

Fig. 4-36 Paraurethral vaginal skin incisions The tape passes through a tunnel 'TU' between the incisions. Perspective: Looking directly into vagina

abdominal wall with the delivery instrument. Cystoscopy is performed. The tapes are pulled up one side at a time and adjusted for tension over a No. 7 Hegar dilator.

Trans-Obturator Approach

In this method, special instruments are used to insert a tension-free midurethral tape. The entry point is from the medial border of the obturator canal. The tape is horizontally disposed and so it is not *strictly* anatomical, as the pubourethral ligaments descend vertically. The major advantage is avoidance of bladder perforation. Potential disadvantages are damage to the obturator nerve or vessels from the 'inside out' approach and to the urethra from the 'outside in' approach.

Anterior TFS Sling

The anterior TFS sling operation (Petros & Richardson 2005) (fig 4-37) has evolved directly from the 'tension-free' tape operations for cure of stress incontinence. A full thickness midline incision is made into the vagina from just below the urethral meatus to midurethra. The vagina is dissected off the urethra laterally and inferiorly with dissecting scissors. The dissection is carried 0.5 to 1cm beyond the perineal membrane. The space created should be just sufficient for the passage of the applicator. The applicator is placed into the dissected space and triggered to release the TFS anchor. The tape is pulled with a short sharp movement to 'set' the prongs of the anchor into the tissues. Adequate 'gripping' of the anchor is tested by pulling on the free end of the tape. The procedure is repeated on the contralateral side. With the applicator providing counter pressure to the anchor base, the tape is tensioned over a urethra distended by an 18G Foley catheter just sufficiently without indenting it, and the free end cut. The vaginal hammock fascia and the external ligamentous attachment of the external urethral meatus are then tightened with 2–0 Dexon sutures, as previously described. No cystoscopy is required. Mean operating time is approximately 5 minutes.

All patients to date have been discharged within 24 hours of surgery. There has been no post operative urinary retention, and only paracetamol analgesia was required in the first cohort of 36 patients (Petros & Richardson 2005). The surgical cure rate for stress incontinence appears to be equivalent to that for the 'tension-free' tape slings.

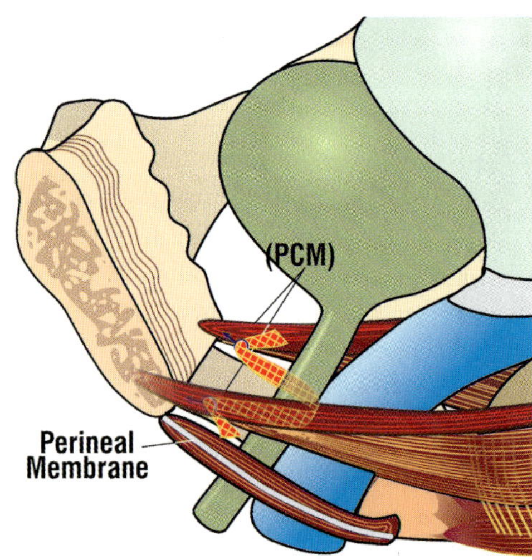

Fig. 4-37 Anatomical position of the TFS anchor. The tape is anchored into the inferior surface of the pelvic floor muscles.

EUL Shortening

With a No. 18 Foley catheter *in situ*, and using a No. '0' or '00' suture on a small needle, sutures are inserted into the ligament on both sides of EUL approximately 1 cm lateral to EUL's insertion into the urethral meatus and brought into the midline. The suture is tied after the hammock suture is inserted. This step is only performed if EUL is loose. Special care should be taken to avoid constricting the distal urethra. In most cases this step can be combined with the hammock suture. If this operation fails to strengthen the EUL, tape insertion may be required (see below).

EUL Reinforcement with a Small Segment of Polypropylene Tape

This operation may be required in patients with very loose external urethral ligaments, especially if urine loss can be controlled by use of the 'simulated operation' technique (see Chapter 3) by applying digital pressure just lateral to the external urethral meatus while the patient coughs with a full bladder. A vertical incision is made into the ligaments, almost to the pubic bone. A rectangle of polypropylene tape, dimensions approximately 0.5cm x 0.8 cm is then inserted into the incision and sutured to close it off. This operation strengthens the EUL very effectively. However, 'slippage' and extrusion of the tape may occur in some cases using the technique described.

Hammock Tightening

With a No. 18 Foley catheter *in situ*, and using the tip of a short needle, the fascial tissue is firmly penetrated on both sides from the inside with a horizontal mattress suture so that the fascial tissue is brought towards the midline (figs 4-34a & b). It is essential to avoid contact with the tape during suturing. By taking the needle into the lower end of EUL it is possible to tighten EUL and hammock using only one suture.

Potential Intra-Operative Complications of Mid-urethral 'Tension-Free' Tape Slings

It is emphasized that inserting a suburethral sling with a delivery instrument is a blind procedure. The small bowel in the prevesical pouch, the bladder, the external iliac vessels and the obturator nerves and vessels all lie within 2 to 4cm of the track taken by the instrument. Creating a hole in the pelvic diaphragm directly below the bone and orienting the delivery instrument so it can only move upwards vastly reduces the possibility of major complications.

Difficulty with Passage of the Delivery Instrument

It is important to open out again with scissors and avoid excessive pressure on the delta wing handle as this may make the point 'dig into' the soft cartilage of the symphysis and obstruct upward movement. Always ensure the delta wing is horizontal on re-entry.

Retropubic Fibrosis from Previous Incontinence Surgery

Where there is excessive retropubic fibrosis from previous surgery, dissecting scissors may be used to create a plane of dissection between periosteum and scar tissue. Once the plane is created, continue the dissection for 2.5 to 3cm upwards. This creates a space between bone and scar tissue for insertion of the delivery instrument. If resistance continues, re-insert scissors and continue further dissection upwards, always angling the scissors towards the bone. Re-insert the delivery instrument. On rare occasions, it may only possible to insert one side of the sling. In such circumstances, attach the other side deep into the pubococcygeus muscles.

Scarring in the Rectus Sheath

If scarring from a previous abdominal operation is preventing abdominal surfacing of the delivery instrument, the surgeon may occasionally need to cut down on to the rectus sheath with a scalpel.

Urethral Constriction by the Tape

Tape constriction of the urethra can be avoided by inserting a No. 7 Hegar dilator into the urethral cavity and press downwards when tightening the second limb of a non-stretch tape. If elastic tape is used, a space must be left between the tape and the urethra.

Bleeding

If there is bleeding from the venous sinuses during insertion, apply digital pressure for 2 to 3 minutes. If bleeding persists, a haemostatic gel may be placed along the tape from below and digital pressure re-applied until the bleeding ceases.

Bladder Perforation

Bladder perforation may occur in the superolateral surface usually between 11 and 1 o'clock. If this occurs, remove the tape and re-insert. Use a cystoscope with sheath and fill bladder with 500 ml fluid. Sometimes, there is no bleeding with perforation. The only sign of perforation may be the finding of a low bladder volume at the end of the operation due to extraperitoneal loss. If bladder perforation is suspected, and can't be identified, inject an ampoule of methylene blue into 500ml of saline, fill the bladder, and look for suprapubic staining at exit of tape.

Urethral Constriction by the Tape

Failure to pass any urine at all within 48 hours generally indicates a tape obstruction which needs to be surgically relieved. In the few cases that have been experienced by the author, microscopic loops were used to identify the shiny fibrils of the tape which is always under tension. The tape retracts immediately when touched gently with a sharp blade.

Slippage of the TFS anchor

In the first cohort of 36 patients, total slippage of the tape occurred on one side, in just one patient. This presented as a large vaginal granuloma (Petros & Richardson 2005) and a recurrence of stress incontinence. The TFS operation was successfully performed on this patient on another occasion indicating that whatever the cause of the previous failure, the surgical methodology was sound.

Testing for Continence at the End of Midurethral Tape Operations

Adjusting tape tension during coughing was previously considered to be an important part of the operation (Petros and Ulmsten 1993). However, because a three point repair (PUL, EUL and hammock) 'spreads the load', it makes testing for continence less critical. This allows the operation to be done more confidently with the patient under a general anaesthetic (Petros 1999).

4.3.2 Surgery of the Middle Zone

The Structures of the Middle Zone

The pubocervical fascia extends as a broad membrane between bladder neck and the cervical ring or hysterectomy scar (fig 4-38). The bladder base sits on this membrane. Collagen and smooth muscle within the vaginal wall provide its main structural components. Herniations caused by lax connective tissue in the midline (cystocoele), laterally ('paravaginal defect'), or at the attachment to the cervical ring ('transverse defect') are not easy to repair using traditional techniques, as up to one third may recur.

A fourth (iatrogenic) defect, excessive tightness from scarring or excessive elevation at the bladder neck, needs plastic surgery techniques to restore tissue elasticity in that area, the 'zone of critical elasticity'.

As there are no transverse ligaments in the middle zone, the pubocervical fascia is the main supporting structure. This is generally considered as the most difficult part of the vagina to repair because it has an inherent tendency to prolapse due to intra-abdominal pressure above and gravity below.

The vagina is suspended between arcus tendineus fascia pelvis (ATFP) laterally and the cervical ring posteriorly. Correct diagnosis of which structures are damaged, central membrane, collagenous 'glue' to ATFP or the ATFP itself, or attachment to cervical ring, is an essential precondition for repair (figs 4-38, 4-39).

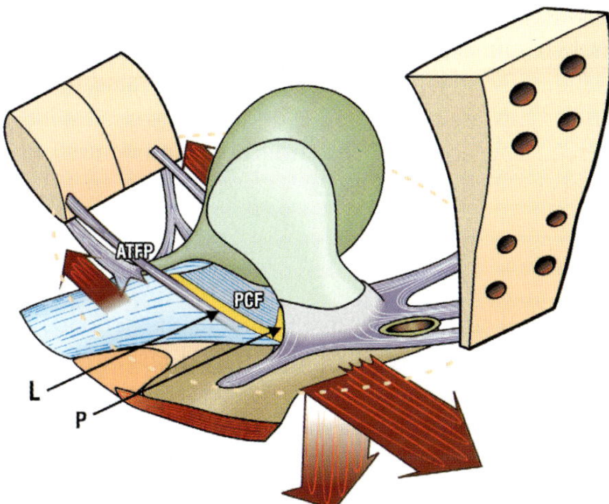

Fig. 4-38 The pubocervical fascia (PCF). The fibromuscular layer of the vaginal wall (PCF) is attached laterally (L) to arcus tendineus fascia pelvis (ATFP) and posteriorly (P) to the cervical ring by collagenous tissue (yellow). Dislocation of 'L' may cause a paravaginal defect and of 'P', a high cystocoele. Muscle contractions (arrows) stretch the pubocervical fascia (PCF) to support the bladder base (as illustrated in the 'trampoline analogy').

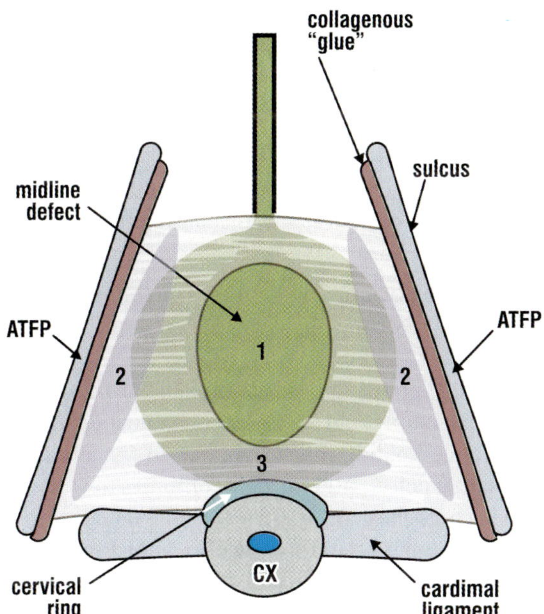

Fig. 4-39 Potential sites of damage: 1. Midline defect (central part of PCF); 2. Paravaginal defect (collagenous 'glue' and ATFP); 3. High cystocoele (attachment of PCF to cervical ring, 'transverse defect'. Schematic 2D view from below. Perspective: looking into the anterior wall of the vagina.

It is helpful to conceptualize the ATFP as two suspended lines extending between symphysis and ischial spine. Dislocation of ATFP from the ischial spine causes a 'dip' in the lines. Excessive stretching of the collagenous 'glue' between vagina and the adjoining muscles appears as a flattening of the paravaginal sulcus. If the central fascial layer is intact, rugae are seen. The surgical technique used needs to address all three components if it is to be successful.

Sites of damaged fascia

The circles in figure 4-41 are simple representations of the foetal head stretching the fibromuscular layer of the vagina ('pubocervical fascia' (PCF)), its principal supporting structure. When dislocated from the cervical ring, a high cystocoele is created. Damage further down creates a mid cystocoele and laterally, a paravaginal defect (figs 4-39, 4-40).

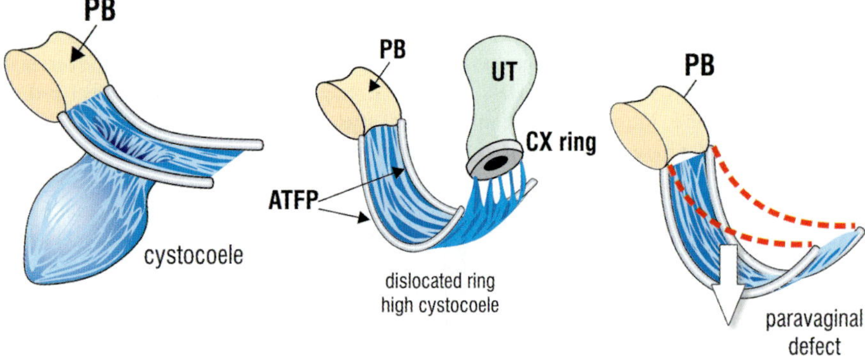

Fig. 4-40 The structural differences between midline (cystocoele), lateral (paravaginal) and cervical ring (high cystocoele) defects. All appear as 'lumps' in the vagina. Sagittal view.

A mid-cystocoele (fig 4-42) is caused by rupture or thinning of the pubocervical fascia (PCF) causing prolapse of the bladder base, giving it a shiny appearance on examination.

With a cystocoele, the supporting fascia is broken (or thinned out) so that the vaginal epithelium appears shiny. With a pure paravaginal defect, transverse rugae are seen. Ring-type sponge-holding forceps applied in the lateral sulci restore the prolapse with a paravaginal defect. A cystocoele continues to bulge when the patient strains. Often both defects coexist (fig 4-43).

Fig 4-43 demonstrates the inferolateral bulging of a central herniation (arrows). Given the wide distribution of the foetal head pressure (broken lines) it is highly likely that the tissues may also be damaged more laterally (arrows) in the paravaginal areas.

It is important to exclude dislocation of PCF from the cervical ring (fig 4-44) as a cause of urgency symptoms. This can be done using a 'simulated operation' technique by gently compressing its lateral edges with Littlewood's forceps and observing the effect on the urge symptoms.

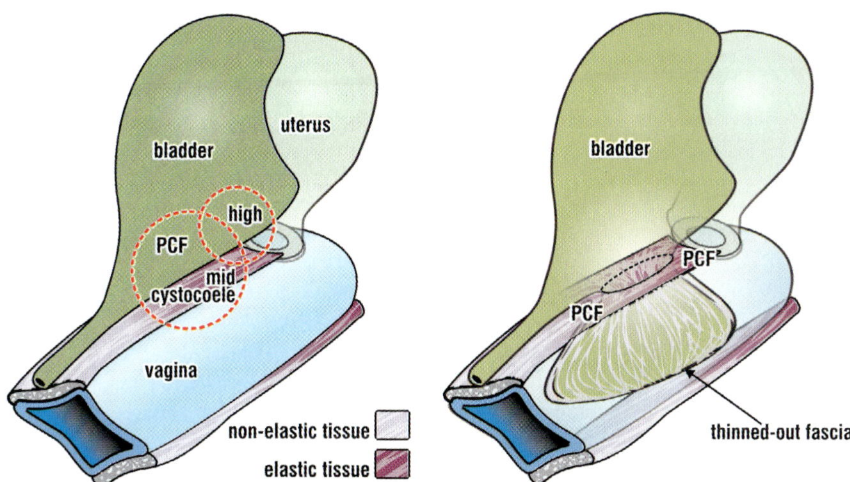

Fig. 4-41 Damage to fascia may cause a central or cervical ring defect. 3D sagittal view.

Fig. 4-42 Thinning of the pubocervical fascia (PCF) causes prolapse of the bladder base. 3D sagittal view.

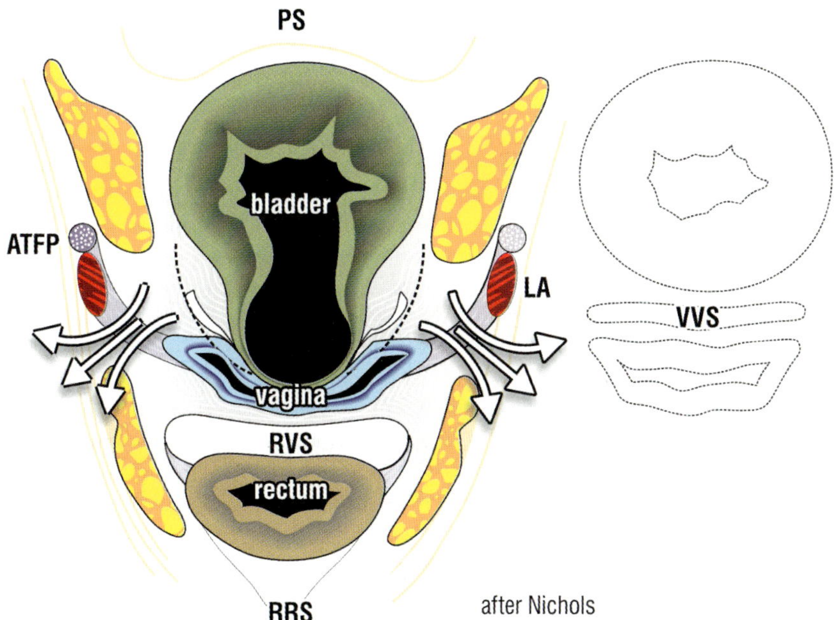

Fig. 4-43 Co-existence of central and lateral defects. The ghost areas to the right indicate the shape of undamaged vagina and bladder (B). VVS = vesicovaginal space; ATFP = arcus tendineus fascia pelvis; LA = levator ani muscle; R = rectum. Broken lines represent pressure exerted by the foetal head.

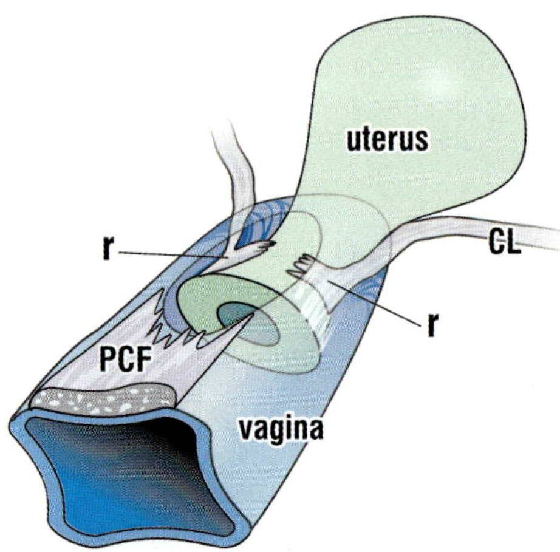

Fig. 4-44 Cervical ring extension. The cervical ring (r) extends laterally to the cardinal ligament (CL). A break in the cervical ring may cause prolapse of the puboservical fascia (PCF) or uterine prolapse due to lateral displacement of CL.

The Relationship between the Middle and Posterior Zones

Figure 4-45 demonstrates the structural relationships between the middle and posterior zones. Repair of vault prolapse may temporarily appear to 'cure' the cystocoele. However, if the fascia is damaged, the condition is likely to recur (fig 4-46). In a functional sense, the apparent 'cure' may provide sufficient structural support to 'N' (fig 4-45) to relieve co-existing urge symptoms for a few weeks, but they are likely to return after recurrence of the cystocoele.

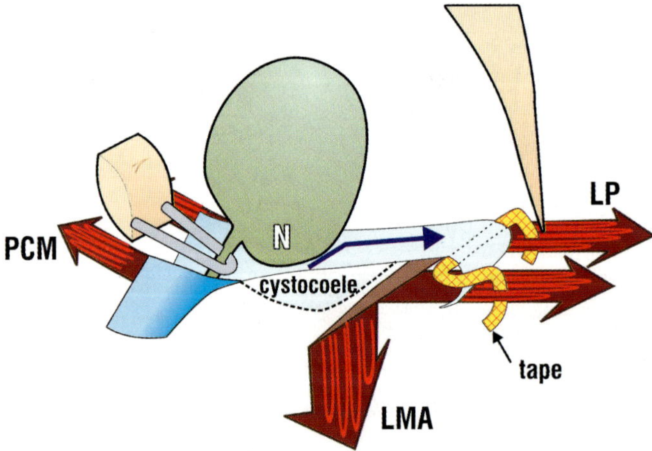

Fig. 4-45 The relationship between middle and posterior prolapse. Backward stretching of the anterior vaginal wall with a Posterior IVS may 'cure' the cystocoele. If PCF is damaged, however, the cystocoele may recur.

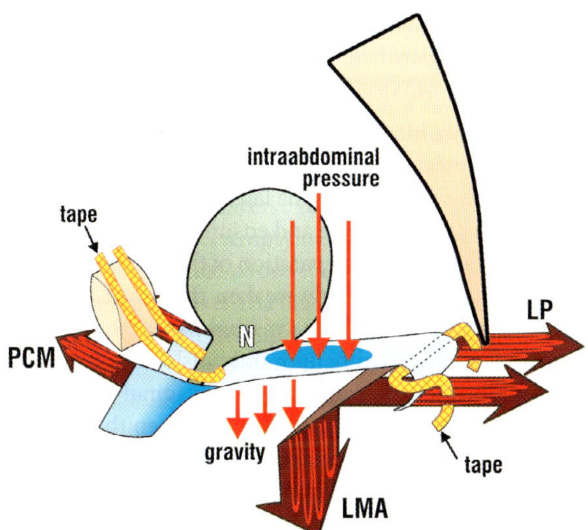

Fig. 4-46 A middle zone prolapse has an inherent tendency to recur if the fascia is damaged. This is because of the dual impact of intraobdominal and muscle forces on a membrane which has no structural support from below.

The Indications for Surgery in the Middle Zone

Structural

Everting anterior wall due to paravaginal, central defects or cervical ring dislocation, may cause dragging pain, discomfort or even ulceration if the eversion is chronic.

Functional

Abnormal emptying is the main symptom associated with middle zone defects. Symptoms of urgency may occur if the patient has sensitive nerve endings.

The Methods - Surgical Repair of the Middle Zone

Surgical Options

The options available are:
1. Direct repair - with maximal conservation of vaginal tissue
2. Recycling excess autologous tissue into a 'double-breast' or 'bridge' repair
3. Reinforcement with mesh sheet or porcine dermis
4. Using the TFS system to repair cystocoele or paravaginal (ATFP) defect directly, or in association with a 'bridge repair, heterologous tissue or mesh sheets.

Direct Repair

Direct repair cannot always adequately restore stretched damaged tissue. Moreover, the site of the surgical operation requires at least 6 weeks to achieve wound strength, rendering the wound vulnerable to dislocation by the intraabdominal and muscle

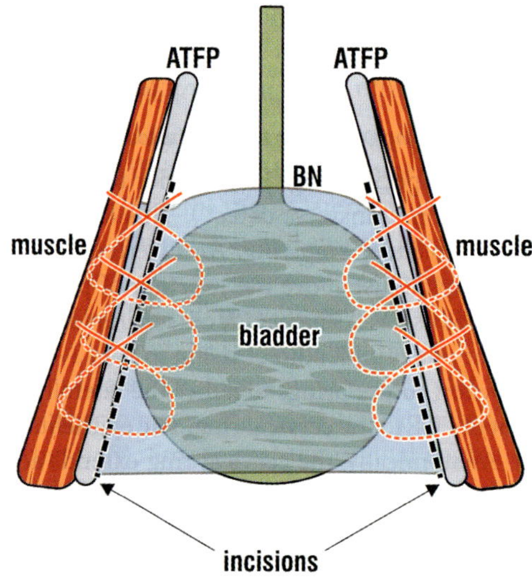

Fig. 4-51 Direct repair - paravaginal defect. Looking into the anterior wall of the vagina. BN = bladder neck

can only be performed in patients with very large herniations. It is emphasized that adequate tissue tension is not always achievable, so some symptoms may persist. These operations work well when used in conjunction with a tensioned TFS sling.

Bridge Repair of Cystocoele

In patients with large herniations it is sensible to create a leaf-shaped incision ('bridge') and to anchor it deeply into the healthy fascia laterally rather than excise tissue (fig 4-53). The main complication is that stretching the vagina medially over the bridge may weaken it laterally causing a paravaginal defect. A retention cyst may occur in up to 5% of patients. The steps for anterior bridge repair are:

- Estimate the width of the bridge.
  Grasp the proposed bridge with Allis forceps distally and proximally, and test by bringing the lateral vaginal walls towards the midline.
- Remember that an excessively wide bridge is more likely to break down.
- Make a full thickness leaf-shaped incision in the anterior vaginal wall, always behind the bladder neck.
- Use minimal dissection to separate the edges.
- Diathermy or excise the surface epithelium.
- Dissect laterally between bladder and vagina and suture the edges of the bridge to healthy fascia laterally. Attach one end of the bridge below the vaginal skin anteriorly, and to firm tissue around cervical ring or vault scar posteriorly. Insert a series of No. 1 vertical mattress holding sutures transfixing the bridge to the rest of the vagina.
- Suture the cut vaginal skin with a continuous 2-0 Dexon suture.
- Avoid an excessively tight bridge.

Constriction Ring Formation During Vaginal Repair

In terms of shape, the vagina is essentially a tube (fig 4-52). Excision of vaginal tissue may shorten and narrow the vagina. Simultaneous repair of the anterior and posterior walls may constrict the tube at segment 'V'. To avoid such 'hourglass' constrictions it is best to *not* excise vaginal tissue.

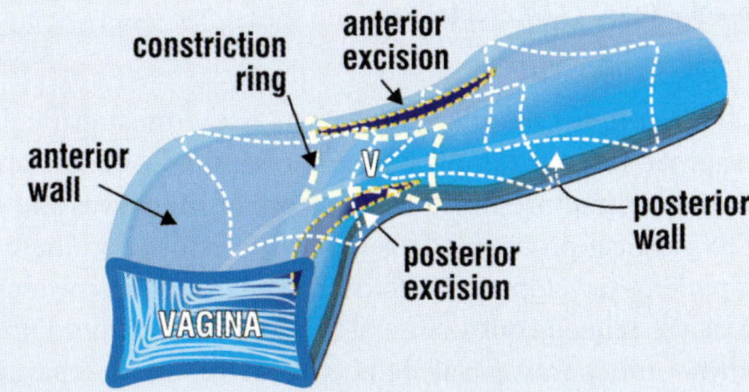

Fig. 4-52 Segmental vaginal narrowing. Perspective: patient lying supine

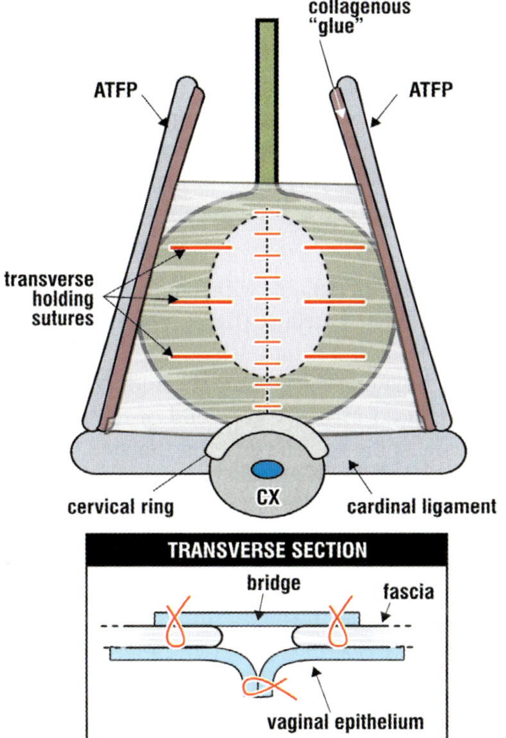

Fig. 4-53 Bridge repair of cystocoele

Double Breasted Repair of Cystocoele

The 'double breast' technique (figs 4-54 to 4-58) is useful in patients with excessive and thin tissues, or with everting cystocoele. It is a simple operation and has great strength. The rationale for a 'double-breasted' repair is that a double layer is far stronger than the alternative, excision and stretching. The flaps are created over the central herniation. The main complication can be the tearing out of one flap if the repair is made too tight.

Reinforcement with TFS or Mesh Sheets

Middle Zone Repair Using TFS

Achieving long term cure for middle zone defects is the most difficult problem in reconstructive vaginal surgery (Shull, B., pers. comm.) Concerns about creating excessive scar tissue contracture using large pieces of mesh was the driving force in developing TFS surgical procedures for repair of cystocoele. There was also the consideration of patients developing the 'tethered vagina' syndrome many years after surgery because of age-related contracture of the scar tissue around the mesh.

Initially, midline and paravaginal defects were repaired separately, then by placement of 3 horizontal tapes. Although effective, this approach was wasteful of tapes and required significant dissection laterally. Because of the risk of bladder perforation this was difficult in patients who had undergone previous cystocoele surgery. The predicament was resolved with the development of the 'U-sling' operation which reinforces both the lateral and midline defects simultaneously using only one tape.

During repair of the cervical ring defect with the lower horizontal tape, it was noted that the cervical ring actually formed part of the cardinal ligament. This has led to the development of a separate 'cervical ring' operation in which the tape is placed laterally along the cardinal ligament. The Transverse (fig 4-60), or 'U'-sling and cervical ring operations used in combination (figs 4-63 & 4-62) can be used and entirely replace sheet mesh. The TFS operations are described below.

Paravaginal TFS Repair

This operation is only indicated in patients with a pure ATFP defect. It has generally been superseded by the 'U-sling' procedure (figs 4-59 & 4-63) which also reinforces central defects.

An incision is made in the lateral sulcus from the midurethra almost to the ischial spine. The bladder is displaced medially. One end of the tape is anchored to the tissues medial to the ischial spine and the other is attached subpubically much like a subpubic TFS sling. The medial part of the incised vagina is then attached deeply to the muscles or ATFP (but not tightly), much like a classical White operation. This technique is much simpler and safer than the abdominal approach for a paravaginal repair, yet takes only a fraction of the time. The main disadvantage is that it does not address the central defects which may co-exist.

Transverse Cystocoele TFS Repair

A full thickness midline incision is made over the length of the cystocoele (fig 4-60). The vagina is dissected off the bladder as laterally as possible, so that the TFS operation is performed in full view. Dissection with a partly full bladder provides built-in safety because any perforation will be quickly recognized by leakage of urine.

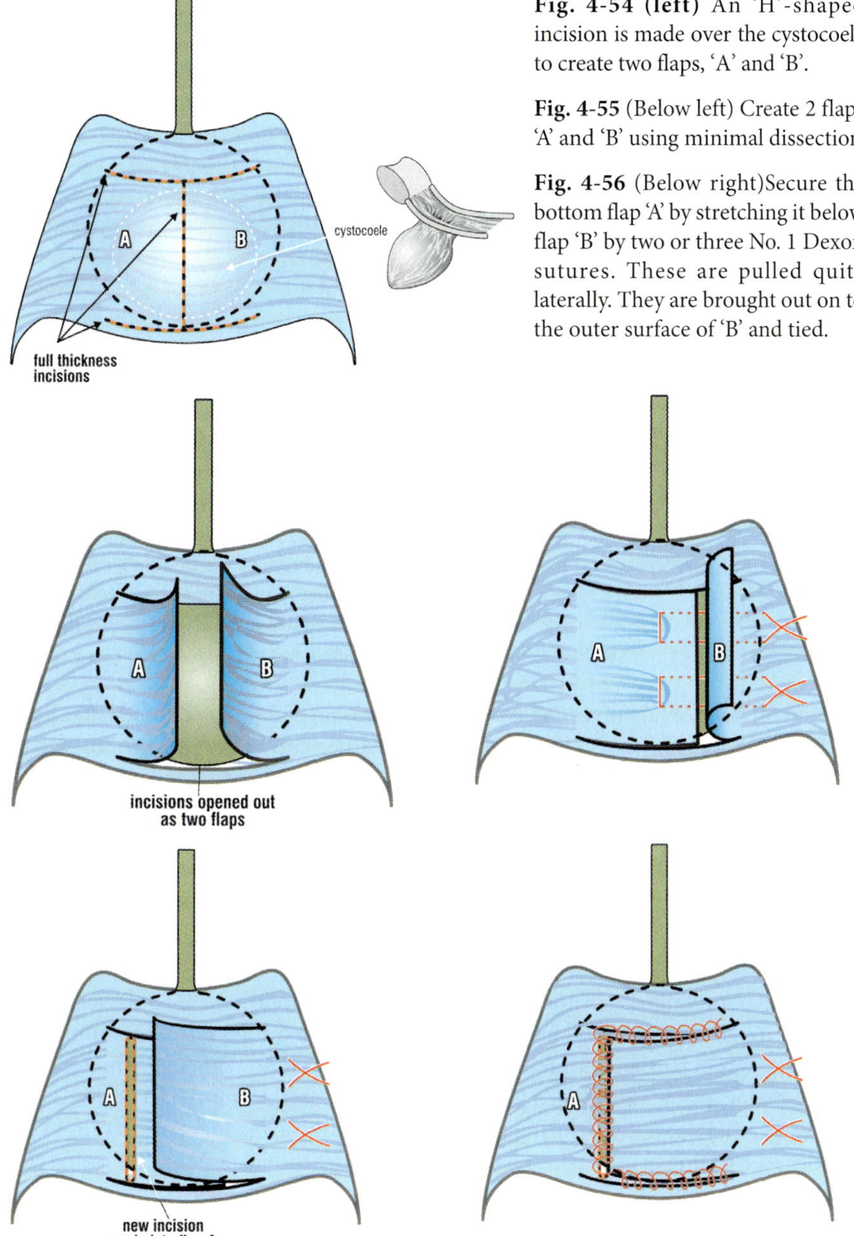

Fig. 4-54 (left) An 'H'-shaped incision is made over the cystocoele to create two flaps, 'A' and 'B'.

Fig. 4-55 (Below left) Create 2 flaps 'A' and 'B' using minimal dissection

Fig. 4-56 (Below right)Secure the bottom flap 'A' by stretching it below flap 'B' by two or three No. 1 Dexon sutures. These are pulled quite laterally. They are brought out on to the outer surface of 'B' and tied.

Fig. 4-57 Make a full-thickness vertical incision into flap 'A', sufficiently lateral to anchor the edge of flap 'B' into the incision without tension.

Fig. 4-58 Suture the cut edges of flap 'B' into cut edges of A. Flap 'B' is stretched minimally across like a double-breasted coat and sutured into that incision with interrupted sutures. The repair is completed by placing sutures to join the horizontal cut ends of 'A' and 'B'.

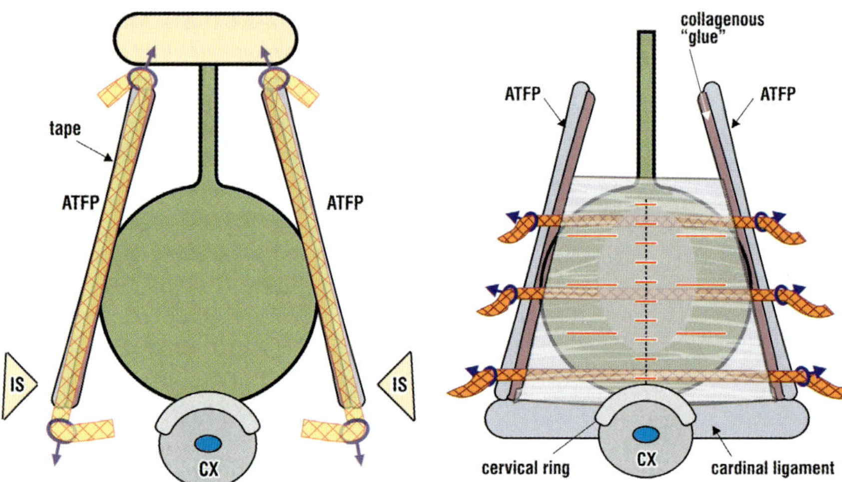

Fig. 4-59 TFS repair of ATFP. The tape reinforces ATFP and 're-glues' the vagina to ATFP by creating a collagenous reaction.

Fig. 4-60 Cystocoele repair by Tissue Fixation System (TFS). The transverse tape reinforces the damaged central fascia much like a ceiling joist supports the ceiling, and the damaged ATFP and paravaginal fascia are like the ceiling beam supporting the joists.

Strips of horizontal polypropylene mesh tape 0.8 cm wide are anchored laterally by the tissue fixation system (TFS), and tightened sufficiently to support the overlying bladder, much like joists of a ceiling reinforcing a plasterboard. One, two, or three tapes may be used)(fig 4-60). The number of tapes required becomes evident to the surgeon during the operation. The advantage of this method is that, unlike large sheets of mesh, antero-posterior elasticity is largely maintained.

This method is minimalist compared to large mesh sheets. Much less scar tissue is formed, and the risk of fistula, tethered vagina, and organ adherence greatly reduced. If a tape is required near the bladder neck, it should not be set tightly as this may prevent the opening out of the outflow tract during micturition. A transverse TFS, set superior to the hysterectomy scar seems to achieve a high cure rate in patients who complain of persisting urgency symptoms after Posterior IVS, and who reported diminished urgency when tested with a 'simulated operation' for defect '4' (fig 3-07). Extreme caution is required during dissection so as to avoid bladder perforation, as the bladder is often thin or adherent. Therefore, the bladder should be completely dissected off the vaginal wall and cervix (or hysterectomy scar) and its fascial layer plicated with interrupted sutures before any tapes are inserted. An inverted 'T' incision may be required to facilitate this dissection in difficult cases.

Cervical ring 'transverse' defect (high cystocoele) repair

This is a common lesion, especially after hysterectomy, which necessarily dislocates the attached facia. As illustrated in figures 4-61 and 4-62, an inverted 'T' incision is made, with the horizontal incision along the lower end of the cervix. The bladder

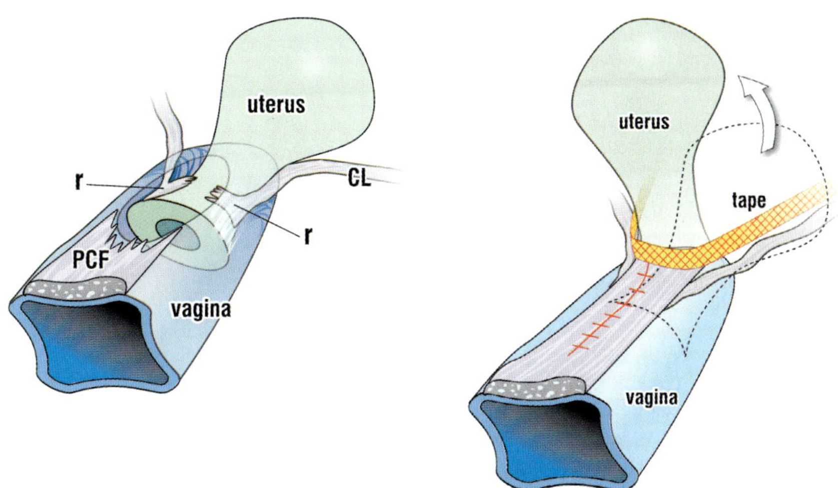

Fig. 4-61 (Left) Cervical ring defect. The cervical ring acts as a bridge between the two cardinal ligaments (CL). A cervical ring tear not only dislocates the attachment of the pubocervical fascia (PCF) to cause a high cystocoele, it causes lateral displacement of the cardinal ligaments. This may cause uterine retroversion and downward displacement of the uterus and/or vaginal apex.

Fig. 4-62 (Right) Cervical ring/cardinal ligament repair. The tape is placed along the anterior lip of cervix and extends along the cardinal ligament. On tightening, the cervix is pulled back, and the uterus anteverts.

is dissected clear of the vagina and cervix, and its fascia layer plicated. Using fine dissecting scissors, a 4-6 cm long channel is made along the cardinal ligament towards, but not necessarily to, the ATFP. The TFS applicator is inserted into the tunnel and the anchor released. After a wait of 30 seconds, the tape is tugged to set the anchor. The procedure is repeated on the contralateral side. The tape is set as before, and tightened, anteverting the uterus and restoring prolapse of the anterior portion of the vaginal apex. Using No. 1 Dexon with a large needle, the laterally displaced fascia is brought across medially to cover the tape. The vagina is sutured without excision.

TFS 'U' sling

The surgical principle underpinning this operation is to mimic the ATFP and to provide a transverse neofascial 'beam' to reinforce the damaged pubocervical fascia.

Where the cystocele is more extensive, a 2nd 'U' sling can be inserted (fig 4-64). The vagina is dissected off the bladder wall and the plane of dissection carried laterally until the muscle behind the obturator fossa is reached. The fascial remnants over the cystocele are approximated. The TFS is placed into the retroobturator space and the anchor displaced adjacent to the muscle and tugged to fix it. This is repeated on the contralateral side and the tape tightened just sufficiently to reduce fascial laxity. Care is taken to avoid excessive tension, as this may pull the sling up towards the bladder neck to cause post-operative urinary retention. At times, the horizontal section of the tape may need to be sutured to the fascia prior to tightening.

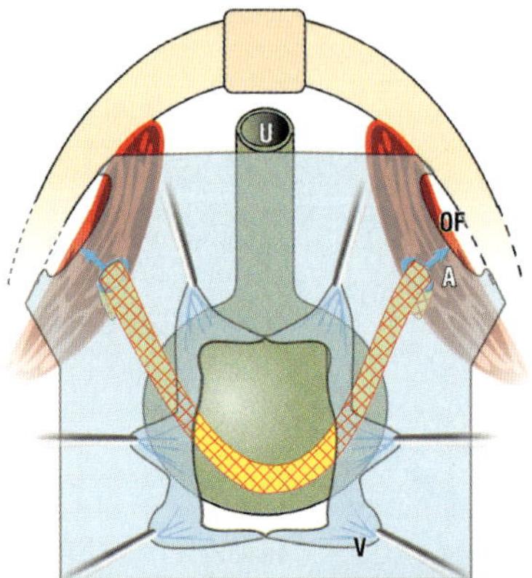

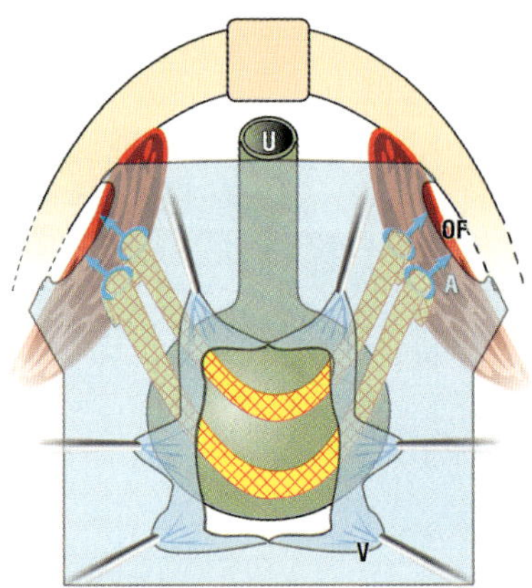

Fig. 4-63 'U' sling. View into the anterior vaginal wall. Vagina (V) is dissected off the bladder wall, and stretched laterally. The TFS tape is anchored (A) just behind the obturator fossa (OF) muscles.

Fig. 4-64 Double 'U' sling. View into the anterior vaginal wall. Vagina (V) is dissected off the bladder wall, and stretched laterally. The TFS tape is anchored (A) just behind the obturator fossa (OF) muscles.

TFS 'U' sling TFS with 'bridge' repair

This operation repairs large herniations more accurately and more easily than 'tape plus mesh' operations. The 'bridge' is prepared as described earlier (fig 4-23)and anchored laterally to the fascia with sutures as per figure 4-65. The tape is placed at the middle or lower end of the bridge as a 'U' sling configuration and tightened.

The suspension bridge analogy (fig 1-08) provides an illustation of how the anterior vaginal wall is supported. If there is a co-existing cervical ring ('transverse defect'), it should also be repaired with a second TFS (fig 4-65) so that the 'bridge' does not 'unzip' from the bottom up and cause the herniation to recur.

TFS 'U' sling with mesh sheet

This operation was originally used in patients with weak thin tissues following previous surgery. Figure 4-66 illustrates how the tape is threaded through the superior and inferior parts of the mesh, then tightened to elevate the anterior wall. Mesh is rarely used now as the 'U'-sling and cervical ring tapes (figs 4-63 & 4-62) have been found to provide sufficient support.

Middle Zone Tightness - The Special Case of the Tethered Vagina Syndrome

The Integral Theory specifies connective tissue laxity as being the predominant cause of pelvic floor dysfunction. The 'tethered vagina syndrome' is an uncommon and entirely iatrogenic condition that is caused by scar-induced tightness in the middle zone of the vagina. As such it forms a special case. This condition needs to be considered in patients with multiple operations and severe incontinence. It is somewhat equivalent to 'motor detrusor instability' (MDI). The classical symptom is commencement of uncontrolled urine leakage as soon as the patient's foot touches the floor, indeed, often commencing as the patient rolls over to get out of bed. The

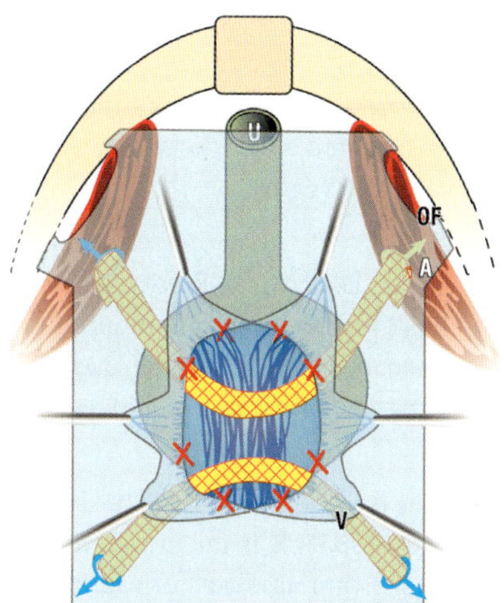

Fig. 4-65 TFS 'bridge' repair. Large cystocoele repaired with bridge secured anteriorly by 'U'-sling and posteriorly by cervical ring TFS.

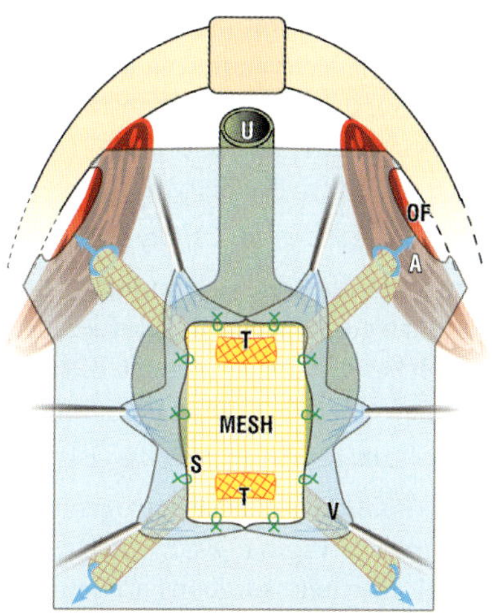

Fig. 4-66 TFS plus mesh. View into the anterior vaginal wall. The TFS tape (T) passes through slits in the mesh and is anchored (A) just behind the obturator fossa (OF) muscles and along the tracks of the cardinal ligament remnants to ATFP. Sutures (S) attach the mesh to the fascia below the vagina (V).

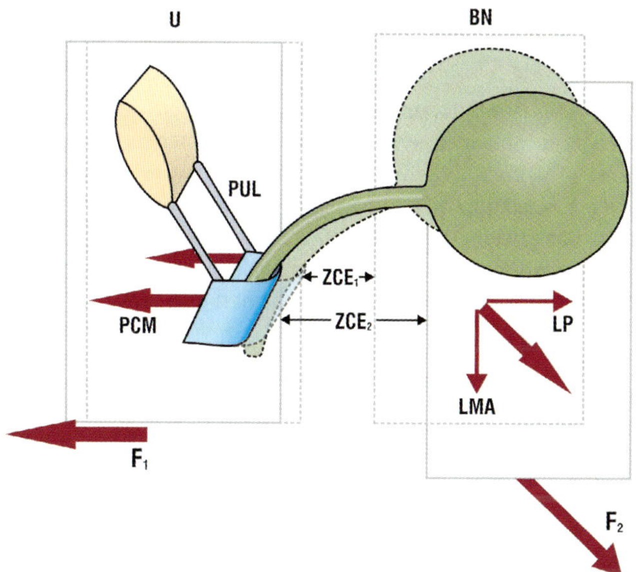

Fig. 4-67 The Zone of Critical Elasticity (ZCE) and the urethral (U) and bladder neck (BN) closure mechanisms. ZCE_1 = ZCE at rest; ZCE_2 = ZCE during effort or micturition. F1 represents the PCM vector and F2 represents the resultant force of the LP/LMA vectors.

patient does not complain of bed-wetting during the night. The symptoms are caused by loss of elasticity in the bladder neck area of the vagina: the 'zone of critical elasticity' (ZCE). Because scar tissue contracts with time, it may present twenty years after vaginal repair or bladder neck elevation. This condition can be cured by plastic surgery whose aim is to restore elasticity to the bladder neck area of the vagina.

Zone of Critical Elasticity (ZCE)

Figure 4-67 illustrates the importance of Zone of Critical Elasticity (ZCE) for the urethral (U) and bladder neck (BN) closure mechanisms. The ZCE stretches from midurethra to bladder base. Scarring across ZCE 'tethers' the muscle vectors F_1 and F_2. Then F_2 overcomes F_1 to pull open the vaginal hammock on effort, causing uncontrolled urine loss.

Pathogeneses of the Tethered Vagina Syndrome

This condition is entirely iatrogenic and is caused by excessive tightness in the bladder neck area of vagina (ZCE) (Petros & Ulmsten 1990, 1993). It is far more common in regions where surgeons are taught to remove significant amounts of vaginal skin during vaginal repairs. Often there is very little stress incontinence. The reason is that cough creates short sharp fast-twitch contractions, and there may be just sufficient elasticity at ZCE to prevent urine leakage on coughing.

Getting out of bed in the morning stretches ZCE far more as the pelvic floor contracts to support all the intra-abdominal organs. The classical symptom is commencement of uncontrolled urine leakage as soon as the patient's foot touches the floor. Often there is no urgency. A scar at ZCE 'tethers' the more powerful backward forces 'F_2' (fig 4-67) to the weaker forward forces 'F_1', so the bladder is pulled open as in micturition. The aim is to restore elasticity in the bladder neck area of the vagina, the 'zone of critical elasticity' (ZCE), so that 'F_1' and 'F_2' can act independently of each other.

Temporary 'Tethering'

Temporary 'tethering' may occur after bladder neck elevation, but can occur occasionally even after tension-free tape surgery where there is poor elasticity in the bladder neck area of vagina, ZCE. The patient presents with *de novo* uncontrolled bladder emptying immediately on getting out of bed in the morning. Generally this is first noticed a few days after surgery. Over the ensuing weeks to months, the patient slowly improves, by gradual natural restoration of elasticity at ZCE, most likely by an 'averaging out' of tissue tension through the walls of the vagina.

Specific Clinical Findings

Generally the tightness in the bladder neck area of vagina is obvious on speculum examination (fig 4-68). Often no urine loss is evident during coughing and even straining. On ultrasound there is generally very little descent of bladder neck, perhaps only 2 to 3mm. One provocative test which may be useful is to grasp the bladder base part of vagina gently with Littlewood's forceps and press backwards while asking the patient to cough. This removes any residual elasticity at ZCE, and very frequently a spurt of urine comes out when there was previously no urine loss on coughing. This test is specific for low elasticity at ZCE, not necessarily for the tethered vagina *per se*. Care must be taken not to clamp the forceps. This may cause severe pain, a consequence of the visceral nerve innervation of the vagina.

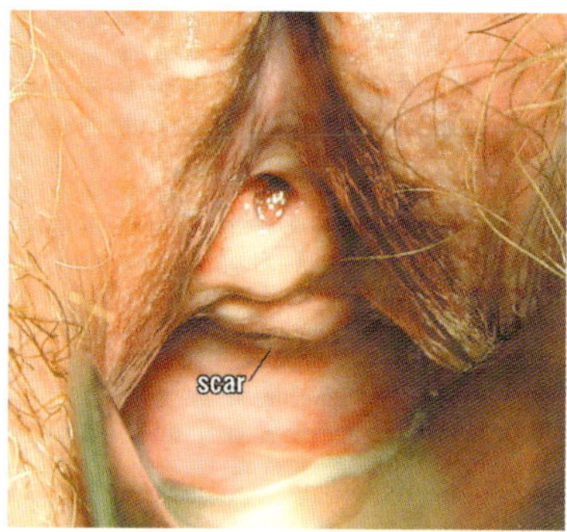

Fig. 4-68 Scar at bladder neck. The scar 'tethers' the anterior and posterior muscle forces, so that the urethra is forcibly pulled open on getting out of bed in the morning.

By permission Goeschen, K.

The Surgical Restoration of Elasticity to the Bladder Neck Area of the Vagina

Preliminaries

No matter what technique is used, it is essential to dissect the vagina from the bladder neck and urethra, and then to free all scar tissue from urethra and bladder neck ('urethrolysis'). There must be no scar tissue anchoring the bladder neck to the pelvic side wall.

Restoration of Elasticity to the Zone of Critical Elasticity (ZCE)

The surgical principle applied is that fresh vaginal tissue must be brought to the bladder neck area of vagina. If there is a severe shortage of tissue, the only solution is a skin graft. This can be a free graft, a Martius labium majus skin graft, or a split labium minus flap graft. A free graft can be problematical as up to one third may not 'take' or shrink excessively. Labium minus or Martius grafts are technically challenging, but bring their own blood supply.

I-plasty

This is the simplest technique and is especially indicated if there is a co-existing cystocoele. I-plasty aims to increase the volume of tissue in the bladder neck area of the vagina, thereby restoring elasticity (fig 4-69). It will not work long term if there is a net deficit of vaginal tissue.

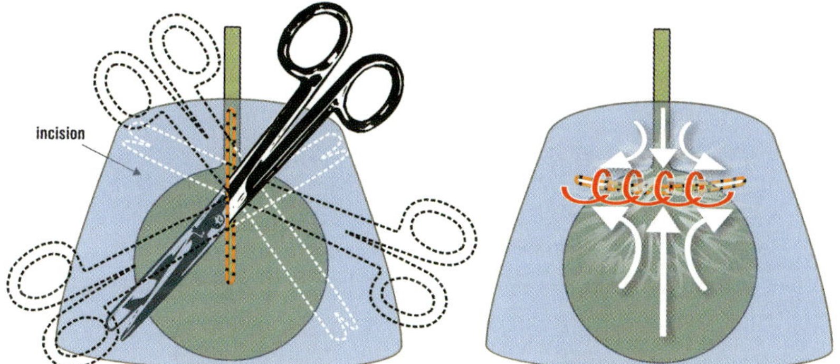

Fig. 4-69 I-plasty. The vagina is widely separated from the underlying tissue (above left). The freed vagina is sutured transversely without tension (above right).

A vertical incision is made from midurethra to at least 3-4 cm beyond bladder neck. The vaginal skin is dissected off the scar tissue and is extensively mobilized, forwards to the edges of the vaginal hammock, backwards as far possible right down to the cervix or hysterectomy scar, and as laterally as possible. The freed tissue is brought into the ZCE and is sutured transversely with interrupted sutures. This increases the quantum of vaginal tissue in this area.

Skin Graft to Bladder Neck

This procedure can be performed either with a transverse or vertical incision at bladder neck, depending on the prevailing geometry. Following the incision, the vagina, urethra and bladder neck are dissected free of scar tissue and widely mobilized, as in the I-plasty operation. Once this is done, the vagina retracts laterally and the tissue deficit becomes evident.

A full thickness skin graft is removed from an elastic area of the body, lower abdomen or buttocks. The former is far less painful post-operatively. It is difficult to gauge the exact size of the graft. Generally a graft which takes well will shrink 50% over the ensuing 6 months. An excessively large skin graft may sometimes cause incontinence within 6-9 months by creating excess laxity in the hammock and adjoining tissues. Ensure a dry bed for the graft. Remove all fat from the skin graft. The graft is then applied to the bladder neck area of the vagina (ZCE) with a series of quilting sutures to the bladder neck and base. The aim is to prevent the possibility of a haematoma dislodging the graft. Finally, the graft is sutured to the surrounding vaginal tissue with interrupted 00 or 000 dexon. The advice and assistance of a plastic surgeon is advisable for the first few cases.

The quilting sutures (fig 4-70) are followed by suturing the graft to the cut edges of vagina, taking care not to devascularize the tissues with excessively tight sutures. Once the skin graft takes it permits the forward and backward closure forces to operate independently of each other.

Complications

The graft may be rejected in one third of the cases. If this happens, more fibrosis may be created at ZCE and this may worsen symptoms. An excessively large graft may loosen the hammock, thereby causing SI.

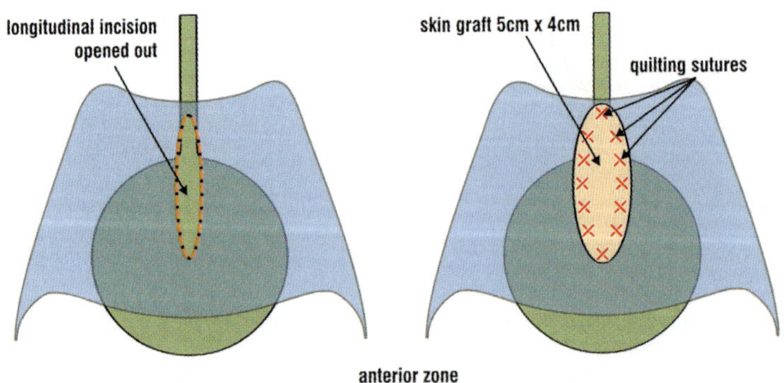

Fig. 4-70 Skin graft to bladder neck area of vagina is attached by quilting sutures.

Labium Majus Martius Skin Graft with Vascular Fat Pedicle

This operation (figs 4-71 to 4-75) was devised by Professor Klaus Goeschen, Hanover, Germany. A 4 x 2.5 cm ellipse of vulval skin is created over the labium majus and is transferred as a Martius fat graft into the dissected area. It is attached to the adjacent vaginal skin taking care to avoid constriction of its vascular pedicle.

Figures 4-71 to 4-75 were kindly supplied by Professor Klaus Goeschen.

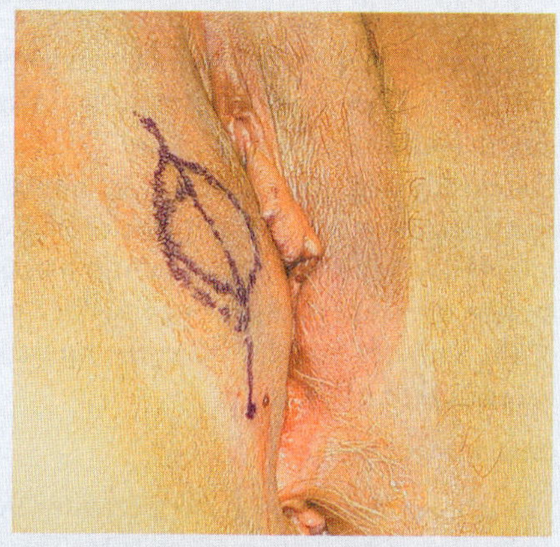

Fig 4-71 Marking of labium majus

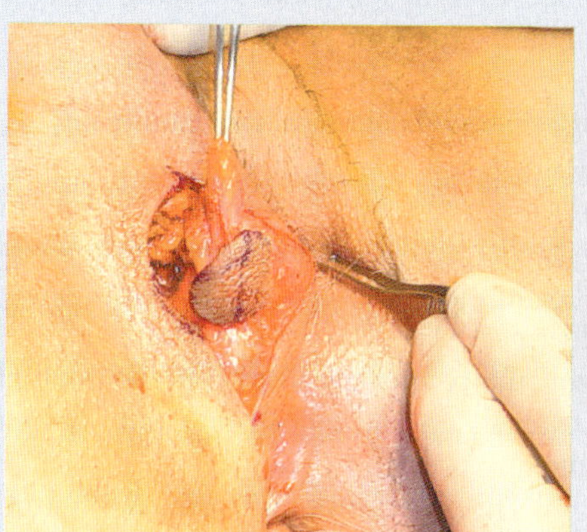

Fig 4-72 Graft freed from underlying tissues

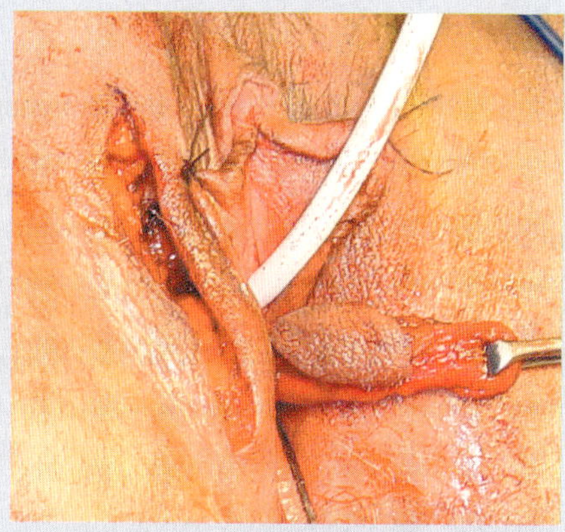

Fig 4-73 Graft brought through to the vagina

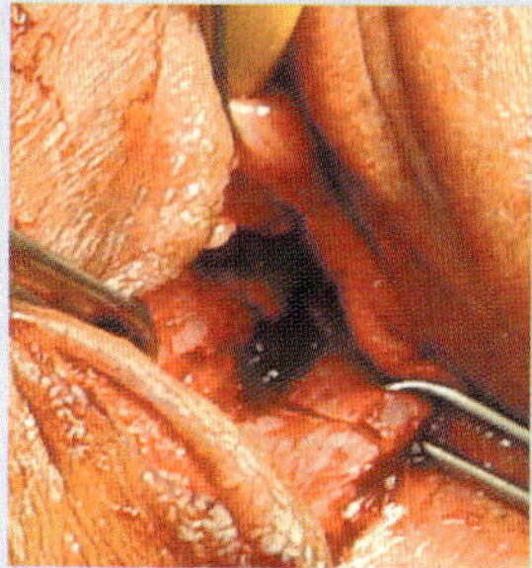

Fig 4-74 Transverse incision at bladder neck. The vagina, urethra and bladder neck are freed from the scar tissue

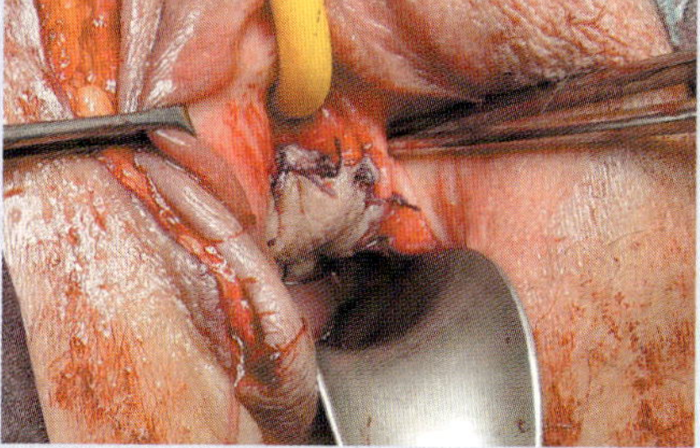

Fig 4-75 Martius skin graft sutured to the edges of the vagina. The wound from the site of the graft is to the left. This is sutured with subcuticular 00 Dexon sutures.

Labium Majus Martius Skin Graft with Vascular Fat Pedicle

Professor Klaus Goeschen reports significantly better results with this technique than with I-plasty or free skin graft (see figs 4-71 to 4-75). He compared three methods for cure of the 'tethered vagina syndromet (n=57): I-plasty (n=13); free skin graft (n=21); bulbocavernosus-muscle-fat-skin-flap from the labium majus.(n=23). At 6 month follow-up, cure rates were 23%, 52% and 78% (urine loss of <10gm/24 hours). The mean operating time was 73 minutes (range 41 – 98 min) for the scar dissection and the flap-repair. No serious bleeding was observed. No patient required a blood transfusion. The mean hospital stay was 5 days (range 2 to 9 days). All patients were mobile at least 4 hours after operation. 3 patients could not pass urine after extraction of the catheter one day after the operation and another permanent catheter was necessary for 1 day.

Labium Minus Flap Graft

The labium minus flap graft operation (figs 4-76 to 4-81) works well in patients with normal or large labia minora (LM). In essence it consists of separating the inner mucosal surface of LM from its outer surface, opening it out and swinging it across to provide new tissue to the urethra area of the vagina. One graft is usually sufficient for the tethered vagina syndrome. It is anticipated that these grafts could be useful for fistula surgery where there is tissue damage around the urethra and bladder neck.

The operation has two stages. Firstly, two flaps 'A' and 'B' (fig 4-76) are created separate from the urethra and swung down towards the bladder neck. Secondly, the labium minus graft is stretched across to cover the bare area left by 'A' and 'B'. Three full-thickness incisions (as indicated in fig 4-76) are made, beginning with a vertical incision extending from external meatus 3-4 cm beyond bladder neck exactly as per an I-plasty incision. Flaps 'A' and 'B' are created with two horizontal incisions: one just below the external urethral meatus, the other at the level of the bladder neck and opened out. Dissect vagina clear of urethra, bladder and where relevant pubic bone from below.

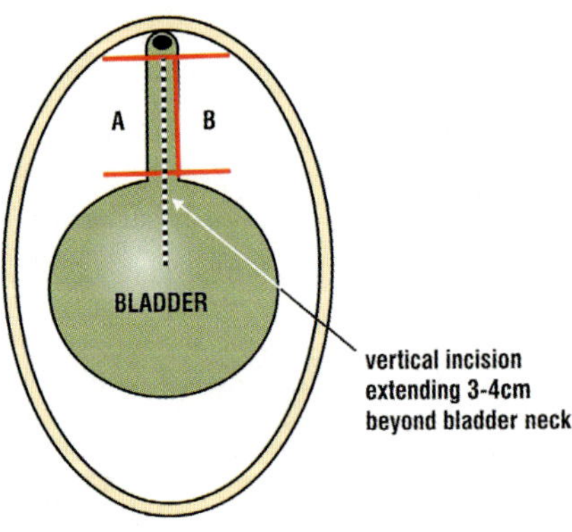

The dissection aims to free vagina from scar tissue, mobilizing it as far as possible inferiorly, laterally and superiorly.

Post-operatively, there is very little pain. The labium minus becomes vestigal and is displaced medially. (The vestigal labium minus is situated just above the label 'flap' in figure 4-81.) There have been no complications recorded thus far with this procedure. Failure rate has been 25% at 12 months due to re-scarring at the operation site.

The limitation of this operation is that it cannot be performed in patients with small labia minors.

Fig. 4-76 Labium minus flap graft. An 'H'-shaped vaginal incision is made to create vaginal flaps 'A' and 'B'.

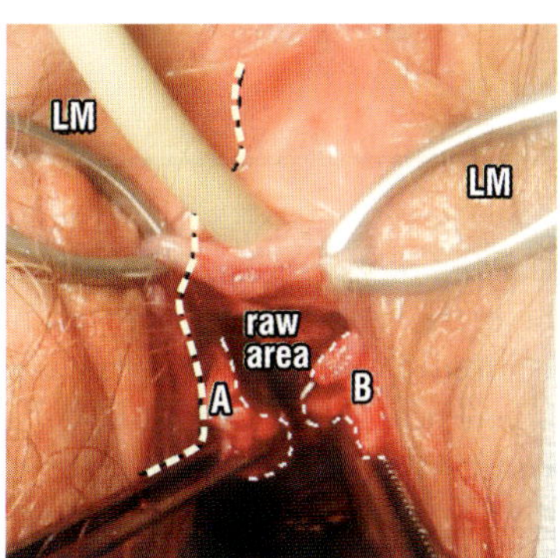

Fig. 4-77 Preparation of flap. 'A' & 'B' are mobilized and swung downwards into the ZCE. Using a sharp scalpel, a transverse incision is made across the base of the inner surface of LM extending up towards the clitoris (broken lines).

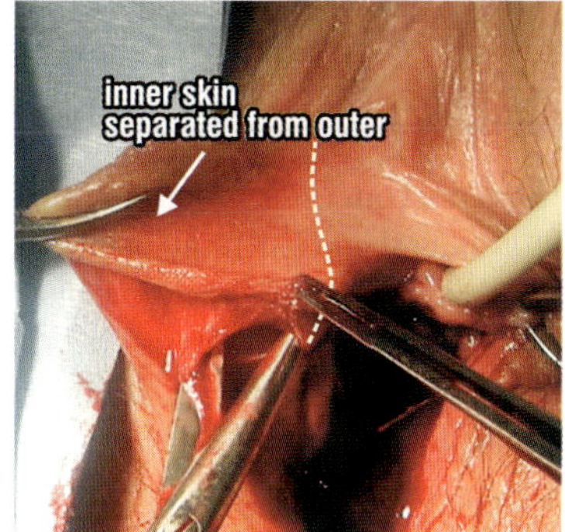

Fig. 4-78 Separation of outer and inner surfaces of LM. Dissecting scissors are used to separate inner and outer surfaces of the LM flap, taking care not to 'buttonhole' the outer surface, as the labium minus tissue is often very thin. Two parallel vertical cuts are made along the sides of the labium minus to the central ridge to open the flap.

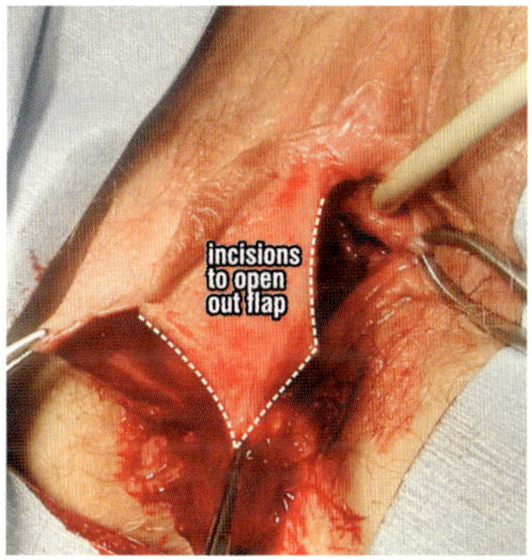

Fig. 4-79 LM flap completed and opened out. The inner (mucosal) surface of LM has been separated from its outer (skin) surface.

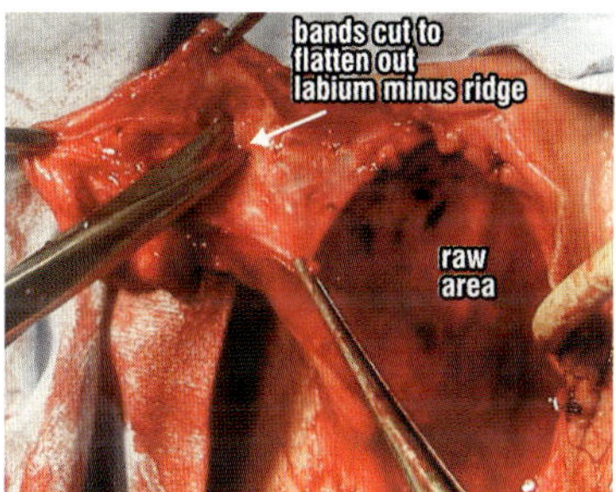

Fig. 4-80 Release of ridge bands to open out ridge. The flap is turned over and the collagenous bands which form the ridge are divided, 'flattening out' the ridge. This greatly increases the available surface area of the graft.

Fig. 4-81 (left) Completion. The LM flap is now attached to the laterally sited pubococcygeus muscles, urethra and the two parts of the hammock, A and B which have now been mobilized and rotated downwards. 'A' & 'B' are sutured to the new tissue brought into the bladder neck area of the vagina. It may be necessary in some patients to insert a midurethral sling if in the opinion of the surgeon, there is a possibility of stress incontinence post-operatively.

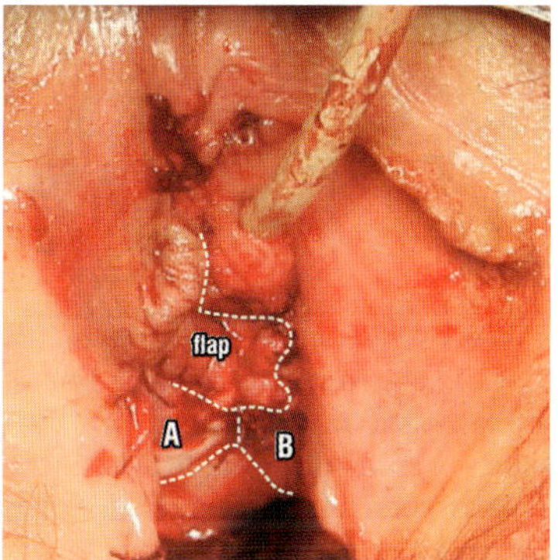

4.3.3 Surgery of the Posterior Zone

The Structures of the Posterior Zone

The posterior zone extends between the cervical ring and perineal body (fig 4-82). It includes the uterosacral and cardinal ligaments, the apical segment of the vagina, rectovaginal fascia, perineal body and external anal sphincter. These structures work synergistically as a subsystem, so that repair of all three is often required. The role of the uterus as a 'keystone' of the pelvic floor, and its conservation where possible is emphasized, as is conservation of the vagina. The vagina is no less an organ than the uterus. Therefore, with rectocoele repair, excision of tissue should be avoided where possible.

The Fibromuscular Supports of the Vagina

Interconnectedness of the Posterior Zone Fascia

In figure 4-82, the cervix is a key anchoring point for the posterior part of the vaginal membrane. Contraction of the smooth muscle components of uterosacral (USL) and cardinal ligaments (CL) help to tension the vagina and to counteract 'F', the force of gravity (fig 4-83).

The inherent strength of the rectovaginal fascia (RVF), together with its backward stretching by the levator plate (LP), are major factors in preventing prolapse - which is really a form of intussusception. Note the importance of the descending branch of the uterine artery as a major blood supply to the apical fascia and uterosacral ligaments (USL). This explains why it is often difficult to locate USLs in patients who have undergone hysterectomy due to atrophy.

In terms of structure, the uterus functions in a similar way to the keystone of an arch (fig 4-84).

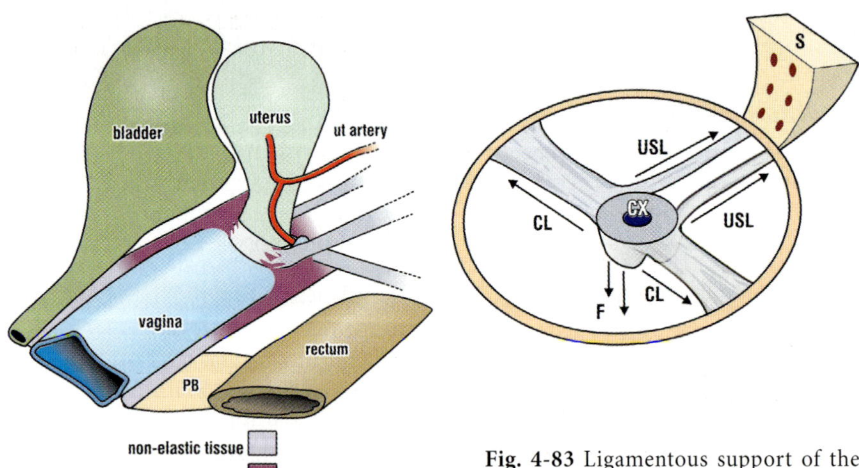

Fig. 4-82 The fibromuscular supports of the vagina. Note the dense fibrous tissue at the distal 2-3 cm of the vagina, urethra and anus. Superior to this area there is less collagen, and more smooth muscle and elastin.

Fig. 4-83 Ligamentous support of the cervix. The arrows indicate the line of tension created by the ligaments. F = force of gravity; CL = cardinal ligament; USL = uterosacral ligament. Perspective: View from above.

Hysterectomy may weaken the fascial side-wall support, and weaken the uterosacral ligaments by removing a major part of its blood supply. Conservation of the uterus is important in the long-term prevention of vaginal prolapse and incontinence (Brown 2000, Petros 2000).

The fascial sheets (fig 4-85) are all interconnected, extending anteriorly (pubocervical fascia) and superolaterally to the arcus tendineus fasciae pelvis, posteriorly (apical fascia) and infero-laterally (rectovaginal fascia (RVF)), between vagina and rectum. Thus BOTH the anterior and posterior fascial supports may need repairing in a patient with uterine or vault prolapse.

The ring around the cervix (fig 4-86) is composed of pure collagen. Therefore it provides a strong anchoring point for the fibromuscular tissue (fascia) which extends forwards below the bladder as the pubocervical fascia, and backwards above the rectum as recto-vaginal (Denonvillier's) fascia to the perineal body. Tearing of the attachment points may present as a high cystocoele, high rectocoele, or enterocoele.

The rectovaginal fascia (or Fascia of Denonvilliers) attaches the posterior vaginal wall to the perineal body (PB) inferiorly and to the levator plate muscle group (LP) superiorly (fig 4-87) (Nichols 1989)). Contraction of LP (arrow) stretches the posterior vaginal wall backwards against the perineal body into the horizontal position shown in figure 4-86. The intra-abdominal and gravitational forces act to maintain this position.

Because the levator plate (LP) stretches the vagina via the rectovaginal fascia (RVF) any fascial repair must be adequately tight to enable the muscle forces to give strength to the system by their tensioning effect. This is evident in the radiograph figures 6-37 to 6-40 (inclusive, see Chapter 6). It follows that a loosely applied mesh sheet cannot enable this system *per se*. The displaced fascia still needs to be restored before the organ can be tensioned sufficiently by the muscle forces to restore function (cf Chapter 2).

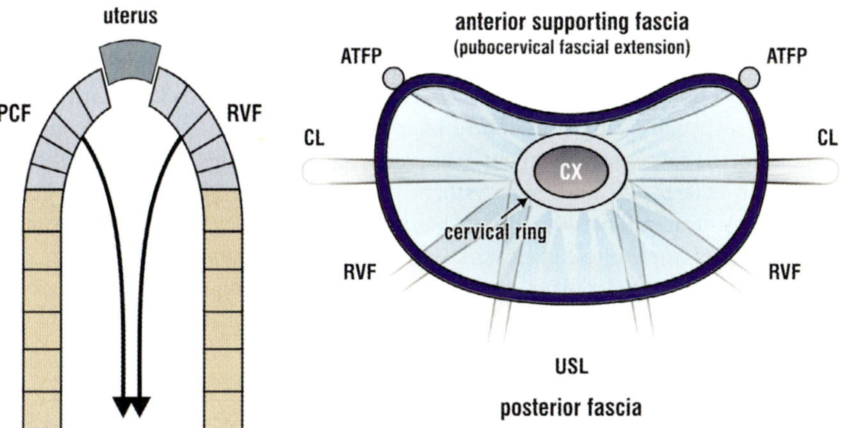

Fig. 4-84 (left) The uterus acts like a keystone of an arch. Adequately tight fascia (PCF, RVF) supports the uterus from below. Therefore PCF and RVF may also need to be repaired.

Fig. 4-85 (right) Interconnectedness of pelvic fascia. Perspective: 3D view, looking into the posterior fornix of the vagina. All fascial and ligamentous structures insert directly or indirectly into the cervical ring.

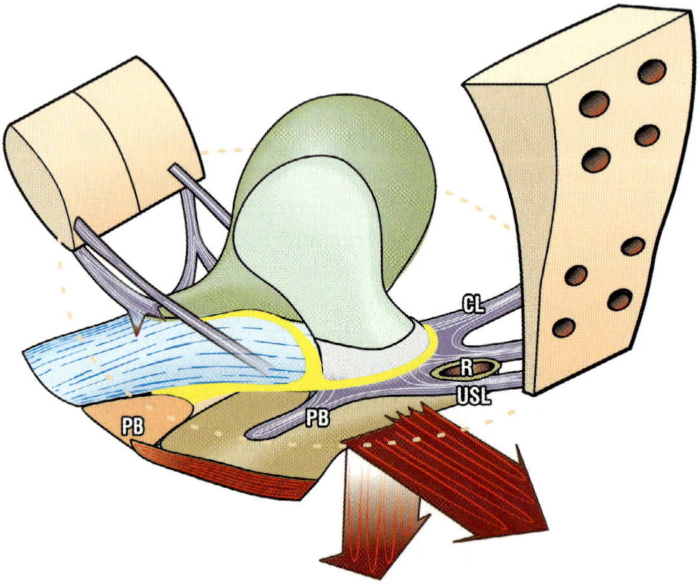

Fig. 4-86 The cervical ring (yellow) is an important attachment point for pubocervical, rectovaginal and apical fascia

Prolapsed Vagina

In the normal patient, the vagina is anchored by the cardinal (CL) and uterosacral ligaments (USL), supported laterally and inferiorly by the rectovaginal fascia (RVF), and superiorly by the pubocervical fascia (PCF). It is tensioned by the levator plate muscles (figs 4-86, 4-89, arrows). Note how the uterus acts as a central anchoring point.

A prolapsed vagina is essentially an intussusception (fig 4-88). Herniations (prolapses) are caused by breaks and lateral displacement of this fascia, and/or stretching of the suspensory ligaments. Frequent accompaniments to the vault prolapse are traction enterocoele and high cystocoele and rectocoele (fig 4-88). Congenital laxity can occur in nulliparous women. For permanent reduction, the side walls may need to be strengthened to a critical mass beyond which the apex cannot progress to eversion, much like repair of an intussusception. This may require repair of anterior (PCF) and posterior (RVF) fascia.

Uterine Prolapse

Uterine prolapse (fig 4-90) is caused by weakened cardinal (CL) or uterosacral (USL) ligaments and is often accompanied by weakening and displacement of the fascial sidewall support, which causes the uterus to descend into the vaginal cavity.

It is clear that as well as a posterior sling, approximation of the sidewall fascial supports (fig 4-91, arrows) is also needed to support the apical repair as well as lengthen the vagina. A significant superior defect (cervical ring/cardinal ligament) should also be repaired as required.

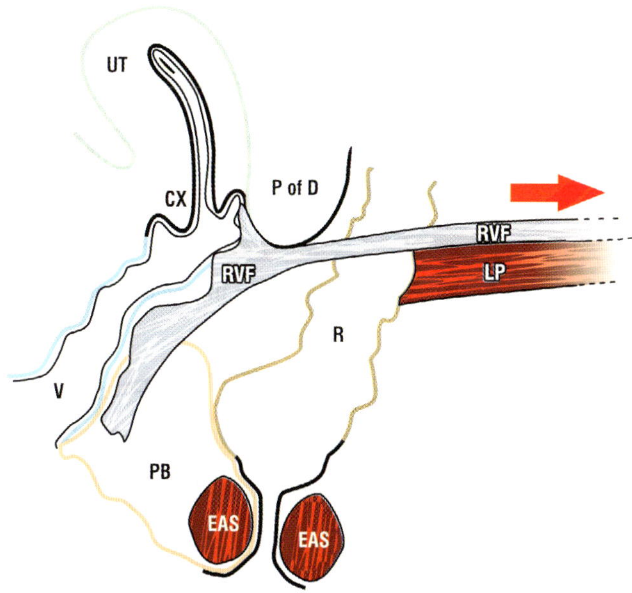

Fig. 4-87 Rectovaginal fascia (RVF) extension (fascia of Denonvilliers) to levator plate (LP). PB = perineal body; CX = cervix; P of D = Pouch of Douglas; UT = uterus; V = vagina; R = rectum; EAS = external anal sphincter. (After Nichols)

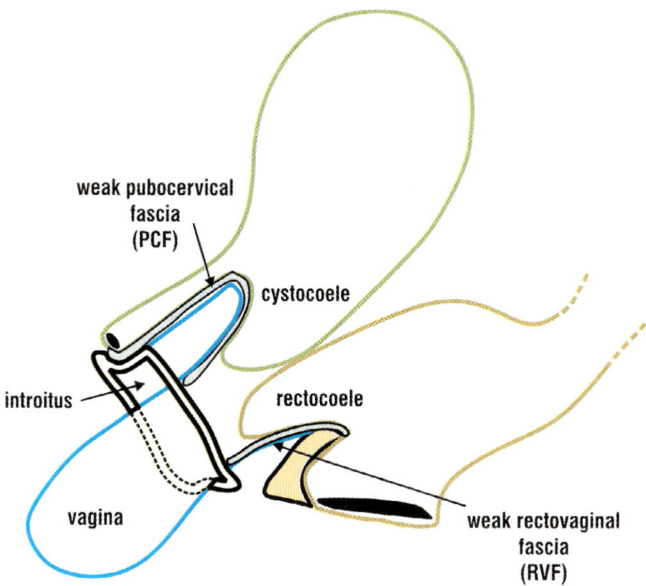

Fig. 4-88 Prolapsed Vagina -'intussusception'. Diagram shows the 'traction' prolapse of adjoining fascia.

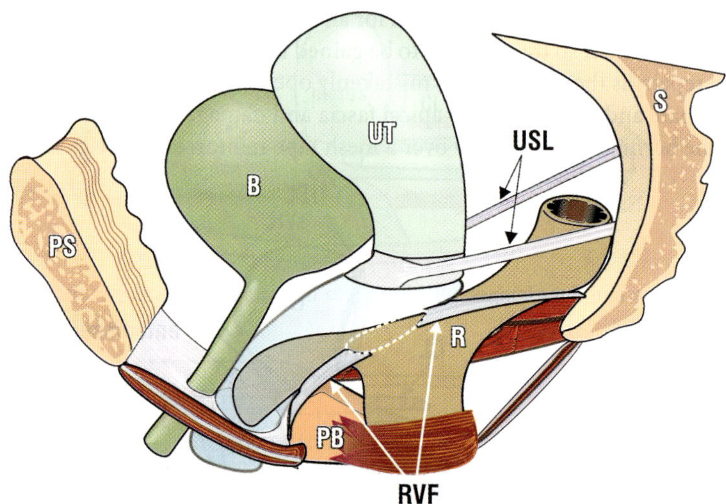

Fig. 4-94 A high rectocoele (RVF fascial defect) may be confused with an enterocoele (apical defect).

Indications for Posterior Zone Surgery: Damage to the Uterosacral Ligaments

Manifestations of damage may be structural or functional.

Structural

Prolapsed uterus or vaginal apex, or posterior vaginal wall defects causing discomfort.

Functional

Symptoms of 'posterior fornix' syndrome: urgency, frequency, nocturia, abnormal emptying and pelvic pain, are the main symptoms associated with posterior zone defects (fig 1-11, chapter 3). Insensible urine loss and mild stress incontinence may also occur with USL defects in some patients. The amount of prolapse may be minimal in patients with the 'posterior fornix syndrome'.

The uterosacral ligaments are usually atrophic (following hysterectomy), or attenuated (in prolapse). With reference to figure 4-87, contraction of levator plate (LP) stretches the vagina (V) backwards and downward in the axial plane so it becomes compressed by the intra-abdominal pressure. Adequately strong rectovaginal fascia is needed for this to occur.

The Methods: Surgical Repair of the Posterior Zone

The posterior zone functions as a subsystem. Therefore it is advisable to repair all damaged parts of the system if there is evidence of damage. That is, uterosacral ligaments, apical fascia, rectovaginal fascia and perineal body should be repaired.

In principle, the same operation is performed for uterine prolapse and vaginal vault prolapse. Generally, uterosacral ligaments and their regional fascia are much thinner in patients with vault prolapse who have undergone hysterectomy.

In the posterior zone, it is primarily damage to the distal part of the uterosacral ligament (USL) which causes dysfunction. However, cervical ring rupture and lateral displacement of the cardinal ligaments (fig 4-61) can, on its own account, cause apical or uterine prolapse. In the author's experience, this damage usually extends to the adjoining upper rectovaginal fascia.

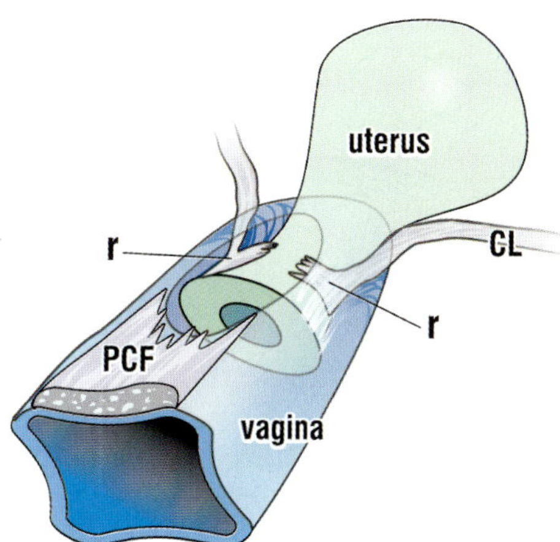

Fig. 4-61 Ruptured cervical ring (r) may induce laxity of the cardinal ligament (CL) causing retroversion or prolapse of the uterus

Posterior IVS Operation for Vaginal Vault or Uterine Prolapse ('Infracoccygeal Sacropexy') - Level 1 Repair

Essentially the same operation is performed for both uterine or vault prolapse (figs 4-95 to 4-99). The posterior sling or 'infracoccygeal sacropexy' works differently to the TFS in that it only reinforces the distal part of the uterosacral ligaments and it anchors the vaginal apex to the posterior muscles of the pelvic floor with a polypropylene tape (Petros 2001). A high cystocoele indicates the cervical ring/cardinal ligament complex has been disrupted (fig 4-61) and needs to be repaired. If the apex is wide (fig 4-95), a transverse full-thickness incision approximately 2.5 to 3 cm wide is made in the posterior vaginal wall 1cm below the hysterectomy scar line. If the apex is narrow, or if the surgeon prefers it, a longitudinal incision is made starting from the level of the scar. Using dissecting scissors with the tip pressed against the vaginal skin, a channel is made in the direction of the ischial spine sufficient to insert the index finger. The ischial spine is located, and the point of entry through the pelvic muscles for the insertion instrument determined (fig 4-98). If an enterocoele is opened it is ligated with a high purse string suture.

With the patient in the lithotomy position (fig 4-96), bilateral skin incisions 0.5 cm long are made in the perianal skin at the 4 and 8 o'clock positions halfway between the coccyx and external anal sphincter (EAS) in a line 2cm lateral to the external border of EAS. The tunneller is pushed 3 to 4 cm into the ischiorectal fossa (IRF) keeping the plastic tip parallel to the floor. The index finger is placed into the tunnel created in the vagina to locate the tip of the tunneller which is then brought to the point of penetration of the pelvic muscle 1 cm medial and caudal to the ischial spine (figs 4-97 and 4-98). At this point, the tunneller is safely sited well away from rectum and peritoneum.

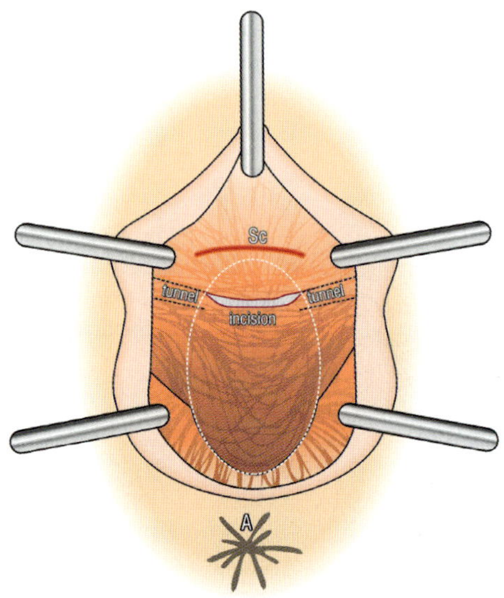

Fig. 4-95 Posterior IVS operation ('infracoccygeal sacropexy') Sc = hysterectomy scar.

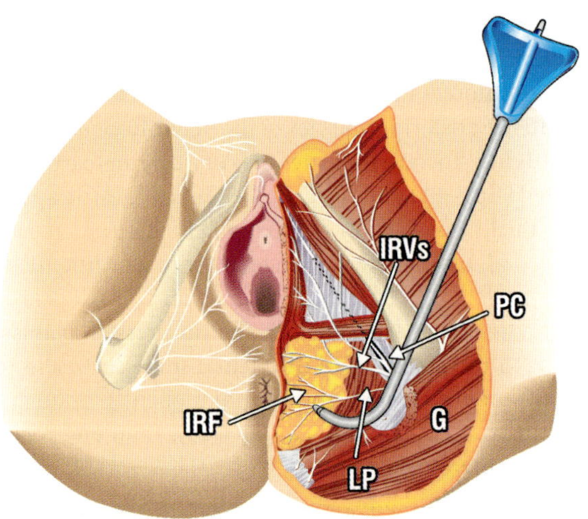

Fig. 4-96 Insertion of the tunneller. IRV = inferior rectal veins; PC = pudendal canal; IRF = ischiorectal fossa; LP = levator plate; G = gluteus muscle.

With the index finger continually applied to the plastic tip (fig 4-98), the tunneller is gently inclined medially, towards the vaginal vault, and pushed through the incision. With uterine prolapse, it is helpful if the tape exits through the uterosacral ligament. A rectal examination is made to ensure there has been no perforation. The insert is reversed. An 8mm polypropylene tape is threaded into the eye of the plastic insert, bringing the tape into the perineal area. The procedure is repeated on the contralateral side, leaving the tape as a 'U' entirely unfixed at the perineal end.

Ensure the tape is kept flat, then suture it securely with interrupted No. 00 Dexon sutures behind the hysterectomy scar or, preferably, uterosacral ligaments. Ensure the tape is positioned well away from the incision, so as to minimize erosion. The remnants of the uterosacral ligaments and attached fascia are brought across to cover the tape. Generally this converts the transverse incision to a longitudinal one, narrowing the apex and lengthening the vagina. If there is excessive tension, suture the vagina as as a 'Y' or transversely. Excessive tension may lead to wound breakdown and exteriorization of the tape. According to surgeon preference, one or two loosely applied No. 1 Dexon transvaginal mattress sutures help to keep the tissues in place while wound healing occurs. The perineal ends of the tape are pulled to full extension and then cut and left free, without suturing. The skin incision may be sutured without tension or apposed with 'steri strips'. If sutures are used, ensure that they are removed in 24 hours as this is usually the most painful part of the operation.

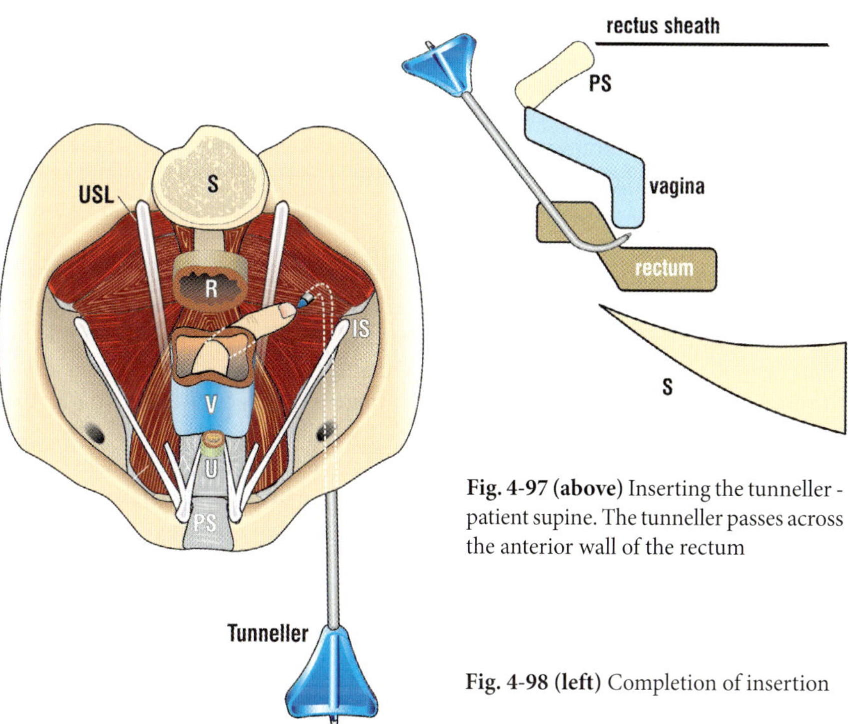

Fig. 4-97 (above) Inserting the tunneller - patient supine. The tunneller passes across the anterior wall of the rectum

Fig. 4-98 (left) Completion of insertion

Choosing Between a Transverse or Vertical Incision

Some surgeons use a longitudinal incision routinely, others only if the vaginal apex is narrow. The laterally displaced fascia at the level of the uterosacral ligaments (USL) should be brought across to cover the tape. This displaces the apex further posteriorly.

Overlying Fascial Repair

A fascial layer not only protects the tape from erosion, it helps reduce the prolapse. The fascia will begin to adhere to the tape by the tenth day. A No. 1 Dexon transvaginal holding suture helps to maintain the tissues in position while healing takes place. A TFS tape better restores the laterally displaced fascia (fig 4-104), and so better restores function.

Posterior Sling Repair of Uterine Prolapse

In this case, similar principles to the Manchester Repair are followed and these are combined with a posterior sling An elongated cervix is amputated.

A transverse incision is made 1.5 to 2 cm below the junction of vaginal skin to cervix and opened out. This brings the uterosacral ligaments (USL) into view.

In patients with a normal cervix, a longitudinal incision in the posterior vaginal wall, starting at the cervix may be preferred.

Once the amputated cervix is reconstituted, the posterior sling is inserted as described previously. If possible, exit of the tunneller is directed between uterosacral ligaments (USL) and cervix. The tape is sutured into the USLs near their insertion to cervix. A temporary 0 Maxon suture is first inserted to approximate the laterally displaced rectovaginal fascia. Taking care not to include the tape, internal approximating sutures are placed as laterally as possible into the vaginal tissue. The purpose is to bring together the USL remnants and the laterally displaced vaginal fascia. Then a series of transvaginal No. 1 Dexon mattress sutures is inserted during repair of the rectovaginal fascia to ensure the fascia stays in a medial position, beginning at the level of USL and ending at the perineal body. The Maxon suture is removed at the end of the operation.

Equally important to the posterior sling in restoring the position of the uterus is adequate approximation of USLs and rectovaginal fascia (Petros 2001). If the prolapse is not adequately restored, it is possible that the transvaginal fascial suture is not lateral enough. It may also be necessary to re-attach the laterally displaced parts of the pubocervical fascia to the cervical ring if there is a high cystocoele. This further reduces the prolapse.

Simultaneous repair of anterior and posterior walls may cause a ring constriction at that point (fig 4-52). Longitudinal vaginal incisions and avoidance of tissue excision help avoid these constrictions.

If the cervix is very wide, a wedge can be resected from 4 to 8 o'clock (fig 100). This simplifies approximation of the uterosacral ligaments and rectovaginal fascia without tension. However, care must be taken to electively ligate the descending branch of the uterine artery as primary post-operative bleeding may occur if the cervical sutures loosen post-operatively. This is always a possibility given the difficulties usually encountered in suturing the cervix.

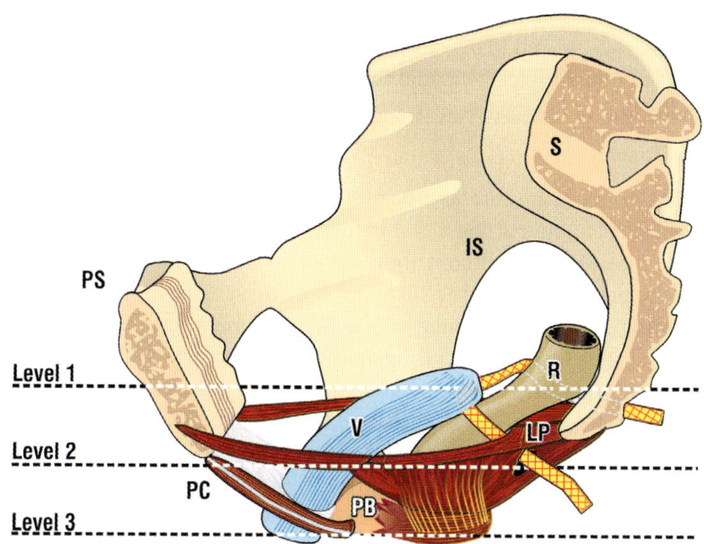

Fig. 4-99 The role of the posterior sling tape in anchoring the apex of the vagina. The posterior IVS operation does not reinforce the uterosacral ligament along its course. It anchors the apex of the vagina to the posterior pelvic floor muscles, which then contract to retain it in position.

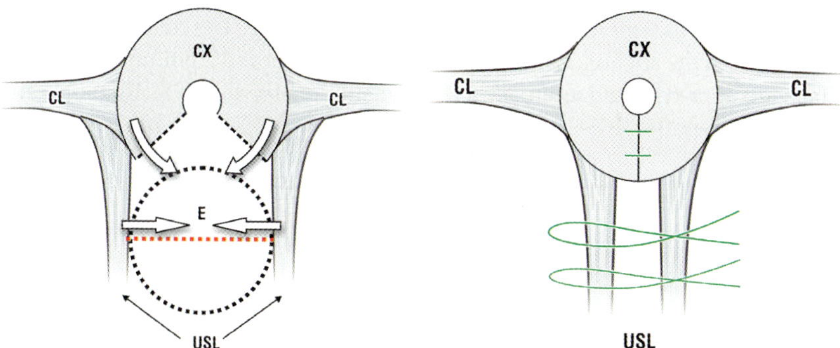

Fig. 4-100 Wedge resection of large cervix. E = enterocoele; CX = cervix; USL = uterosacral ligaments

Posterior Sling with Apical Defect Repair (enterocoele) (Level 1 Repair)

The apical defect follows the same surgical principles as vault prolapse repair. A longitudinal or transverse incision is made at the apex of the enterocoele, usually between 1.5 to 2 cm posterior to the cervix or hysterectomy scar. Care is taken to free the enterocoele sufficiently so as to locate the cardinal and uterosacral ligaments. The enterocoele is not routinely opened. With a large prolapse, the enterocoele is dissected clear. If entered, closure is effected with a purse string suture. A Posterior sling operation is performed, and the tape is anchored to the uterosacral ligaments or behind the hysterectomy scar. The uterosacral ligaments and attached fascia are approximated to close the enterocoele and to cover the tape using internal and transvaginal sutures as described previously. Excess vaginal tissue is not excised, rather it is sutured into the fascia. Excision of the vagina will only narrow or shorten it.

The Posterior TFS sling

It is important to assess the anterior apical supports (figs 4-61 & 4-62) and the upper rectovaginal fascial supports (fig 4-92) before proceeding to a posterior TFS sling. Both of these make important contributions to the structural integrity of the total structure of the pelvic floor (cf. the suspension bridge analogy, fig 1-08).

The posterior TFS sling is similar to the McCall operation insofar as it anchors the apical fascia into the uterosacral ligaments (USL) (fig 4-101). A full thickness, 2.5cm transverse incision is made in the vaginal apex, 2 cm below the cervix, or just below the hysterectomy scar. The uterosacral ligaments or their remnants are identified and grasped with Allis forceps. If an enterocoele is present it is reduced. Fine dissecting scissors angled at 30 degrees created a 4-5 cm space between the ligamentous remnants and the vaginal skin just below the insertion point of the USLs, just sufficient to accommodate the TFS delivery instrument. At the required depth, the instrument is triggered, and the anchor ejected. The instrument is removed, and 30 seconds allowed to elapse so as to allow for restoration of the tissues. The anchor is 'set' by pulling on the tape. The insertion is repeated on the contralateral side. Maintaining the instrument to support the anchor base, the tape is tightened along the instrument axis, and inspected for adequate tightening. The free end of the tape is cut 1cm from the anchor. The lax uterosacral ligaments and adjoining fascia above the tape are approximated as an extra layer of support for the TFS. Total operating time for this operation is 5-10 minutes.

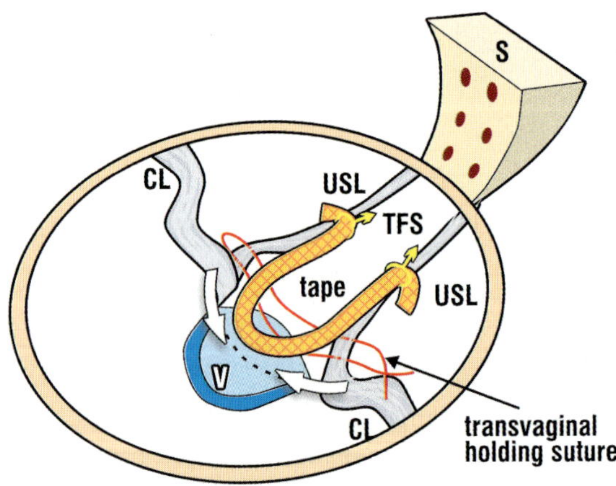

Fig. 4-101 Posterior TFS. Perspective: View from above. The tape is placed along the exact position of the uterosacral ligament (USL). The arrows indicate that the remnants of USL and also the cardinal ligaments (CL) need to be approximated if the apex is wide, so as to prevent enterocoele formation.

Posterior TFS Sling at the Time of Vaginal Hysterectomy

Vaginal vault prolapse is a major long-term complication of hysterectomy. Posterior TFS sling during vaginal hysterectomy is simple, takes only a few minutes to perform, yet provides strong vaginal vault support at 12 month review (Petros and Richardson, unpublished data).

Repair of Rectovaginal Fascia (level 2) and Perineal Body (PB) (level 3)

Traditional vaginal repairs approximate the laterally displaced fascia by sutures only. Damaged tissue is approximated to damaged tissue. The rectovaginal fascia is subjected to powerful stretching forces (fig 1-05). The healing wound has little strength in the first few weeks. The high recurrence rate of this type of surgery can be attributed to tearing of sutures, causing the wound to be stretched.

The perineal body acts as an anchoring point for the perineal muscles, and also, for the external anal sphincter (fig 4-94). It, too, is subjected to powerful muscle forces. A thin "stretched out" perineal body is difficult to repair using sutures only as damaged tissue is sutured to damaged tissue (cf figs 4-104 a & b).

Rectovaginal Fascia Repair (Level 2 Repair)

There are six main options for this technique:

1. Traditional Excision of Vagina and Re-approximation of Cut Edges.

This is the worst of all options and offers no advantages to the direct repair option described below. The surgeon is guessing the position of the laterally displaced fascia. If excess tissue is excised, then the vaginal edges must be stretched, or dissected clear of the fascia so that they may be approximated. In either case the vagina is weakened further, and either shortened or narrowed. This repair can be very painful, due to excess stretching of the vagina.

2. Direct Repair without Excision of Vagina

This technique works well if the displaced tissues appear strong. If the fascia is reasonably good, it can be brought to the midline. A midline incision is made. Adherent rectum is freed from vagina. Laterally displaced fascia is approximated. Excess vagina is attached to the deeper fascia rather than excising it (fig 4-49). Apparent excess of tissue usually shrinks by the post-operative visit. A temporary transvaginal Maxon suture placed as laterally as possible is helpful in bringing healthy fascial tissue more medially, where it is accessible to repair.

3. 'Bridge Repair'

A 'bridge repair' (figs 4-102 & 4-103) uses autologous fascia ('bridge') to reinforce the middle part of the herniation. This creates a strong central bridge over the centre, the weakest part of the herniation. It should only be used with very large herniations which would usually require excision of vaginal tissue.

'Creation of the Bridge'

Full thickness parallel longitudinal incisions are made along the posterior vaginal wall. These are carried down to within 1 cm of the introital skin to create a 'bridge' of tissue generally between 1.0 and 1.5 cm wide (fig 4-102). The borders of the incisions are separated with minimal dissection. Adhesions between vagina and rectum are separated. The surface epithelium of the bridge is destroyed by diathermy, and the edges of the bridge attached with interrupted sutures into the fascia below the adjoining vagina tissue.

The bridge is anchored distally to the perineal body (fig 4-103), and also proximally to the uterosacral ligaments or posterior sling. Interrupted mattress sutures bring the laterally displaced fascia towards the midline. The bridge is anchored into this fascia.

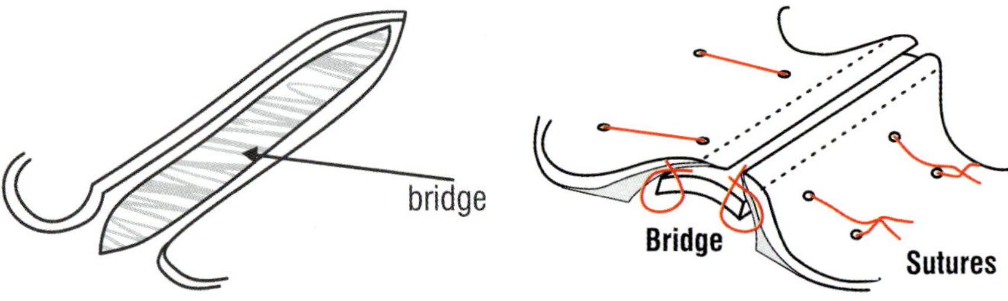

Fig. 4-102 Creation of the bridge   Fig. 4-103 Suturing the 'bridge' 'B'

Potential Complications of 'Bridge' Repair

a. Excessive width of the bridge may narrow the vagina or break down post-operatively.
b. A retention cyst may form in 5% of patients. This is filled with sterile yellow fluid and it can be located with transperineal ultrasound. It is easily treated by excision.

4. Use of Sheet of Mesh to Cover the Whole Posterior Wall

In patients with previous vaginal repairs and especially if the lateral fascia is weak, there may be little option but to reinforce the weakened epithelium with polypropylene mesh. Erosion rates from 3% to 28% have been reported. The erosion rate may be related to technique. A general rule is to approximate the fascial layer over the rectum as much as possible, and use a mesh large enough to extend towards the lateral attachments of the vagina. Some surgeons prefer to suture the mesh laterally, others not.

5. Mesh Sheet or 'Bridge' plus Posterior Sling

Structurally and anatomically, this technique is superior to unattached mesh or 'bridge' as they are anchored into the posterior muscles by the sling. This creates a better backward displacement of the vagina during micturition and defaecation. Anchoring the mesh or sling also to the sacrospinous ligament needs to be avoided at all times:
a. It is not anatomical, and would prevent the backward stretching of vagina which occurs during straining and micturition (figs 2-17 and 2-19).
b. There is a significant danger of damaging pudendal nerves and vessels.
c. It is not necessary. The posterior sling was invented to avoid the complications associated with fixing the vagina to the sacrospinous ligaments.

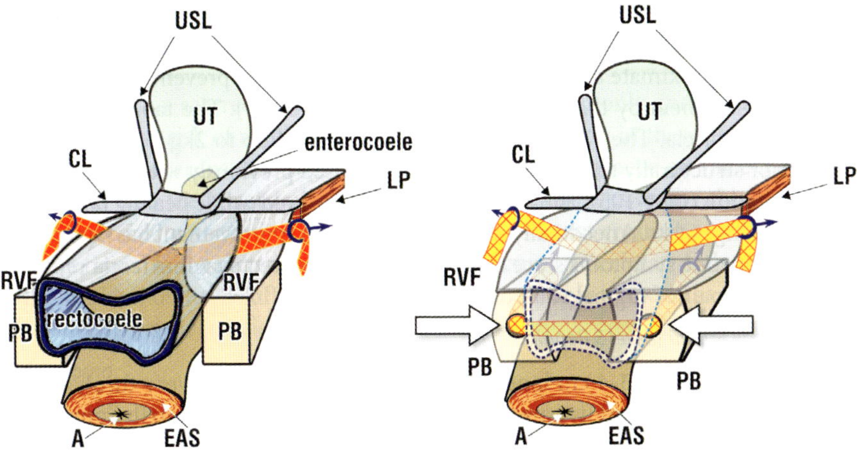

Figs 4-104a Approximation of laterally displaced rectovaginal fascia (RVF). In **fig 4-104b** The TFS is inserted vertically 3 to 4 cm into the perineal body (PB) and approximated. In both cases, the healing wound is less likely to be disrupted by the continued action of the levator plate muscle forces (LP).

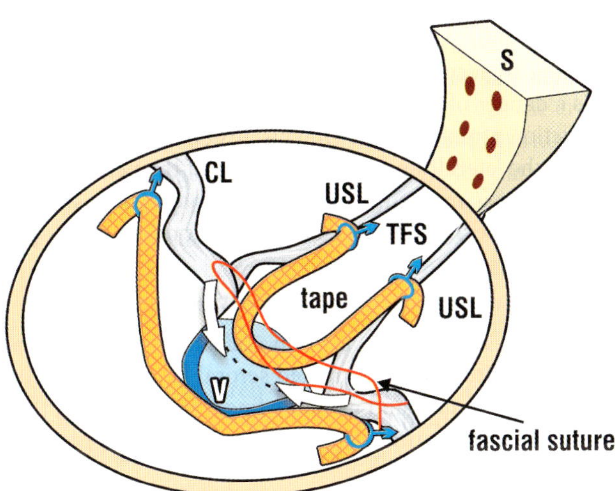

Fig. 4-105 Repair of laterally displaced rectovaginal fascia. A second TFS tape inserted below and laterally to the posterior sling will more strongly restore the laterally displaced fascia than a transvaginal 'holding' suture. Perspective: View from above.

4.4   Post operative Monitoring: Strategies for Managing Recurrent or New Symptoms

In the application of the Integral Theory surgical system, the surgeon needs to address post-operative symptoms from the perspective of 'ongoing management and cure' rather than 'single fix' surgery.

In some cases, more than one operation may be required before sufficient improvement is achieved because of weak tissues, multiple sites of damage, or because the structure of the pelvic floor readjusts after surgery to expose new weaknesses. Because the Integral Theory surgical system emphasizes conservation of tissue, minimal invasiveness and relative absence of pain, repeat operations can be performed in patients with recurrent or new symptoms without harming the patient. It is important to explain all this to the patient before surgery is performed especially as it is difficult for a patient to distinguish between new or persisting symptoms. Neither are they likely to volunteer improvement in some symptoms but not others. They mostly state: 'I am not cured'.

The best way to reassure such patients and give renewed hope is to demonstrate improvement in urgency or stress symptoms by use of 'simulated operations' (Chapters 3 and 6).

Unravelling the anatomical basis for 'failure to cure' may be a complex issue. From the surgeon's perspective, 'failure to cure' may be due to wrong diagnosis, decompensation of other connective tissue structures caused by the intervention itself, or surgical failure.

The author's approach is outlined below. This approach is based on the surgeon having a good knowledge of the connective tissue structures (fig 1-10) and the Integral Theory Diagnostic system, particularly how to diagnose minor degrees of connective tissue damage (because these may be the cause of major symptoms). These understandings are critical in any assessment of recurring or emerging symptoms and are described in detail in Chapters 3 and 6 (section 6.2.4).

The pre-operative protocol set out in Chapter 3 (questionnaire, 24 hour urinary diary, cough and 24 hour pad tests (Appendix)) are particularly useful as a benchmark for patients with ongoing problems.

The Origins of Subclinical Damage - How One Zone May Decompensate After Repair of Another Zone

In the normal pelvis, the pelvic forces are absorbed by the elastic component of the ligaments, muscles, and fascia, all of which act as 'shock absorbers'. Figure 1-09 shows how it is likely that multiple zones may be damaged - each to a different extent - if the foetal head cannot pass easily through the canal. Because the structures of the pelvic floor are interdependent, the three zones may 'balance' the structural defects so that the full extent of the damage is not necessarily reflected by the full expression of symptoms.

Thus, repairing one part of the vagina may cause the pelvic and abdominal forces from the zone that was repaired to be diverted to the other two zones. The weakest zone may give way, either as a total herniation (prolapse) or as a minimal but symptomatic herniation. The author has observed such decompensation ('blowouts') in 16% of patients after the posterior sling operation.

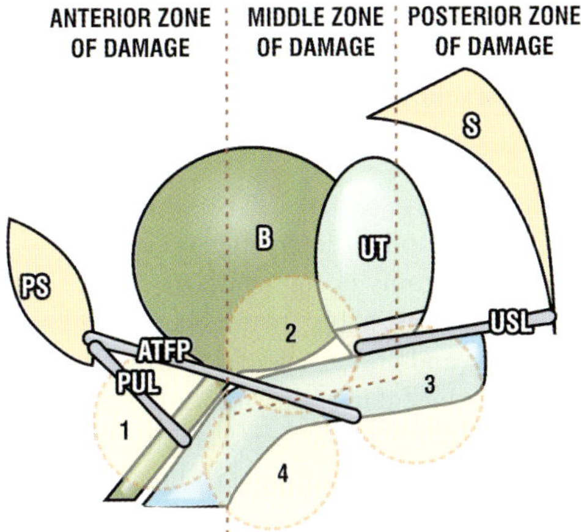

Fig 1-09 The foetal head (circles) may rupture or weaken (subclinically damage) ligaments or fascia in one or more zones of the vagina.

The Dynamics of Symptom Formation

The anatomical cause of new symptom formation is not always clear. Symptom formation is a dynamic process. It is secondary to the interaction of muscles, connective tissue and sensory nerves. The diagnosis of zone damage may not be clear in up to 20% of cases. However, a sound knowledge of dynamic anatomy (Chapter 2), the techniques of 'simulated operations' (Chapters 3 and 6), and the awareness that some neurologically based symptoms such as nocturia, urgency and pelvic pain may be caused by minor anatomical defects, is very helpful in working out the anatomical basis of symptoms.

Persistence of symptoms, in particular urgency, may 'camouflage' a connective tissue decompensation in another zone that causes similar symptoms to emerge. In such cases, the physician needs to compare the post-operative symptoms with the pre-operative symptoms, using the Pictorial Diagnostic Algorithm (fig 1-11) as a guide.

The appearance of new, different symptoms gives a strong indication as to the site of damage. A standard semi-quantitative questionnaire (Appendix) used pre- and post-operatively, and in collaboration with the Pictorial Diagnostic Algorithm (fig 1-11), can provide comprehensive insights. However, use of the Pictorial Diagnostic Algorithm does not help diagnose the 'tethered vagina syndrome' which should always be suspected in patients with multiple vaginal repairs who report large losses of urine. In the 'tethered vagina syndrome', the scar tissue 'tethers' the directional muscle forces so that the posterior urethral wall is pulled open by the posterior muscle forces during prolonged slow-twitch effort (see Chapter 4).

Example 1: Persistence of Symptoms

Persisting urgency after surgical repair of one zone may not always be caused by surgical failure: it may be caused by connective tissue decompensation ('blowout') in another zone. The physician needs to always be aware that symptoms merely reflect the changing dynamics of structure caused by surgical intervention. In this situation, the first step is to meticulously compare the post-operative symptoms against the pre-operative symptoms, preferably by using a standard semi-quantitative questionnaire (Appendix).

Example 2: New Symptoms

The occurrence of neourgency and difficulty in bladder emptying are the best known 'new' symptoms. These symptoms occur in up to 20% of patients after a Burch Colposuspension and may be reasonably attributed to a tight elevation activating the stretch receptors from below, and prevention of active opening out of the outflow tract (fig 2-19). Subsequent improvement in both symptoms can be explained by restoration of normal vaginal tension by viscoelastic creep. Patients with post-Burch urgency and abnormal bladder emptying who also develop an enterocoele are more likely to have suffered connective tissue 'blowout' to the posterior zone. Often such patients have other posterior zone symptoms such as pelvic pain and nocturia (fig 1-11).

Example 3: Stress Incontinence Cure After a Posterior Sling

Many patients report improvement in their stress incontinence symptoms after a posterior sling. This can be attributed to improved function of the downward rotational muscle force (LMA) which acts against the uterosacral ligaments.

Example 4: Post-cystocoele Cure of Stress Incontinence

Many patients report improvement of their stress incontinence symptoms after they develop a cystocoele. This can be explained by backward stretching of the vaginal hammock by cystocoele distension; the pubococcygeus closure muscles grip better and close the urethra from behind. Digitally supporting the cystocoele prevents this distension; the patient loses urine during coughing.

Managing Persisting Symptoms - An Anatomical Approach

Step 1. Diagnose Zone of Damage.

The diagnostic protocol as described in Chapter 3 is used to identify the zone of damage: questionnaire, examination, and where relevant, 'simulated operations' and perineal ultrasound examination.

In some cases, especially with posterior zone symptoms, (fig 1-11) there may be no evident prolapse on clinical examination. However, if there are two or more posterior zone symptoms, some degree of posterior zone prolapse is almost invariably found when in the operating theatre.

Step 2. Distinguish Between New and Old Symptoms - A Question of Timing.

Pre- and post-operative symptoms need to be compared. The scenarios are:

a) Appearance of New Symptoms

It is likely that the connective tissues in another zone have decompensated. Generally any new symptoms will appear weeks or months after surgery, but they may even appear within days.

b) The Same Symptoms Persist Immediately After Surgery

Persistence of symptoms immediately after surgery may be due to wrong diagnosis of zone of damage, or surgical failure due to wound disruption. In patients with symptoms of urgency, causes such as fibroid, vesical cancer, post-operative infection, etc, need to be excluded.

c) Same Symptoms Reappear After a Period of Improvement

If the same symptoms reappear, the cause may be longer-term surgical failure due to poor tissue condition. Symptoms such as urgency which are shared between all three zones may be presented by the patient as 'persisting symptoms'. Detailed questioning of the patient is especially important here.

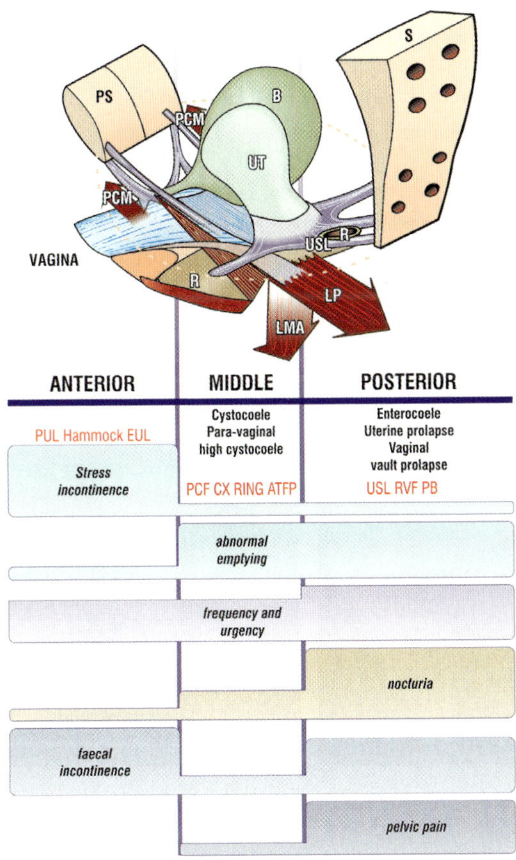

Fig. 1-11 Referring to the Pictorial Diagnostic Algorithm helps guide the physician as to the site of damage.

There are only two possible diagnostic possibilities if a patient reports recurrence of a symptom after a period of weeks or months: recurrence of the original defect, or decompensation ('blowout') in another zone. Because even minor anatomical defects may cause major symptoms, a careful examination of each zone is required (fig 1-11).

'Simulated operations' (Ch3) are especially useful in patients with minor degrees of damage. The physician needs to ensure that a patient's bladder should be sufficiently full to elicit urge symptoms in the supine position. This may require a period of waiting in the consulting rooms until the patient reports that she has urge symptoms. Some surgeons insert a catheter to fill the bladder until the patient reports urgency. The 'simulated operations' procedure is then undertaken, as outlined in chapter 3 and chapter 6 (section 6.2.4).

Step 3. A Zone By Zone Approach

Post-operative Anterior Zone Symptoms - Persisting Stress Incontinence

One of the main causes of failure of a midurethral sling is excessive laxity of the sling. However, the individual contribution of other structures to stress incontinence control needs to be assessed by performing simulated operations: the external ligament, pubourethral ligament, vaginal hammock, and posterior ligaments (see Chapters 3 and 6).

In patients who have had a midurethral sling and who leak unpredictably on sudden movement, but not during coughing, lax external ligaments (EUL) should be suspected, especially if the patient complains of a 'bubble' being released from her urethra. A gaping external meatus or urethral mucosal prolapse, is suggestive of EUL laxity. Transperineal ultrasound can identify the rotation and descent of the bladder base in the post-operative ultrasound (fig 4-106). This signifies an excessively loose pubourethral anchoring mechanism. By applying a haemostat unilaterally to the midurethra, as shown in figure 4-107, the urethrovesical geometry and continence is restored, indicating that this patient requires another midurethral sling.

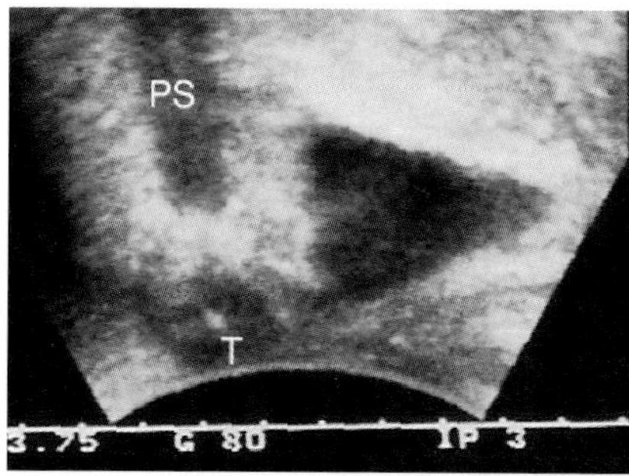

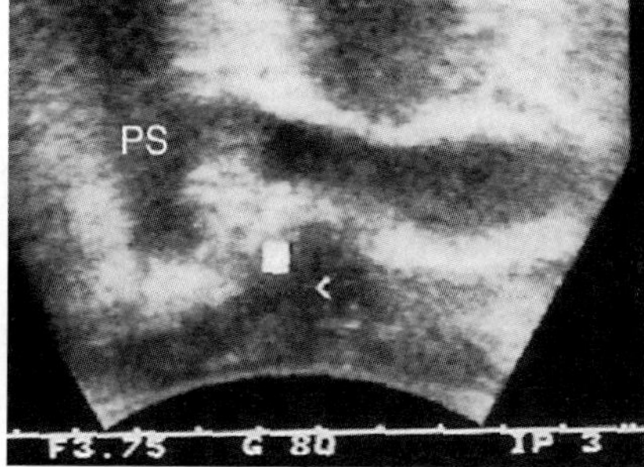

Fig 4-106 Failed sling, sagittal view, straining. Note rotation, funnelling and distal position of the sling 'T'. PS = pubic symphysis.

Fig 4-107 Same patient as 4-106, straining, midurethral anchoring with haemostat (<) restores urethrovesical geometry and continence. The distal urethra remains in the 'open' position.

In the case illustrated in figure 4-107, closer examination reveals that the bladder neck has closed but the distal urethra remains open. In this case, this patient would almost certainly require tightening of the suburethral vaginal hammock fascia, and possibly external urethral ligaments as well, for optimal cure.

As demonstrated previously, (Petros 2003), in patients with previous bladder neck elevation surgery, urine can leak without rotation and descent; these patients exhibited significant changes in their urethral closure pressure with a midurethral simulated operation (figs 6-08 and 6-12). A high percentage of these patients were cured with a midurethral sling and hammock repair. In rare occurrences, post-operative tape slippage may result in the tape holding the urethra open, analogous to the historical description of a fibrotic 'pipestem' urethra. This can be diagnosed by using a transversely applied ultrasound probe. In this case, the urethra does not close, or may even be pulled open during straining by a fibrous attachment to the posterior urethral wall, much as happens during micturition (fig 2-21).

Stress incontinence is mainly an anterior zone symptom. However, in patients with failed anterior sling surgery, who have had hysterectomy, and who continue to leak with coughing even during a midurethral 'simulated operation', lax uterosacral ligaments may be a contributory cause to their stress incontinence. This possibility can be verified by supporting the posterior fornix during a cough stress test (Chapter 6, section 6.2.4).

Multiple Operations, and a Failed Midurethral Sling Operation

In cases with multiple unsuccessful stress incontinence operations an exploratory/curative operation may be performed. The first step is to perform a careful full thickness midline incision to examine the urethral anatomy. If the tape is attached to the urethra, distending it into the open position, the urethra needs to be freed from the scar tissue, and as much tape as possible needs to be excised. If the urethral wall is thin, stretched and dilated, the cylindrical shape of the urethra may need to be restored by suturing the external surface with 3-0 dexon sutures.

If possible, these operations should be performed under local anaesthetic/sedation. Each of the structures contributing to continence control can be repaired and checked, one by one. This is done by installing 300ml saline in the bladder. The patient is asked to cough before and after each stage of the operation:

- reinsertion of a new tape,
- tightening the tape,
- then the hammock, and
- repair of the external ligaments.

If the patient is still leaking urine after this sequence, it may be necessary to test the contribution of the posterior ligaments. The posterior fornix is infiltrated with 1% Xylocaine, the right and left parts of the apex are grasped by Allis forceps and gently approximated to the midline, and the patient asked to cough. If this maneouvre controls urine loss with stress, the posterior ligaments may need to be tightened, preferably with the aid of a posterior sling.

Especially after multiple vaginal repairs and/or Burch colposuspensions, 'tethered vagina syndrome' (Chapter 4) should always be excluded in patients reporting large losses of urine. In this case, it is the operation itself which has caused the problem. The cardinal symptom is large loss of urine every morning as soon as the patient's foot touches the floor on getting out of bed in the morning. The cardinal sign is scarring and immobility in the bladder neck area of the vagina. Stress incontinence is not a major feature of this condition.

Post-operative Middle Zone Symptoms

Post-operative cystocoele may occur in up to 16-18% of patients after posterior zone surgeries (Shull 1992, Petros 2001). Consulting the Pictorial Diagnostic Algorithm, (fig 1-11) and undertaking a speculum examination helps diagnose the exact site of middle zone damage - central, paravaginal, or cervical ring attachment. 'Simulated operations' performed for urgency (see Chapters 3 and 6) help to confirm how much the middle zone defect is contributing to causation. Given that the middle and posterior zones are related anatomically, the posterior zone should always be examined in patients with post-operative urge symptoms.

In patients who report large losses of urine on getting out of bed in the morning, and who have a tight scar across bladder neck, 'tethered vagina syndrome' should be suspected.

Post-operative Posterior Zone Symptoms

If neourgency occurs after a stress incontinence operationthe physician should consult the Pictorial Diagnostic Algorithm (fig 1-11) to check for *de novo* occurrence of pelvic pain, abnormal emptying, and nocturia. The presence of any of these symptoms strongly suggests posterior zone laxity. Sometimes there may be minimal uterine or vault prolapse on vaginal examination. To confirm the characteristic posterior fornix bulge often seen with such patients, the surgeon may need to apply upward pressure on the anterior vaginal wall with ring forceps, while asking the patient to strain downwards. Pelvic pain can be reproduced digitally by pressing into the posterior fornix. This needs to be done with great care, and once only, as it can cause significant pain to the patient. Slow emptying time (>60 seconds) and raised residual urine may help confirm the diagnosis of posterior zone laxity. Slow urine flow rate (<20ml/sec) is an unreliable parameter in the individual patient. See chapters 3 and 6 (section 6.2.4) for further details.

Future Directions for the Objective Diagnosis of Zone of Connective Tissue Damage

Using higher resolution ultrasound machines, and by developing more advanced diagnostic techniques, it may be possible in the future to diagnose breaks or weakness in the fascia, and, therefore, earlier stages of organ prolapse. At this stage, ultrasound is preferable to MRI because of access, cost, and the dynamic nature of the image. Emerging technology such as elastometers or piezo-electric instruments able to measure tissue stiffness may all contribute to the objective diagnosis of abnormally lax or damaged tissue.

4.5 Summary Chapter 4

This chapter discusses the concepts, principles and practice of the Integral Theory system of pelvic floor surgery.

The most important concepts are that: restoration of form will also restore function; that the repair of connective tissue damage in the nine structures, three in each zone, will restore prolapse as well as function; and that major symptoms may occur with only minor structural defects.

Certain surgical principles need to be followed: conservation of the uterus and vaginal tissue where possible (because of long-term effects); and the use polypropylene mesh tapes to reinforce damaged ligaments (as they cannot be otherwise repaired). Basic rules which need to be observed so as to achieve day surgery are:

1. Avoid tension when suturing the vagina
2. Avoid vaginal excision
3. Avoid surgery to the perineal skin
4. Avoid tightness in the bladder neck area of the vagina

Surgical practice has two major elements:

1. Use of special instruments to minimize the surgery.
2. Site specific insertion of tapes to repair damaged connective tissue structures in each zone.

These structures are described in order of the significance for pelvic floor function:

- anterior zone: pubourethral ligament, vaginal hammock and external urethral ligament;
- middle zone; pubocervical fascia (cervical ring attachment, central, and paravaginal);
- posterior zone: uterosacral ligaments, rectovaginal fascia/perineal body.

Two systems for reconstruction of the pubourethral and uterosacral ligaments are described: the 'blind', 'tension-free' tape techniques, and the newer, safer, direct vision 'tissue fixation system'.

The issues, and techniques concerned with repairing damaged fascia as a tensioning adjunct to these methods, or even as an alternative, are discussed: Mesh, autologous 'bridge' repair, use of heterologous tissue, and TFS mesh tapes.

The final section presents a framework for addressing recurrent or new symptoms following surgery. This framework is based on the three zone diagnostic approach, but includes strategies for assessing some possibly confounding anatomical issues arising from the intervention itself.

Pelvic Floor Rehabilitation

5.1   Introduction

The Integral Theory System for pelvic floor rehabilitation (PFR) differs from traditional methods in four major ways:
1.   It addresses symptoms of urgency, nocturia, frequency, abnormal emptying and pelvic pain in addition to stress incontinence
2.   It introduces two new techniques, squatting and reverse pushdown exercises so as to strengthen the 3 directional muscle forces.
3.   It combines electrotherapy, hormones, fast and slow twitch exercises.
4.   It is designed to seamlessly fit into a patient's daily routine.

The scope of traditional pelvic floor rehabilitation methods is mainly confined to Kegel exercises for improvement in stress incontinence, and 'bladder drill' to improve urgency symptoms. 'Bladder drill' can be explained as a 'training' of the neural inhibitory circuits from the cortex to all the inhibitory centres to maximal efficiency. Although urge symptoms are not addressed with conventional pelvic floor exercises, anecdotal reports of patients controlling urge symptoms by 'crossing their legs and squeezing' are consistent with the pelvic muscles having a role in control of urgency symptoms. This can be explained by the pelvic muscles stretching the vaginal membrane to support the stretch receptors (cf. the trampoline analogy).

Current pelvic floor rehabilitation (PFR) methods in the female address mainly stress incontinence. 'Squeezing', upward pulling of the pelvic diaphragm as described by Kegel (1948) is the core element of all traditional methods.

All organs and even levator plate (LP) are actively pulled upwards and forwards with 'squeezing' (fig 5-01). Only voluntary contraction of puborectalis can explain these movements. This movement does not pull directly against any of the pelvic ligaments, although it is likely that PCM reflexly contracts to pull the hammock forwards against the pubourethral ligament. The unbroken lines (fig 5-01) represent the resting position and the broken lines the squeezing position. Vascular clips have been applied to the anterior vaginal wall: '1' to midurethra; '2' to bladder neck; '3' to bladder base.

Acknowledgement: The routine presented is that practised by Dr Patricia M. Skilling, Kvinno Centre, Perth, Australia.

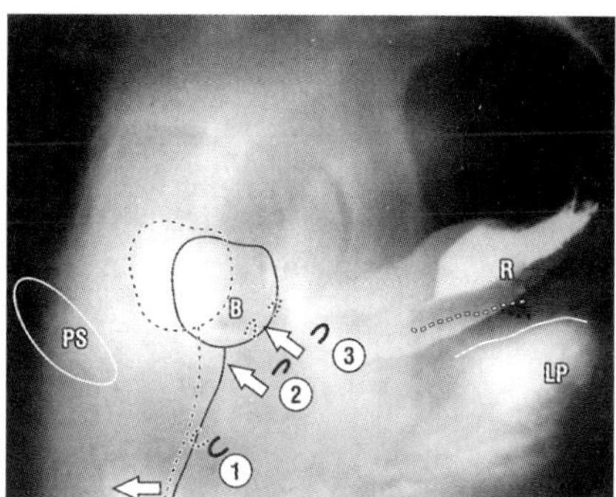

Fig. 5-01 The muscle movements during 'squeezing' are upwards and forwards. LP = levator plate; B = Foley balloon; R = rectum. Note the difference with the movements in figure 5-02. Because 'squeezing' is not the natural mechanism, it must be learned (fig 5-02). (Kegel 1948)
Rest = unbroken lines
Squeeze = broken lines

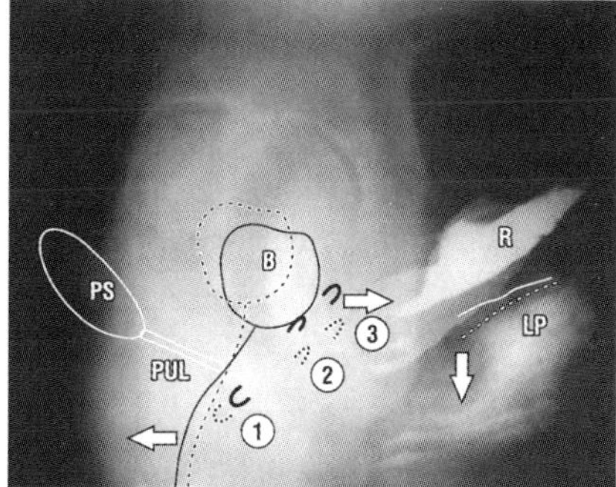

Fig. 5-02 Reflex muscle movements during coughing and straining. Same patient and labelling as figure 5-01. Note how the 3 different directional movements and downward angulation of levator plate pull against the pubourethral and uterosacral ligaments.
Rest = unbroken lines
Strain = broken lines

5.2　The Integral Theory System for Pelvic Floor Rehabilitation

Every part of the pelvic floor system contributes to function. The Integral Theory approach to rehabilitation emphasises the need to strengthen all the parts of the system that contribute to continence: muscle, connective tissue and neuromuscular transmission. In particular, exercises such as squatting, 'reverse push-downs' and electrotherapy in the posterior fornix are included in the protocol so as to strengthen the three directional muscle forces and their ligamentous attachments. The Integral Theory system for pelvic floor rehabilitation was specifically designed for busy women with commitments to home, children, jobs and careers. Minimal time outlay and weaving every element of treatment seamlessly into a daily routine were important goals in the protocol.

5.2.1　Indications

There were no exclusion criteria in the descriptions below. Any patient, regardless of the seriousness of her condition, was accepted for PFR. Patients who lost less than 2 gm urine with the cough stress test, or less than 10 gm in a 24 hour period, were particularly encouraged to do PFR. Also, patients with successful surgery were encouraged to learn PFR so as to maintain their good results.

5.2.2 Design

The regime consists of four visits in three months. The Pictorial Diagnostic Algorithm (fig 1-11) guides diagnosis of anatomical defects in the anterior, middle and posterior zones of the vagina. Hormone replacement therapy (HRT) is administered to thicken epithelium and prevent collagen loss. Electrotherapy is given for 20 minutes a day for the first four weeks to improve neuromuscular transmission. The patients do slow twitch muscle exercises - squatting or sitting on a rubber 'fit' ball - for a total of 20 minutes per day.

First Visit

The patient is instructed in a Kegel exercise routine, two lots of twelve, three times per day. The exercises are performed in bed, face downwards, morning and night with legs apart, according to the methods of Bo (1990). The remaining 24 squeezes are performed at lunchtime or during visits to the toilet. It is helpful for the patient to visualise squeezing the sides of a lemon inwards, or to pretend she is cutting off her urine stream. Endocavity electrical stimulation of 20 minutes per day is prescribed for four weeks. With any anterior zone defect, the probe is placed just inside the introitus on alternate days and in the posterior fornix every other day. The aim is to strengthen both PCM and LP. With pure posterior zone defects, the probe is placed in the posterior fornix only. Squatting or sitting on a 'fit ball' for a total of 20 minutes per day if possible is encouraged as a universal slow-twitch exercise. The aim is to integrate this activity into the patient's daily routine. For instance, the patient is encouraged to substitute squatting for bending at all times. If a patient has arthritis, she may sit on the end of a chair with legs apart or on a fitball. Compliance is vastly improved by explaining the principles behind the exercises, and encouraging patients to plan and record their daily routine.

Second Visit

In patients without a cystocoele, a reverse downward thrust is taught on the second visit. The patient presses upwards with the probe or a finger placed approximately 2 cm inwards from the introitus, and strains downwards. The downward thrust is now alternated with the Kegel squeezes, each three times per day. The downward-acting exercises strengthen the fast twitch fibres of all three directional muscle forces.

Third Visit

The attendant checks the patient compliance (diary), discusses how she has incorporated the programme into her daily routine, and reinforces the aims and principles of the programme.

At the three month review (fourth visit), in consultation with the patient, a decision is made whether to proceed to surgery, or continue with Maintenance PFR.

Maintenance PFR

By the end of three months, it is assumed that the patients have incorporated the exercises into their normal routine. Squeezing is alternated with the downward thrust, a total of six sets of 12 exercises per day. Squatting is by now an acquired habit. Electrotherapy is performed five days per month. The patient is advised to continue this routine for the rest of her life.

Comments

Almost 70% of patients who completed the treatment seemed unwilling to perform the reverse pushdown exercises. Squatting, Kegel and electrotherapy were well received.

Results of the First study (Petros & Skilling, 2001)

Sixty patients completed the study. Improvement was defined as >50% improvement in their symptoms (see Table 1).

Table 1	
Fate of Individual Symptoms (n=60)	
condition	**>50% improvement**
stress (n=42)	78%
urge (n=39)	61%
frequency (n=53)	62%
nocturia (n=24)	75%
pelvic pain (n=20)	65%
leakage (n=50)	68%
bowel problems (n=28)	78%

Table 2	
Fate of Individual Symptoms (n=78)	
condition	**>50% improvement**
stress incontinence (n=69)	57 (82%)
urge incontinence (n=44)	33 (68%)
frequency only (n=12)	10 (83%)
nocturia (n=32)	29 (90%)
pelvic pain (n=17)	13 (76%)

Results of the Second Study (Skilling, PM and Petros PE (2004))

Of 147 patients (mean age 52.5years), 53% completed the programme. Median QOL improvement reported was 66%, mean cough stress test urine loss reduced from 2.2 gm (range 0-20.3 gm) to 0.2 gm (range 0-1.4 gm), p=<0.005 and 24 hour pad urine loss from a mean of 3.7 mg (range 0-21.8 mg) to a mean of 0.76 mg (range 0-9.3 gm), p=<0.005.

Frequency, nocturia were significantly improved (p=<0.005). Residual urine reduced from mean 202 ml to mean 71 ml(p=<0.005) (See Table 2 for improvement in individual symptoms).

5.2.3 Conclusions

The pelvic floor rehabilitation method extends indications for nonsurgical therapy beyond stress incontinence to include posterior zone symptoms. Two major studies of the efficacy of the Integral Theory PFR have been published to date (Skilling, PM & Petros PE 2001, 2004). The results are promising and appear to sustain the theory on which the method is based.

5.3   Summary Chapter 5

The Integral Theory system for pelvic floor rehabilitation expands the indications for treatment beyond stress incontinence to include urgency, frequency, nocturia, pelvic pain and abnormal empytying. An improvement rate greater than 50% is achieved in such symptoms in at least two out of three patients.

Mapping the Dynamics of Connective Tissue Dysfunction

6.1   Mapping Function and Dysfunction of the Pelvic Floor

In 1976, the International Continence Society (ICS) introduced the first definitions for urodynamic testing. This was a seminal step in the history of pelvic floor science, as it established the principle of objective assessment of the lower urinary tract. Moreover, by creating standard definitions, a common language for investigators was created. Subsequent advances in ultrasound, radiology, MRI and biomechanics have provided additional tools for the clinician to identify damaged structures, and to proceed some way towards quantification of the damage. This section shows how such tools may be used to more accurately identify damaged structures. Accurate mapping of function and dysfunction (as opposed to diagnosing specific structural defects) is a far more difficult problem, as not all apparently damaged structures necessarily cause dysfunction. For example, not all patients with 'funnelling' during straining (anterior zone defect) necessarily have stress incontinence: Some patients with major degrees of prolapse (posterior zone defect) have no symptoms associated with lax posterior ligaments, yet others with minor degrees of prolapse may 'complain bitterly' of their symptoms (Jeffcoate 1962). 'Detrusor instability' may be found in up to 70% of normal patients (Van Doorn 1992), yet it is absent in up to 50% of patients with bladder instability symptoms. In order to overcome such problems, the concept of 'simulated operations' is introduced. This technique helps the clinician to more accurately assess function by observing the change following anchoring of a specific connective tissue structure.

Although all urodynamic tests are objective, they only provide a 'snapshot' of the system at that particular point in time. Even with the same test, the result may be different just half an hour later. The reason for this is that the control mechanisms of the pelvic floor behave in a non-linear (chaotic) manner, i.e., even a small change in a minor component of the system may have a major outcome as a result. Non-linear control helps to explain why symptoms (and even objective test results) may vary widely from day to day. It is essential that the basis for variability in test results be understood if objective tests are to make a meaningful contribution to 'mapping' of function and dysfunction of the pelvic floor (Petros & Bush 1998, Petros 2001).

6.1.1 Urodynamics - An Anatomical Perspective

The dysfunctions of the pelvic floor described in this book are all potentially curable by using the simple day-care techniques (as described in Chapter 4) to repair the nine causative defects identified in figure 1-10. The primary aim of 'mapping' techniques is to objectively assess which of these nine defects are the causal agents for the dysfunction that is occurring in the patient. The preceding pages have emphasized the physical properties of the urethra and anus. In simple terms, these are smooth muscle tubes linked by connective tissue to the pelvic muscles which activate opening or closure. The resistance generated within these tubes is perhaps the most critical factor in determining normal function and dysfunction of the bladder or rectum to which they are connected. Very important insights can be obtained by measuring the physical expressions of this resistance, that is, pressure and flow. Urodynamics is a means of measuring pressure within the bladder and urethra and also urine flow parameters. The Integral Theory approach to urodynamics can only be applied to the female at this stage.

The main emphasis of the ICS system in the female is on the cystometric diagnosis of 'detrusor instability' (DI), the presence of DI being a contraindication for surgery. However, this approach overlooks anatomical defects as causal phenomena. In the Integral Theory system, the presence of DI is not a contraindication for surgery: non-neurological patients with DI are potentially curable by repairing the anatomical defects which may be causing the DI. In particular, patients with no SI, but with urge frequency, nocturia, and perhaps other symptoms of posterior zone defect, are curable in 80% of cases following reconstruction of the posterior ligaments (Petros 1997, Farnsworth 2001).

There is no set technique for urodynamic measurement. Controversies exist for almost every aspect of measurement, especially as the act of measurement itself may significantly alter any result obtained. The aim of this section is to give the anatomical and biomechanical basis for urodynamic measurement, and to explain how these measurements relate to symptoms. This involves developing an understanding of the neurological feedback mechanisms. By observing real-time changes in urodynamic and ultrasound parameters following the anchoring of key ligaments, the Integral Theory concept of 'simulated' operations emerges. In this context, the patient's cortex functions as the urodynamic 'machine' which sensitively discriminates the impact on, say, urgency sensations, after each anchoring action of the 'simulated operation'.

The Basis of Urodynamics: Urethral Resistance

In its most basic form, the urethra is a tube which links the storage organ, the bladder, to the outside. The bladder contracts and pushes the urine out against the intra-urethral resistance. (As the x-ray studies show, the urethral tube is *narrowed* along its length by three directional muscle forces during *closure*, but *opened* along its length by two directional muscle forces during *micturition*. The intra-urethral resistance is inversely proportional to the 4th power of the radius (r^4) (fig 6-02) and directly proportional to the length. Therefore, the inability to actively close or open out the urethra because of lax connective tissue may have a disproportional effect on continence or emptying (i.e. bladder emptying times, peak flow and residual urine).

The Anatomical Basis of Urodynamic Measurement

Pressure transducers are used to measure pressure in the bladder, urethra and rectum. The rectal pressure is equated with the abdominal pressure and is subtracted from the bladder pressure to give the 'detrusor pressure'.

However, this methodology is inherently flawed. Like the bladder, the rectum is a receptacle surrounded by smooth muscle, and this may confound measurement. If the transducers are sited below the level of the pelvic diaphragm, pressure readings will be affected by the external anal sphincter (EAS) and puborectalis muscle (PRM) contraction. Only an intraperitoneal transducer can accurately reflect intra-abdominal pressure. Clearly this is not an acceptable methodology. A more valid approach to pressure increase for diagnosing DI is to seek a phasic pattern in the bladder channel because this will accurately reflect an activated micturition reflex.

In the normal patient during filling cystometry, the three directional muscle forces reflexly stretch the vagina to support the hydrostatic pressure of the urine. This relieves pressure on the stretch receptors (N). At the same time, the urethral tube is stretched and narrowed, so that the urethral pressure rises, a common observation during filling.

In the patient with lax ligaments, the vagina cannot be easily stretched (see the 'trampoline analogy'). Inability of the lax vagina to support 'N' may prematurely activate the micturition reflex. PCM relaxes, the urethral pressure falls, the detrusor contracts and this is recorded as 'detrusor instability'. Inflammation or pressure on N (e.g. cancer, uterine fibroids, excess bladder neck elevation) may create the same sequence of events by stimulating the stretch receptors directly.

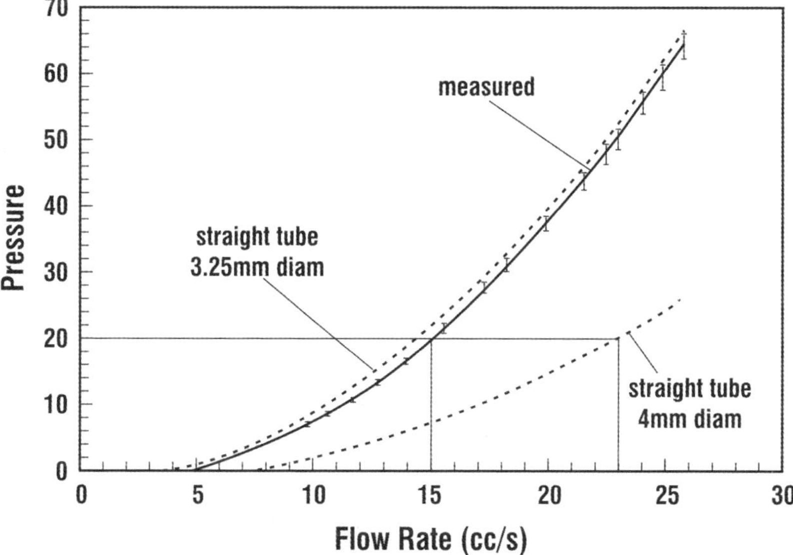

Fig. 6-01 The pressure/ flow relationship as measured experimentally. Note that a 0.75mm increase in tube diameter increased the flow 50% (15 to 23 ml/sec). After Bush et al. (1997).

Urethral Resistance and the Pressure-Flow Relationship

Urethral resistance is the key variable influencing bladder function and urodynamic measurements. The urethral resistance is governed by the musculoelastic mechanism which opens and closes the urethral tube. The diameter of the urethra determines pressure and flow during micturition and also effects closure. In simple terms, the bladder contracts and expels the urine through the tube (fig 6-02).

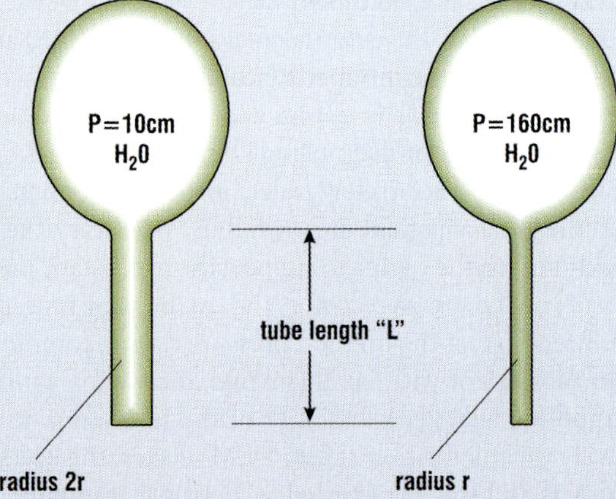

Fig. 6-02 The effect of urethral radius on expulsion pressure. Three directional muscle forces alter the urethral resistance by the 4th power during closure, and two muscle forces alter it during micturition.

Hagen-Poisseuille's Law - the Pressure/Flow Relationship

Hagen-Poisseuille's Law is fundamental to understanding the anatomical basis of urodynamics. It explains what happens during closure (continence) and opening of the urethral tube (micturition). It states that "the pressure 'P' required to expel a liquid through a tube varies according to the resistance within that tube". It can be simplified to: 'the resistance to flow within a tube varies directly with the length of the tube *and* inversely with its radius (to the 4th power)'. Thus, in figure 6-02, if the urethral tube can be opened out from radius r to 2r then the micturition pressure required *reduces* by a factor of 16 (i.e. 2^4).

Failure of the two muscle forces to open out the urethra (i.e. increase r) means that the bladder has to expel the urine against a higher resistance. This may be experienced by the patient as 'obstructed micturition'. Conversely, if during coughing, the urethra can be closed from 2r to r by a Kegel contraction, then leakage will only occur with a pressure greater than 160cm H_2O.

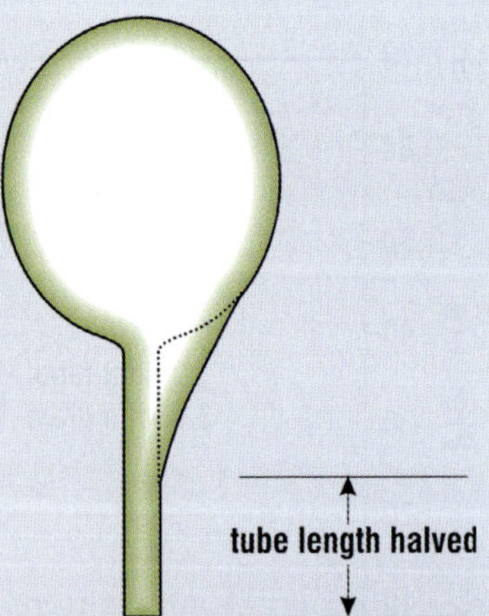

Fig. 6-03 Effect of length on expulsion pressure. During micturition 'funnelling' effectively shortens the urethral tube, further reducing resistance and, therefore, expulsion pressure.

The Origin of Intra-Abdominal Pressure

As the pelvic and abdominal muscles share a common embryological origin (Power 1948), pelvic muscle contraction reflexly activates an abdominal muscle contraction. This proportionately increases the intra-abdominal pressure. This explains observations by Enhorning (1961) and Constantinou (1985) that during coughing, rise in urethral pressure frequently precedes the rise in bladder pressure. The former is activated by pelvic floor contraction, and the latter by abdominal contraction.

The Dynamics of Urethral Pressure Changes

The pressure measured at every point along the urethra by a pressure transducer is determined by the forces acting at that point and the intra-urethral area. (Pressure is force per unit area.)

'Closure Pressure'

'Closure pressure' (CP) is bladder pressure subtracted from urethral pressure. At 0 cm CP there is no resistance to urine leakage. However, many patients with 0cm CP do not leak during testing. Even at 0 cm, CP dynamic and frictional resistance factors may impede urine loss.

The 'Cough Transmission Ratio'

The 'cough transmission ratio' (CTR) is the ratio of the rise in urethral pressure divided by the rise in bladder pressure during coughing. The CTR is expressed in percentage terms.

An adequately tight hammock and pubourethral ligament (PUL) are required to close both 'd' and 'p' parts of the urethra during effort (coughing) (fig 6-04). The downward vector LMA also acts around PUL. Observations from surgeons of SI improvement after the Posterior IVS operation indicate there is also a role for the uterosacral ligament (USL) during urethral closure, USL being the insertion point of the LMA vector.

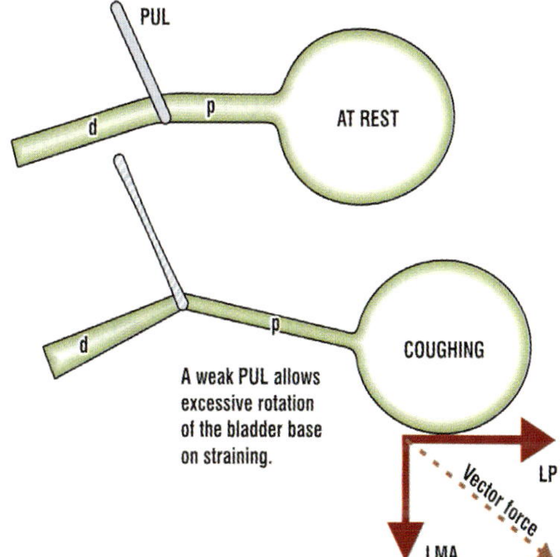

Fig. 6-04 Pubourethral ligament length affects urethral pressure. A weak pubourethral ligament may be stretched excessively by the LP/LMA vector. This may stretch and narrow the proximal urethra 'p'. A weak PUL cannot anchor the PCM force required to close the distal urethra 'd'.

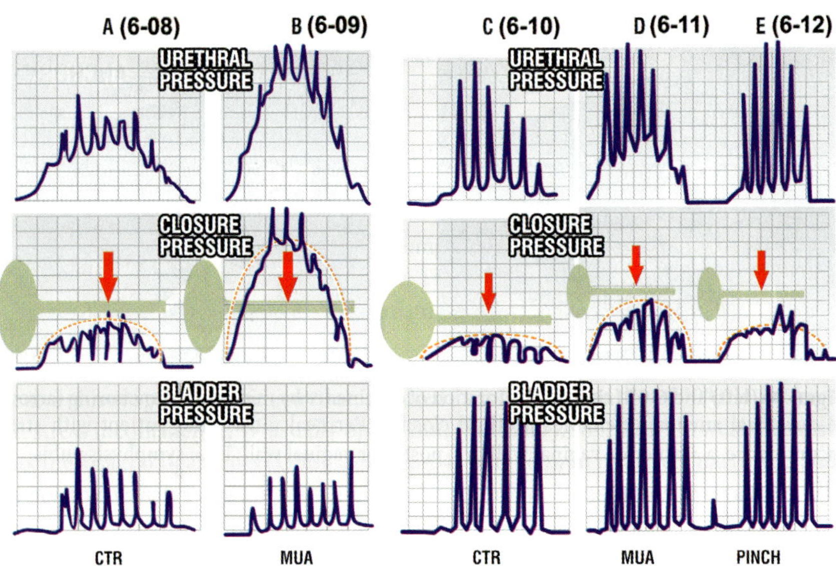

Figs 6-08 to 6-12 (Graphs A-E) The anatomical basis for urethral pressure measurements. 'A' - Note the decrease in closure pressure with each cough. 'B' - Mid urethral anchor (MUA), same patient as 'A'. Note the rise in resting profile and the much higher closure pressure with each cough. 'C' (different patient) - Note the low resting urethral pressure, and the zero closure pressure on coughing. 'D' (same patient as 'C') - Mid urethral anchor (MUA). There is some rise in the resting urethral pressure, but the closure pressure remains at zero. 'E' - Unilateral fold of vagina, taken at the distal urethra ('pinch test'). Same patient as 'C'. Note the rise in closure pressure. (For detailed biomechanical analysis of these events see Petros PE Neurourol. and Urodynamics (2003).)

The Urodynamics of Micturition

The bladder has two stable modes, closed and open ('micturition'). In figures 6-13 and 6-14, the closed mode (continence) circuits are shown as red, and the open mode circuits ('micturition') are shown in green. Both modes have central (neurological) and peripheral (musculoelastic) components.

The open mode requires activation of the micturition reflex. As the bladder fills, the hydrostatic pressure activates the stretch receptors (N) to produce afferent impulses. These impulses are shut off by the inhibitory centre (which acts much like a trapdoor to shut out the afferent impulses), and by the contraction of the three directional muscle forces (PCM, LMA and LP) which stretch the vaginal membrane to support the hydrostatic pressure of the urine. This process stops 'N' 'firing off'. The red lines in figure 6-13 represent the closed mode (C), and the green lines the open mode 'O'.

Beyond a critical mass, the afferent impulses saturate the inhibitory centres and pass information directly to the cortex to be perceived as 'urgency'. Valuable information on the unstable bladder may be obtained from a provocative handwashing test. This test works by interrupting the cortical inhibition of the micturition reflex.

In the open ('micturition') mode ('O' in fig 6-14), central inhibition ceases and the 'trapdoor' opens allowing the afferent impulses to pass through the pons. The forward muscle PCM relaxes, allowing LP and LMA to stretch the vagina backwards to open out the urethra. The detrusor contracts. Several seconds must elapse before this process can be reversed. This explains the wave forms seen in detrusor instability graphs.

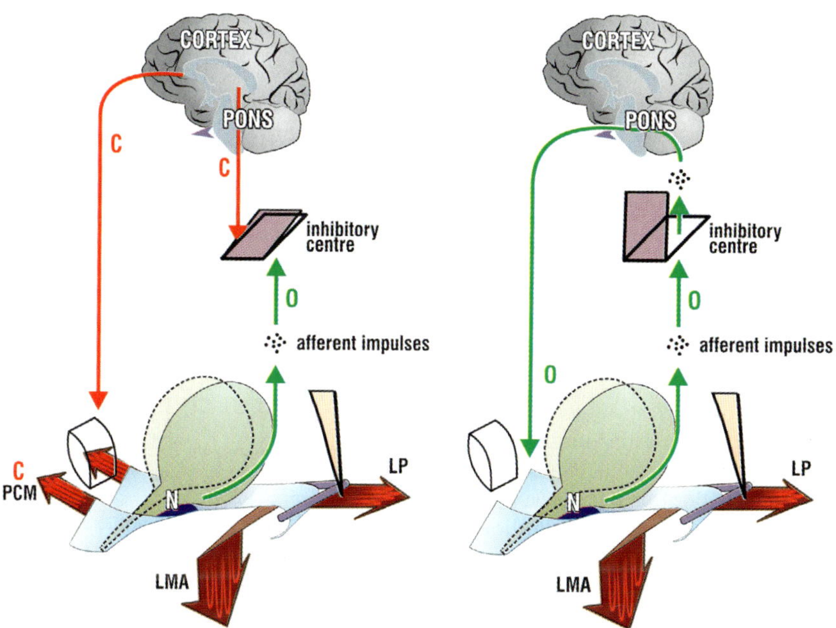

Fig. 6-13 Closure: the anatomical system for control of urgency (premature activation of the micturition reflex.)

Fig. 6-14 Opening: the anatomical system for micturition

Urodynamic Bladder Instability – Premature Activation of the Micturition Reflex

The peaks (small arrows, fig 6-16) denote the closed phase and the troughs the open phase of the micturition reflex. Closed and open phases alternate and produce a sinusoidal curve because of the time taken to switch from one mode to the other. Figure 6-15 represents these events according to Chaos Theory as two competing 'attractors'. An 'attractor' is a phase state which occurs as a result of certain conditions. Normal elasticity in the tissues is one essential condition contributing to the 'closed' attractor. Without elasticity, the urethra is like an open tube and forms the 'open' attractor. Loss of elasticity may initiate a cascade of events which combined with sensitive stretch receptors may cause the bladder to swing between 'open' and 'closed' phases (fig 6-15). With reference to figure 6-16, the open phase overcomes the closed phase only in the centre where 16.6 gm urine loss is recorded.

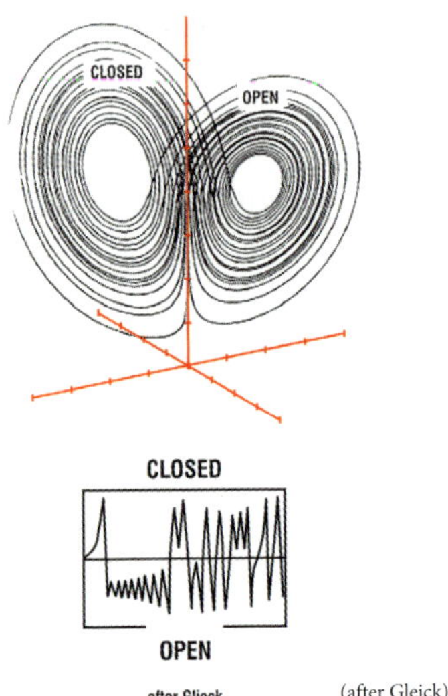

Fig. 6-15 (above) Detrusor instability explained as two attractors, open and closed. Inability of tissue elasticity to maintain the closed position causes the unstable bladder to oscillate between closed (continence) and open (micturition) phases. Because of the time delay in switching between these two phases, the pressure curves are sinusoidal. This is clearly illustrated in both 'U' and 'B' in figures 6-16 and 6-17. The process is similar to the feedback systems described in Chaos Theory (Gleick).

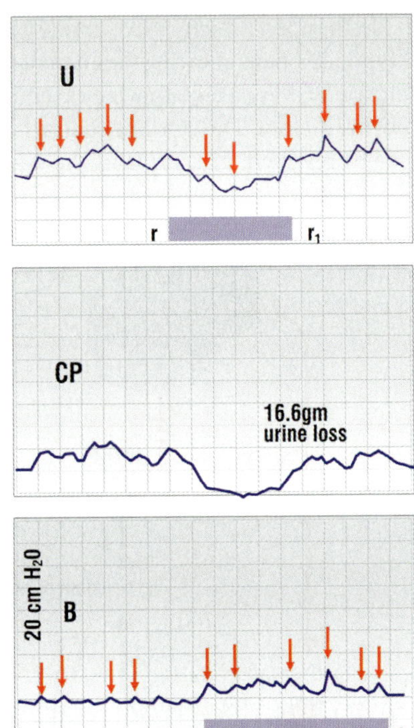

Fig. 6-16 Urodynamic bladder instability - premature activation of the micturition reflex. Microtransducers in bladder (B) and midurethra (U). CP=closure pressure (U-B). Note how urethral relaxation (r-r_1) precedes detrusor contraction (c-c_1).

Voluntary Control of the Micturition Reflex

A common history is of the patient who is shopping, stops, crosses her legs and controls her urgency by 'squeezing' (fig 6-18). 'Squeezing' stretches the vaginal membrane to support the stretch receptors and it is this which controls the afferent flow of impulses from the bladder base stretch receptors - which are perceived by the patient as urgency symptoms.

Figure 6-17 is a urodynamic graph of a patient with a full bladder who is subjected to a handwashing test. At 'X' sensory urgency is experienced and the urethral pressure begins to fall. However, urine loss is controlled by voluntary pelvic floor contraction 'squeezing' ('holding on'). On 'letting go' the urethral pressure falls dramatically, the detrusor contracts (Y, 'd') and urine is lost (red arrow).

Figure 6-18 is the anatomical representation for the situation illustrated in figure 6-17. 'Squeezing' (yellow arrow) has lifted the levator plate (LP) and stretched the vaginal membrane forwards. This provides support for the stretch receptors (N). The 'resting' radiograph of the same patient is figure 2-15.

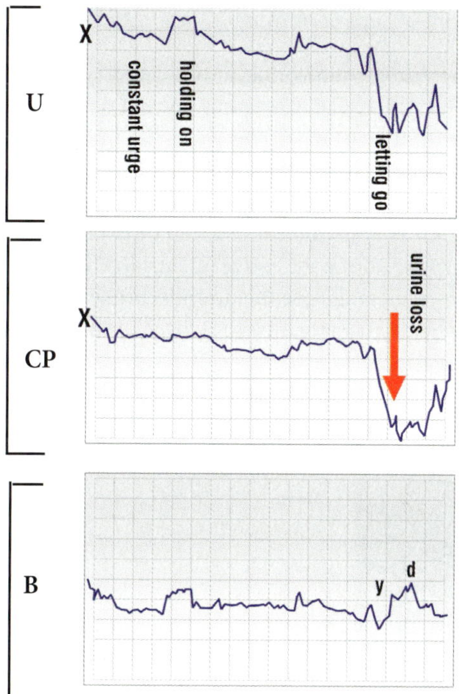

Fig. 6-17 Control of detrusor instability by pelvic floor contraction. X = start of urethral relaxation; Y = start of detrusor contraction 'd'.

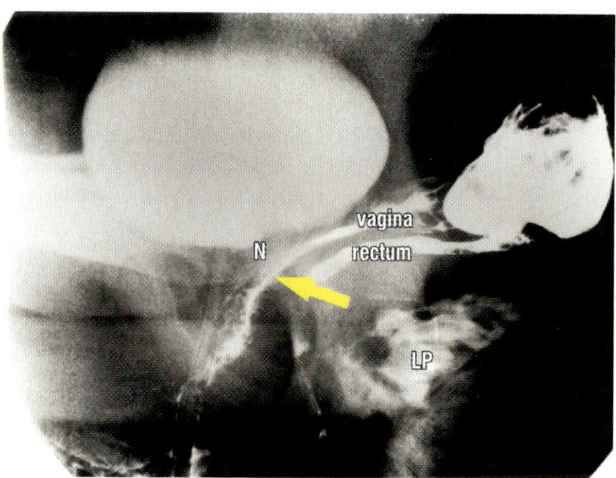

Fig. 6-18 Control of detrusor instability by voluntary pelvic floor contraction (arrow). The levator plate (LP), vagina, rectum and bladder are pulled upwards and forwards - probably by contraction of m. puborectalis.

Normal Micturition and 'After Contraction' - A Sign of Normal Tissue Elasticity.

Figure 6-20 shows a normal micturition curve conforming to the outlet geometry as shown in figure 6-19. During peak flow, the vesical cavity has opened out almost to the midurethra, vastly decreasing urethral resistance. There is a rise in detrusor pressure ('after contraction') which occurs after the end of micturition. This is evident on comparing the cessation of urine flow in the third graph 'FLOW' with the second graph 'DETRUSOR' pressure, figure 6-20. An 'after contraction' can be explained as occurring when a relaxation of the backward vectors at the end of micturition (diagonal arrows, figure 6-19) causes the vagina to recoil and close the urethra (broken yellow lines, fig 6-19). Ongoing contraction of the detrusor against the closed urethra leads to a rise in detrusor pressure 'after contraction'.

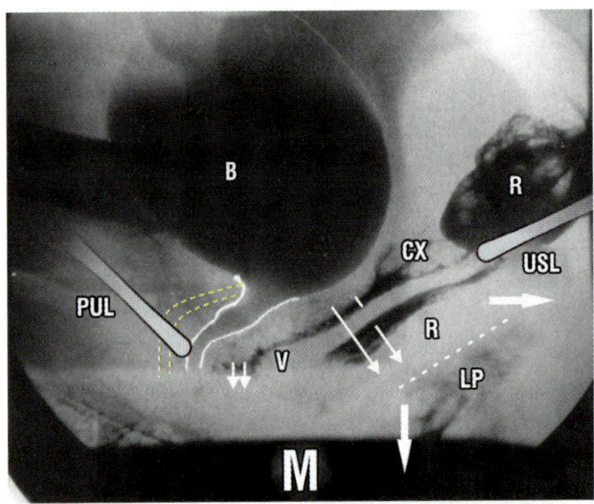

Fig. 6-19 Micturition x-ray showing external opening of the posterior urethral wall. The broken yellow lines indicate the position of the closed urethra at rest.

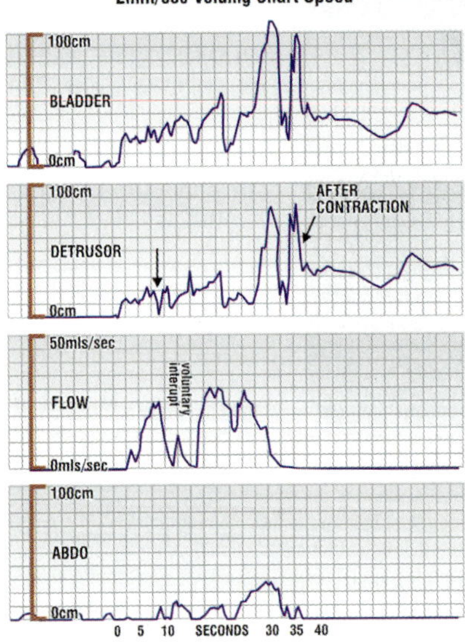

Fig. 6-20 Normal micturition and 'after contraction'. The detrusor continues to contract against a urethra closed by elastic recoil.

'Outflow Obstruction'

If the urethra is 'collapsed' because lax connective tissue does not allow its expansion during micturition, the patient may be diagnosed as having an 'obstructed urethra'. However, obstruction is rarely found on urethral dilatation. The 'obstruction' is functional, caused by the bladder's attempts to expel urine through a narrower tube with high resistance.

Figure 6-21 is a flow chart in a patient with an EMG electrode in the posterior fornix of vagina, recording contraction of the levator plate muscles (LP). The EMG is activated before urine flow commences, indicating that LP contraction precedes urine flow. It can be seen that there is constant activation of the pelvic floor muscles together with a slow prolonged urine flow because of fast-twitch muscle tiring. The geometry of the outflow tract is closer to the closed position (yellow broken lines) (fig. 6-19).

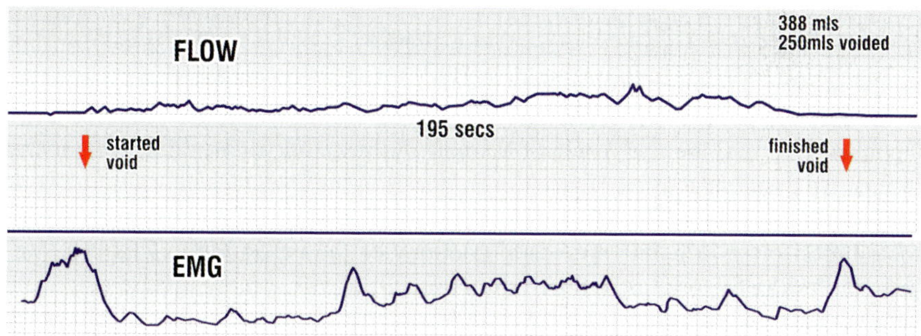

Fig. 6-21 'Outflow obstruction' in the female - Connective tissue laxity requiring constant activation of the LP/LMA vectors.

Limitations of Existing Tests: The Need for a Finite Element Model for urodynamics

Existing tests rely on a single group of measurements taken at a point in time. However, this is only a 'snapshot' of a highly complex and variable system. Even a minor variation in the diameter of the urethral tube may cause major changes in micturition pressure and flow rates (fig. 6-01).

Conceptually the flow graphs in figures 6-20 and 6-21 can be explained in terms of tissue elasticity. Thus measurement of tissue quality with some type of elastometer is an important future development. Lose has developed a system for testing urethral elasticity by distending the urethra with a balloon (Lose 1990, 1992). This is an important contribution, but it is elasticity in the *whole system* which needs to be measured. Using parameters of tissue strength and elasticity, pressure and flow measurements, and measurements of muscle bulk, it may be possible, (in conjunction with a large data base), to develop a finite element model to apply to each patient (Petros 2001). This may provide a model of the continuum of forces and events contributing to the dysfunction, rather than reliance on a mere 'snapshot', as at present.

6.1.2 The Chaos Theory Framework – Its Impact on the Understanding of Bladder Control and Urodynamic Charting

One of the most exciting scientific advances in the 20th century has been the clear exposition of 'Chaos Theory' (Gleick 1987). Chaos Theory states that every biological organism consists of a series of interrelated systems. Each system has several components working synergistically (such that the whole is greater than the sum of the parts). A change in any component of the system, no matter how minor, may have profound consequences for the system and the organism itself.

The pelvic floor is such a system. With regard to bladder and rectum, the pelvic floor has just two functions, opening (micturition, defaecation) and closure (continence). Its components are the pelvic bones, striated muscles, smooth muscles, ligaments, fascia, organs, and the sympathetic and parasympathetic nerves which link all parts of this system to the central nervous system. As every person is different, each component will have a different significance, and so it will contribute differently to normal function within that system. The significance of each component and therefore each contribution will follow a probability curve.

Within the Chaos Theory framework large scale symptoms (such as urge incontinence) may be the result of a small dysfunction (disequilibrium) in the connective tissue structures. Hence the emphasis in the Integral Theory framework on obtaining a clear and precise understanding of how each component structure contributes to the dynamic structural anatomy of the pelvic floor. This is a vital stage in finding the origins of the dysfunction. Only with a more precise diagnosis can a surgeon obtain the best clinical results from the minimalist surgical techniques described in Chapter 4.

In particular, there are two aspects of Chaos Theory which have had profound ramifications for the Integral Theory: fractals and the 'butterfly effect'.

Fractals

Fractals explain the relationship between macro and micro domains, and the self-similarity in the components. Good examples are the lung and arterial systems. Each microdomain (alveolus) reflects the major domain (the lung). In the pelvic floor, one macrodomain is laxity in one or more of the three zones; with component fascia and ligaments, collagen and proteoglycans forming even smaller microdomains. This relationship is exploited therapeutically. Hormone treatment aims to decrease collagen loss with age. Pelvic floor exercises, strengthen the muscles, the ligamentous insertion points of these muscles, the periosteal attachment of these ligaments, and may even change the muscle metabolism. Another example of fractals is the sinusiodal shape of a detrusor instability curve, and its fractal-like subsections.

Extreme Sensitivity to Initial Conditions (The 'Butterfly Effect')

The 'butterfly effect' is used in Chaos Theory to illustrate the phenomenon of extreme sensitivity to initial conditions. It explains how a minute disturbance or change (such as the flapping of butterfly wings) can disrupt a system (such as the weather) in dynamic equilibrium and manifest as huge changes elsewhere in that system (such as a hurricane). In the pelvic floor several systems exhibit this behaviour. Minor degrees of posterior zone laxity may cause pelvic pain and multiple symptoms in the bowel and bladder. Detrusor expulsion pressure and urine flow vary according to the intra-urethral resistance, which varies (in simple terms) inversely with the 4th power of the radius. Thus a urethra which can be actively opened out ('funnelled') so that it doubles its width lowers the urethral resistance by a factor of 16 (i.e. 2^4) (fig. 6-02). Micturition then requires only 1/16th the expulsion pressure than one where lax tissues entirely prevent this action. This is an example of 'non-linearity', and it explains why it is very difficult to replicate results from 'objective' tests such as flow rate (fig. 6-01). Slight variance in any of the components contributing to active opening of the outflow tract will affect exponentially the intra-urethral resistance encountered during a particular test and, therefore, the flow rate. In analysis using a linear system framework, halving the resistance would halve the expulsion pressure required, not decrease it 16 times as one finds when a 'non-linear' system framework is used. The dynamics within a non-linear system vastly shorten the opening and closure intervals and the threshold for incontinence is raised exponentially for a normal patient. In a linear system, the dynamics would be such that, as the urine entered the bladder, it would stimulate the stretch receptors and the patient would leak at low volumes.

Detrusor instability is another example where Chaos Theory provides a useful framework to help us unravel the complex interactions between bladder function and the cortex. With Chaos Theory, for the first time, there is a theoretical framework that can describe how a small structural defect can lead to a neurological response that creates further instability in the overall system. Micturition has both 'mechanical' and neurological dimensions, but the relation between the two is not simple. Bladder function is not a 'hard wired' network linked to the cortex. Incontinence, by definition, involves some type of malfunction, or 'false' urge. And even in a normally functioning system, the handwashing test can 'bring on' micturition urge.

In a patient with very sensitive nerve endings, only minor alterations in the tension of the vaginal membrane may cause the stretch receptors to 'fire off' (cf. the 'trampoline analogy') and activate the micturition reflex. There is a cascade of events which may culminate in uncontrollable urine loss or urge incontinence. This phenomenon explains how minor degrees of 'prolapse' may cause major symptoms, and supports the idea that surgical reinforcement using polypropylene tapes be used to improve symptoms as described in the Pictorial Diagnostic Algorithm (fig 1-11) even in patients with minimal prolapse.

Using Chaos Theory as a basic framework, the author was able to interpret the apparently contradictory data which followed a handwashing test to link low compliance to 'detrusor instability' (Petros 1999).

By using a basic feedback equation $X_{next} = cX(1-X)$, where X represents the number of afferent impulses, with 1 being the maximum possible number of impulses and 'c' represents the inverse of cortical and peripheral suppression mechanisms, it was possible to mimic all states of the bladder, acontractility, normal response to a full bladder, 'low compliance' (a micturition reflex activated but controlled) and instability (fig 6-25).

6.1.2 A Non-Linear Perspective of the Neurological Control of the Micturition Reflex

Normal Function

The control of the micturition reflex is essentially by a feedback system. The squares containing dots (fig 6-22) represent neurological impulses, afferent (Oa) or efferent (Oe). As the bladder fills, the stretch receptors (N) 'fire off' and afferent impulses 'Oa' are transmitted via the spinal cord. This is the initiating part of the micturition reflex. If inconvenient, the cortex activates the closure reflex (C). This has two stages. Firstly, the inhibitory centres all along the brain and spinal cord are activated. These function like trapdoors to shut off afferent and efferent impulses. Secondly, the pelvic floor muscles contract (Cm) to close off the urethra and stretch the vaginal membrane to support 'N'.

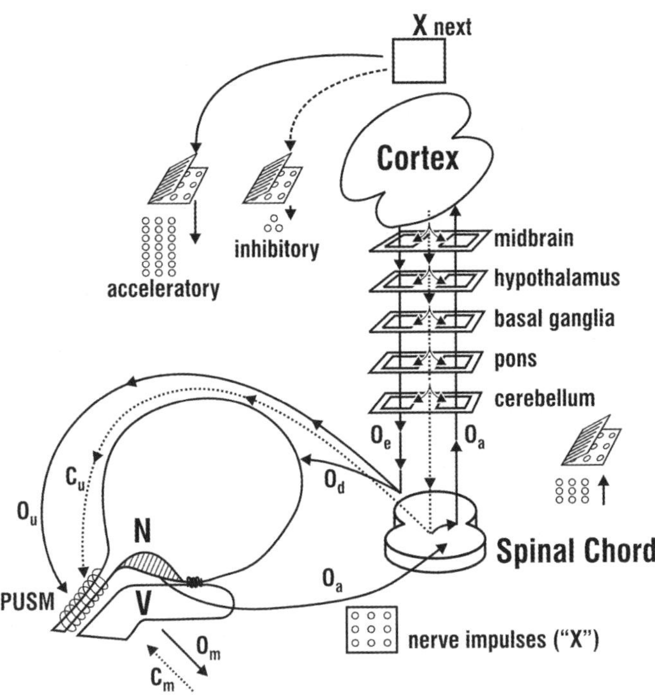

Fig. 6-22 The neurological control mechanisms for micturition. 'O' (unbroken lines) represents the 'open' (micturition) phase and 'C' (broken lines) the closed (continence) phase. N = stretch receptors; V = vagina; PUSM = periurethral striated muscle (a thin muscle sited mainly on the superior wall of the middle third of the urethra); Cm = anterior part of pubococcygeus muscle (reflex contraction) or puborectalis muscle (voluntary contraction); Om = LP/LMA vector. The dots 'X' (small circles) represent nerve impulses. The paired oblong squares along the brain and spinal cord represent the acceleratory and inhibitory centres. These work like 'trapdoors'. Ou = urethral relaxation; Cu = urethral closure; Od = detrusor contraction.

Conversely, if it is convenient to micturate, the acceleratory nuclei are stimulated. The inhibitory centre is suppressed, so its 'trapdoors' open. The anterior part of 'Cm' relaxes and 'Om' contracts to open the urethra. 'Om' contraction further stimulates 'N' to produce more afferent impulses.

Dysfunction

If the vaginal membrane 'V' is lax, 'N' may 'fire off' at a lower bladder volume. 'C' may not be able to control the micturition reflex 'O' and the patient may wet. Similarly, any neurological lesion along the path of 'C' (e.g. in multiple sclerosis) may prevent the closure reflex so that the afferents pass directly through the pons to cause incontinence. Transection of the cord will not allow 'Oe' to pass through, so the patient may have retention of urine (fig 6-22).

Note: The 'trapdoor' system has only two phases, open ('O') and closed ('C') (cf. the binary system of a computer).

Bladder Instability - A Struggle between the opening (O) and Closure (C) Reflexes

Figure 6-23 is a urodynamic graph which reflects the events illustrated in figure 6-22. The interpretation given below correlates the urodynamic traces in figure 6-23 with the dynamic events described in figure 6-22. With reference to figures 6-22 and 6-23:

Fig. 6-23 Detrusor instability- a premature activation of a normal micturition reflex. This is a urodynamic graph of a patient with a full bladder undergoing a handwashing test.

The sequence of events is:
(1) a feeling of urgency,
(2) a fall in urethral pressure at X (graph 'U'),
(3) a rise in bladder pressure at Y (graph 'B') then
(4) urine loss arrow, (graph 'CP').

U = urethral pressure graph;
B = bladder pressure graph;
CP = closure pressure graph (U minus B)
C = closure (continence) reflex
O = opening (micturition) reflex, with its components being:
Ou = urethral relaxation;
Od = detrusor contraction;
Om = opening out of the outflow tract.

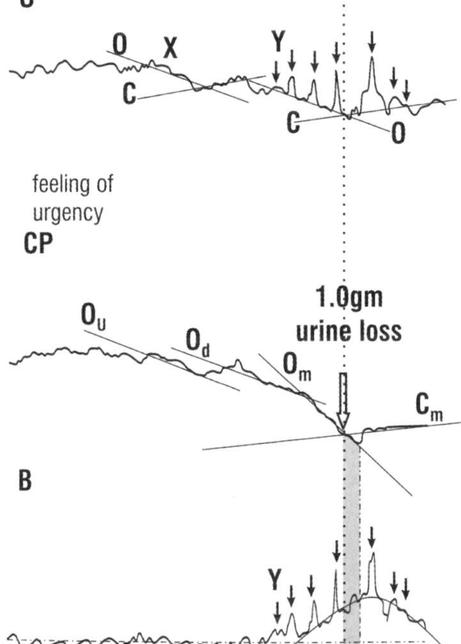

- The afferent impulses from the stretch receptors reach cortical consciousness as feelings of urgency. These pass through the pons to cause a fall in urethral pressure (X, graph U), by causing relaxation of Cm and the PUSM (fig 6-22).
- However, this is soon counteracted by assertion of the closure reflex ('C' on graph U) and so urethral pressure rises.
- This correlates with contraction of the forward arrow, Cm and PUSM, in figure 6-22. The micturition reflex 'O' is too strong, however, and it dominates.
- Thus the closure pressure falls dramatically (graph CP) and detrusor pressure rises (Y graph B) with urine loss (white arrow, graph CP).
- Note the precipitous fall in CP (Om, graph CP). This correlates with opening out of the urethra by the posterior muscle forces Om, in figure 6-22.
- As bladder smooth muscle contracts by muscle-to-muscle transmission (Creed 1979), it effectively 'spasms'. This 'spasm' is denoted by a curve starting at 'Y' in figure 6-23. The small downward arrows (graph U) are consistent with efforts of fast-twitch striated PCM muscles ('Om' fig 6-22) contracting ineffectively against this 'spasm'.

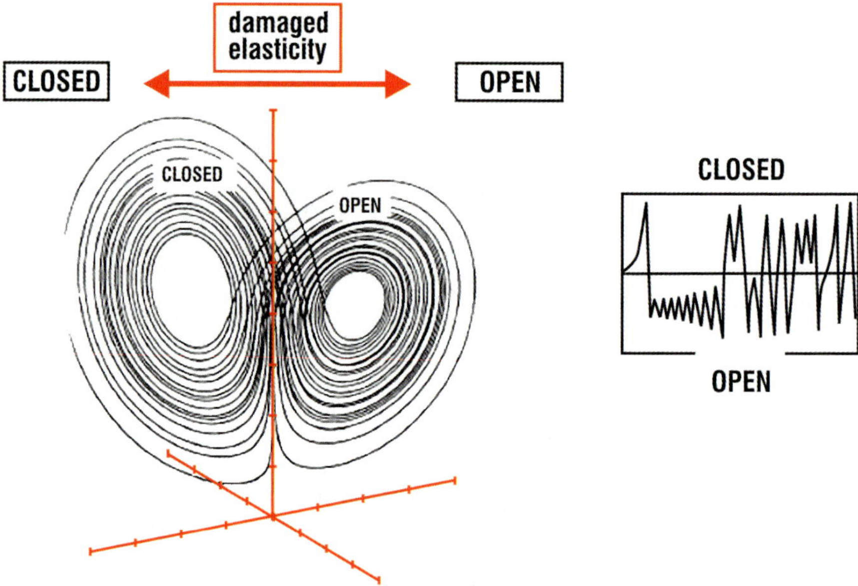

Fig. 6-24 (after Gleick 1987). Unstable opening and closure of the bladder - two competing 'attractors'. With damaged tissues, passive elastic closure is diminished and so the bladder may not be able to either close or open properly. In a continent patient, the 'open' phase (micturition) is a temporary state created by a normal micturition reflex. Damaged connective tissue may prevent passive elastic closure such that the patient now has two competing 'attractors', 'open' and 'closed'. With urgency, the loose vaginal tissue cannot support the hydrostatic pressure of urine and the stretch receptors may fire off at a lower bladder volume: 'detrusor instability'.

Mathematical Testing of Feedback Control of the Micturition Reflex

The graph (fig 6-25) represents iteration of the classical feedback equation, $X_{next} = Xc(1-X)$, where 'X' represents the afferent impulses and 'c' represents the central and peripheral control mechanisms. The maximum number of impulses which can be carried by the system is 1, and $X<1$. As the bladder fills, afferent impulses 'X' travel to the cortex, and these are controlled by 'c'.

When 'c' is small, iteration of the equation shows the impulses are extinguished. This can be correlated with the state of urinary retention.

When 'c' is between 2 and 3, the system is stable and it remains closed. As 'c' becomes larger than 3, the system splits into 2 phases. As 'c' increases further, the phases become a geometric progression, 4, 8, 16, etc., and reach the chaotic zone (Gleick 1987).

In this urodynamic context, low compliance is explained by bladder contraction which is controlled by 'c'. The upper part of the graph (fig 6-25) explains the often seen conversion of low compliance into detrusor instability, a phasic pressure variation in the bladder.

To illustrate the above mathematical testing procedure, the iterations of a simple feed back equation, viz $X_{next} = Xc(1-X)$, are presented below. These are taken from an actual experiment, in which a group of patients were subjected to a handwashing test during fast-fill cystometry. A full account of the experiment and a more detailed analysis on which the above is based is available in Petros (1999).

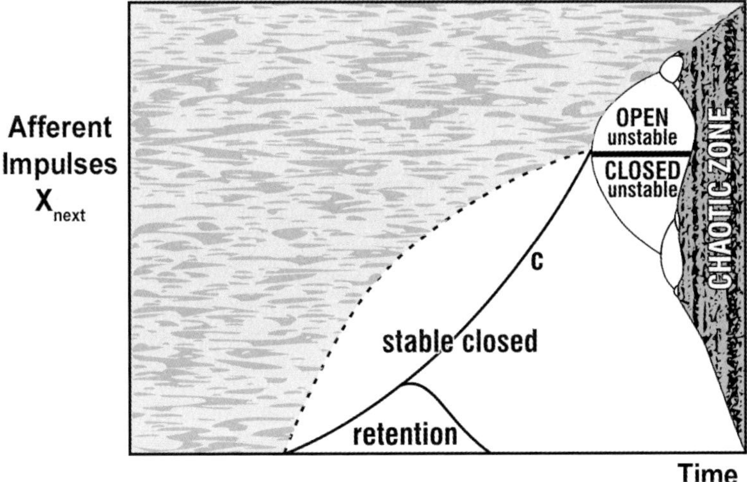

Fig. 6-25 (after Gleick 1987). Feedback control -bladder instability as a manifestation of Chaos Theory. The line 'c' represents the sum of cortical and perpheral inhibition by the musculo-elastic system (two variables). The broken line represents the course plotted when there is only one variable. X_{next} can be equated to the number of afferent impulses and also the detrusor pressure. x axis = time; y axis = X_{next}.

Example of Iterations of a Simple Feedback Equation (as per figure 6-25)

Taking a nominal bladder volume of say, 300ml, and the maximum number of impulses originating from the stretch receptors to be 0.5 (i.e. 50% of the possible maximum), then, based on observed results, (no urgency in a normal patient, a low compliance pattern in some patients, and detrusor instability (DI) and urine loss in others), one can postulate that inhibition of the micturition reflex is working:

- successfully in the normal patient,
- partially in the low compliance group, and
- unsuccessfully in the detrusor instability group.

By equating degrees of inhibition of the micturition reflex with the central and peripheral control mechanisms (c), it is possible to calculate what happens in each system when it is subjected to the feedback process. This is done by using the formula $X_{next} = Xc(1-X)$.

Normal Patient

In figure 6-22, all control systems are assumed to be functioning perfectly, stimulation of 'N' is controlled, and the equation is iterated with a low 'c' value of 0.2.

1st iteration: $X_{next} = 0.5 \times 0.2\ (1 - 0.5) = 0.05$
2nd iteration: $X_{next} = 0.05 \times 0.2\ (1 - 0.05) = 0.019$
3rd iteration: $X_{next} = 0.019 \times 0.2\ (1 - 0.019) = 0.0037$

'X' is almost extinct by the 3rd iteration. This is the 'retention' area in fig. 6-25.

Low Compliance Group

As bladder contraction is an accepted cause of low compliance, and no urine was lost during filling, 'c' needed a value that reflected an activated, but 'stable closed' state, as shown in figure 6-25. The equation was iterated with a 'c' value of 2.0 to reflect a constant 'X' value.

1st iteration: $X_{next} = 0.5 \times 2\ (1 - 0.5) = 0.5$
2nd iteration: $X_{next} = 0.5 \times 2\ (1 - 0.5) = 0.5$
3rd iteration: $X_{next} = 0.5 \times 2\ (1 - 0.5) = 0.5$

'X' remains at 0.5, a steady state at the 3rd iteration. (The 'stable closed' area in fig. 6-25.)

Bladder Instability Group

The patterns of urethral and bladder pressure shown in figure 6-22 are clearly much less controlled, indicating more numerous afferent impulses from the bladder stretch receptors. As 'c' needed to be in the region of >3.0 to reflect fluctuation between the 'unstable open' and 'unstable closed' states, the equation was iterated with a 'c' value of 3.6.

1st iteration: $X_{next} = 0.5 \times 3.6\ (1 - 0.5) = 0.9.$
2nd iteration: $X_{next} = 0.9 \times 3.6\ (1 - 0.9) = 0.324.$
3rd iteration: $X_{next} = 0.324 \times 3.6\ (1 - 0.324) = 0.788.$
4th iteration: $X_{next} = 0.788 \times 3.6\ (1 - 0.788) = 0.601$
5th iteration: $X_{next} = 0.601 \times 3.6\ (1 - 0.399) = 0.864.$
6th iteration: $X_{next} = 0.864 \times 3.6\ (1 - 0.136) = 0.423.$

'X' is oscillating between two states, 'unstable open' and 'unstable closed', as shown in figure 6-25.

6.1.3 Transperineal Ultrasound

Ultrasound uses reflected sound waves to detect soft tissue structures. It is a relatively inexpensive office tool which allows the clinician to determine the dynamic geometry of the pelvic organs, urethra, bladder, vagina, anus and rectum, at rest, during effort and during anchoring of specific connective tissue structures. It can also identify the pelvic muscles, their movements relative to rest, and the location of implanted tapes and meshes. This section explains how the physician can use ultrasound to assess funnelling and rotation of the bladder neck (anterior zone), then proceed to assessment of the other zones. Using the 'simulated operations' of anchoring specific ligaments and observing the changes in urethrovesical geometry, it is possible, over time, for the clinician to gain a greater understanding of the importance of adequately tight ligaments for pelvic floor function. These techniques are also a means of directly testing predictions of the Integral Theory.

The image must be oriented in the sagittal position to obtain accurate data. A 3.5 or 3.75 MHz curvilinear abdominal probe is applied to gently touch the perineum, pointing upwards into the vagina. A split image is used to allow comparison of the geometry of the resting and straining positions. The bladder and urethra are located

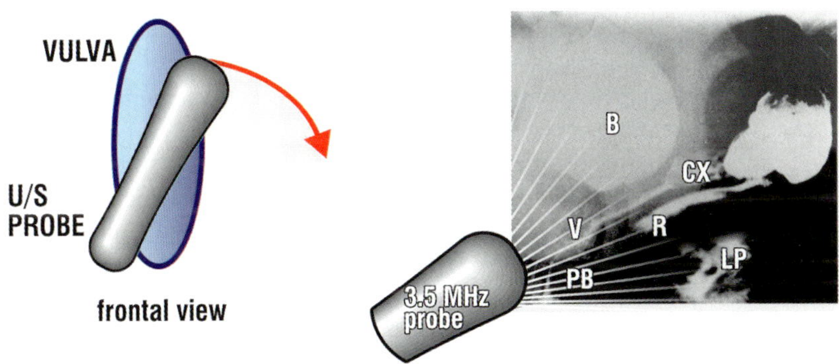

Using the ultrasound probe (above):
Apply probe at an angle of 5 - 10 degrees until the urethra and bladder are outlined. Rotate slowly so as to keep the urethra in focus. To visualise the levator plate, turn the probe at a greater angle until the rectum and posterior muscles come into view. Then follow the movements by angulating the probe.
X-ray (above right) shows the anatomical relationships of the organs in resting position.

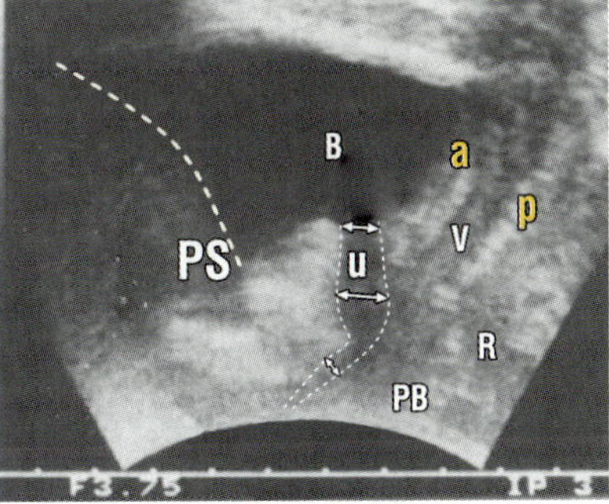

Fig. 6-26 Ultrasound at rest - sagittal view. Patient semi-recumbent. The arrows at bladder neck, mid and distal urethra show the positions used for measuring diameter change from the resting to the straining position. PS = symphysis pubis; a = anterior vaginal wall; p = posterior vaginal wall; U = urethra; V = vagina; R = rectum; PB = perineal body.

at rest. Then, the probe is rotated slightly during straining so as to retain a picture of the urethra as the bladder base descends from the bladder during straining. The three directional forces are easily identified during coughing and straining. Upward movement of all the organs and levator plate are seen when the patient 'squeezes'. The technique is easily learned.

Ultrasound Assessment of the Anterior Zone

Changes in urethral diameter during straining (fig 6-27 right) may be used to assess the integrity of the urethral and bladder neck closure mechanisms. Bladder base descent greater than 10 mm and funnelling during straining might suggest a pubourethral (PUL) defect. Gross rotation and funnelling during straining is evidence of gross laxity in the PUL. Repeating this manoeuvre after unilateral anchoring at midurethra restores geometry and continence (Petros & Von Konsky 1999).

Ultrasound Assessment of the Middle Zone

Knowledge of the middle zone and its relationship to the anterior and posterior zones can be obtained by observing changes in morphology during straining, coughing and after anchoring various connective structures, such as the pubourethral ligament (PUL), arcus tendineus fascia pelvis (ATFP) or uterosacral ligaments (USL). Stretching (and therefore) tightening of the suburethral hammock can sometimes be observed as the cystocoele moves downwards (Petros 1998).

A cystocoele is easily recognized just behind bladder neck. On straining it balloons downwards. Often it is irregular in shape (fig 6-30). A paravaginal defect is not so easily recognized. To detect it, the transducer must be directed more laterally. It is more curved. If there is also some degree of vault prolapse, anchoring the posterior fornix during straining may often result in a marked diminution of the size of the cystocoele. This demonstrates the interconnectedness of the middle zone with the posterior zone.

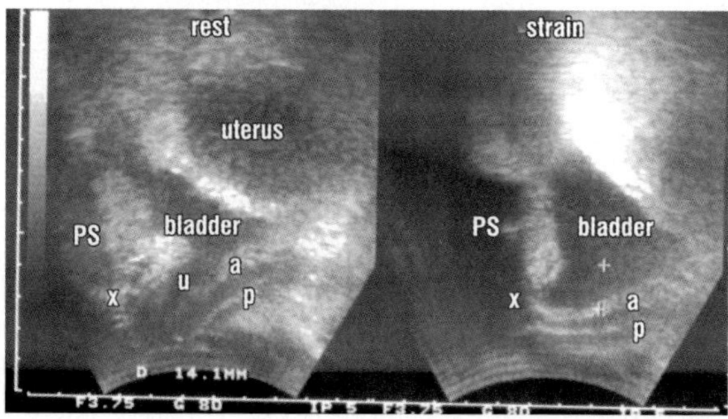

Fig. 6-27 Patient with SI. Left = resting; Right = Straining; The anterior and posterior vaginal walls are stretched backwards to open out the bladder neck.
U = urethra; a & p = anterior and posterior vaginal walls; X = lower border of pubic symphysis (PS). The same directional movements occur during coughing as when straining.

Lateral Attachment of Mesh (M)

After cystocoele repair lateral attachment of mesh can be accurately identified by turning the transducer horizontally and pointing it posteriorly (fig. 6-31). If there is a discrepancy in the level of attachment between the two sides if the attachment, one will be sited lower than the other.

Identification of mesh is very useful. Any detachment from its lateral inserts is readily identified.

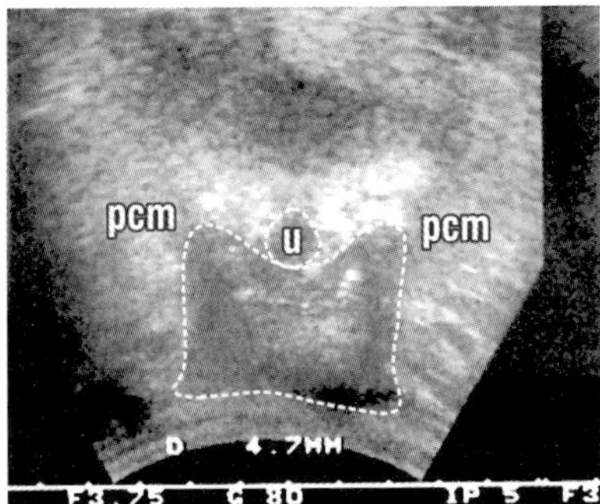

Fig. 6-28 Anterior zone - transverse position of 3.5 MHz probe- focus on midurethra. Note the 'H-shaped' vagina and urethra (U) sited above the anterior vaginal wall. On straining or coughing the angles move sharply upwards as does the distal urethra. When focused more posteriorly, the bladder neck and proximal urethra are pulled downwards.

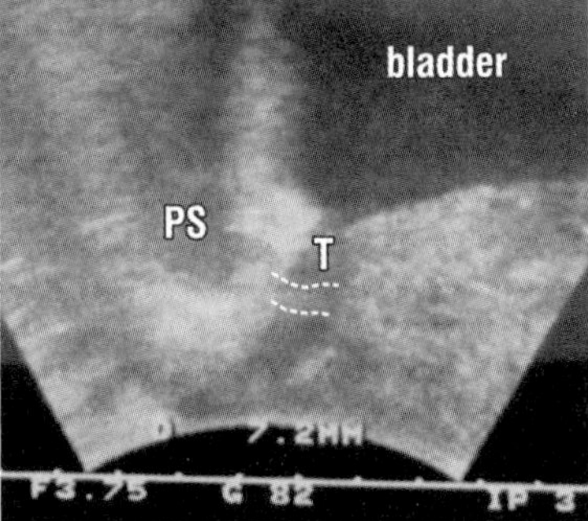

Fig. 6-29 The tape sited at midurethra appears as an opaque strip which passes behind PS. As polypropylene is opaque to ultrasound, it is quite easy to locate. This technique is especially useful for locating the tape in patients with post-operative urethral obstruction after an anterior sling procedure who may require incision of the tape.

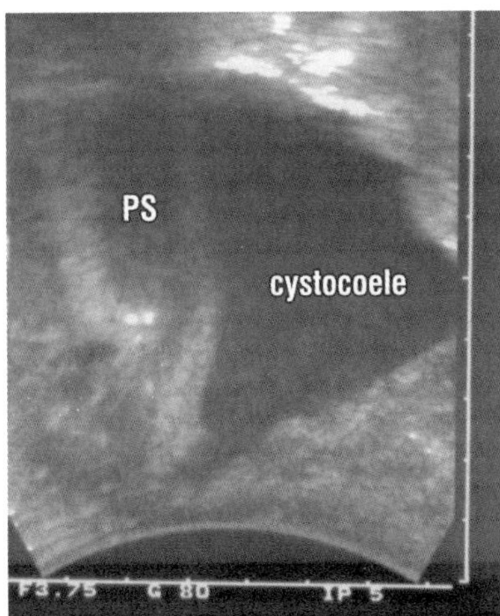

Fig. 6-30 Middle zone cystocoele, 3.75 MHz probe axial

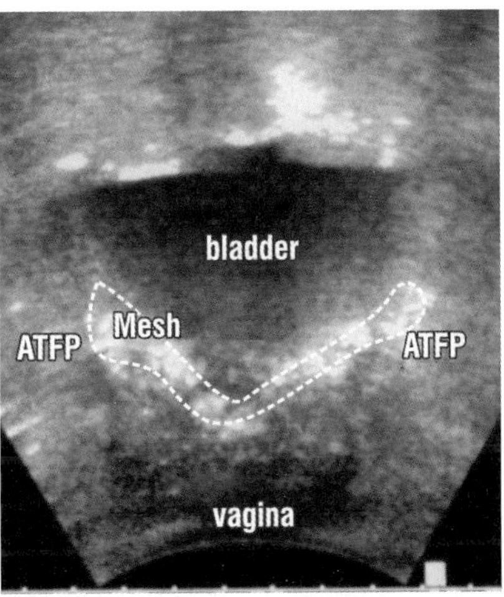

Fig. 6-31 Middle zone ultrasound - identifying mesh. 3.75 MHz probe transverse.

Ultrasound Assessment of the Posterior Zone

With ultrasound it is possible to visualize almost all the structures seen with more invasive or costly techniques, such as video x-ray and MRI, and in a dynamic way. Anchoring vital structures such as perineal body, PUL or USL while testing can give profound insights as to how these structures contribute to pelvic floor geometry and function. Pointing the probe more posteriorly, one can visualize the anus and rectum. Behind the rectum, a thickened vertical muscle mass is sometimes seen. This corresponds to the longitudinal muscle of the anus (LMA). The LMA is separated from the rectum (R) by a space. LMA connects LP to the external anal sphincter. More posteriorly, horizontal collagenous fibres indicate the position of levator plate (LP) and its attachment to the posterior wall of the rectum (fig 6-33). In the normal patient, during straining or coughing, LP moves backwards and upwards, with downward angulation of its anterior border. With a lax perineal body (PB), there may be a momentary downward flicker followed by an upward pull. Digitally anchoring PB restores downward angulation of the anterior border of LP. This sequence of events

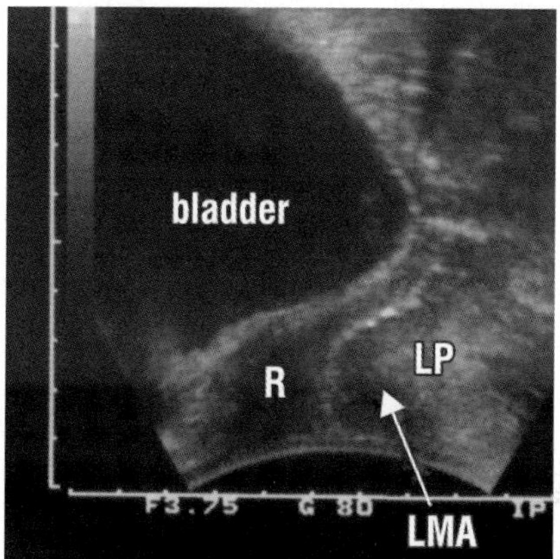

Fig. 6-32 Posterior zone - probe axial

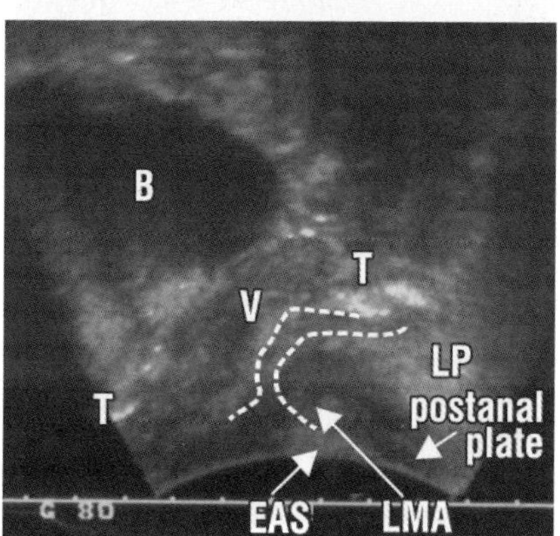

Fig. 6-33 Posterior zone - probe axial

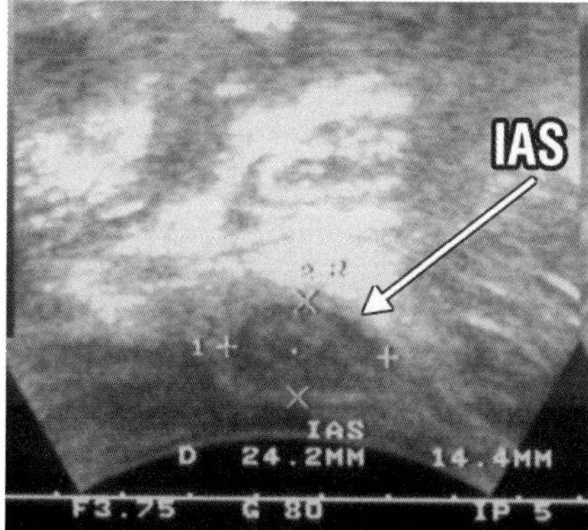

Fig. 6-34 Internal anal sphincter location - probe transverse

convincingly demonstrates that the role of the perineal body is to help anchor the external anal sphincter, the insertion of the downward muscle force (LMA).

The two limbs of the posterior tape 'T' (fig 6-33) attached behind the apex of the posterior vaginal wall 'V' are visible as two thick short opaque lines sitting just above the horizontal part of the rectum (broken lines) and pointing towards the superior surface of levator plate (LP). A midurethral tape 'T' can be seen just above the distal part of the vagina. There is a first degree enterocoele just above 'V' (fig 6-33).

The internal anal sphincter is easily assessed from the perineum, preferably with a 5.5 MHz probe.

The probe is placed on the perineal body and turned backwards (fig 6-34). This is a far less painful method than using the endoanal probe. The thickness of the anterior and posterior parts of the internal anal sphincter muscle can be measured.

6.1.4　The Role of X-rays in the Diagnosis of Ligamentous and Connective Tissue Defects

Although x-rays have been largely supplanted by transperineal ultrasound, insertion of radio-opaque dye into the organs and the levator plate gives valuable information about function and dysfunction.

Anterior Zone X-rays

An intact pubourethral ligament (PUL) is a prerequisite for directional stretching of the vagina by the pelvic muscles. The following x-rays demonstrate organ prolapse occurring due to the inability of PUL to anchor the muscle forces.

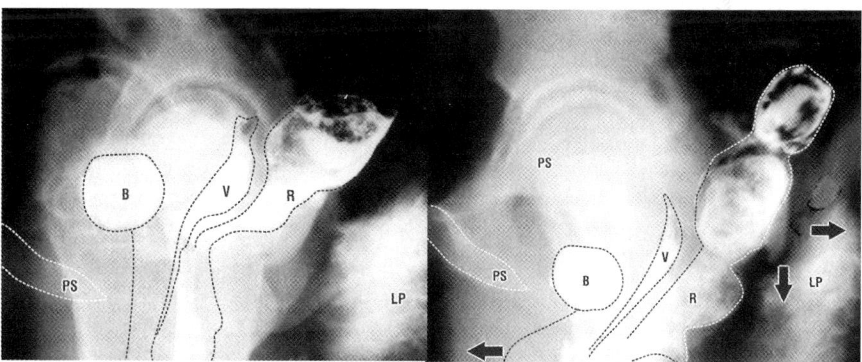

Fig. 6-35 At Rest
PS = pubic symphysis; B = Foley balloon in the bladder; V = vagina; R = rectum; LP = levator plate.

Fig. 6-36 Straining - Pubourethral ligament defect. Note the apparent collapse downwards and backwards of vagina, bladder base and rectum. However, the three directional forces (arrows) appear to be functioning normally. Note the downward angulation of the levator plate (LP).

Middle and Posterior Zone X-rays

The following sequence of x-rays is presented to demonstrate the role of adequately tensioned connective tissue in maintaining normal geometry as well as how an inadequately angulated vagina may predispose to prolapse of the middle and posterior zones.

The Normal Patient

In the normal patient, the proximal vagina (V) is nearly horizontal (fig 6-37). It is compressed on to the rectum (R) during straining (fig 6-38).

Figure 6-37 is a standing lateral x-ray in a normal nulliparous woman at rest. The anatomical relationships are essentially normal. '1', '2' and '3' delineate the three levels of the pelvis (cf. anatomy section). The angle 'a' is the angle of the proximal vagina (V) to the horizontal.

Figure 6-38 shows a downward angulation of the vagina around perineal body (PB) and midurethra. Note the obvious stretching backwards of vagina and rectum, and the downward angulation of the levator plate (LP). The angle 'a' becomes almost zero as the vagina is stretched virtually to a horizontal position. Note the compression of level 2.

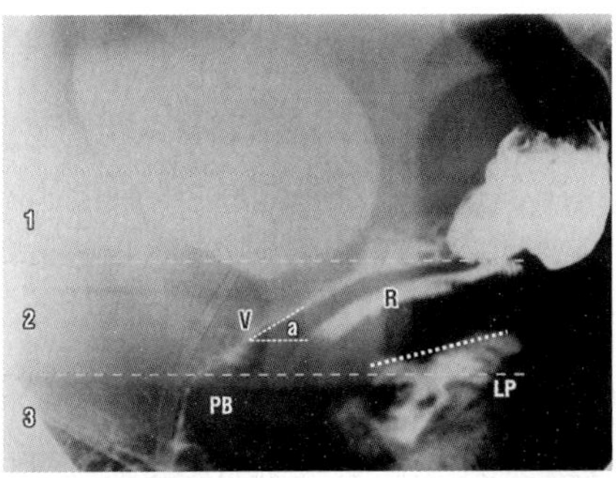

Fig. 6-37 (above) The role of the posterior zone - at rest. R = rectum; LP = levator plate.

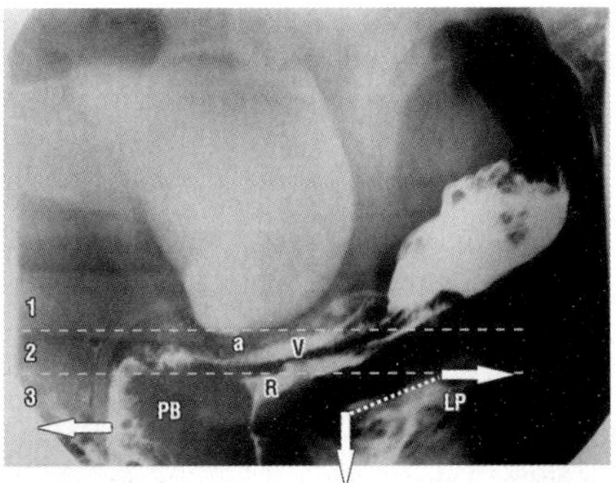

Fig. 6-38 (above) Role of the posterior zone - Straining.

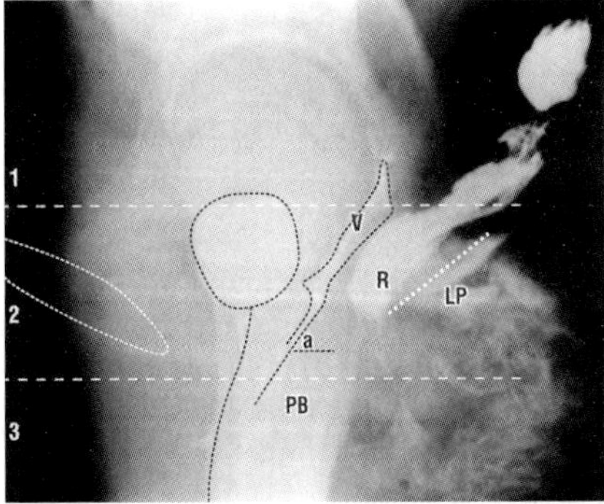

Fig. 6-39 At rest

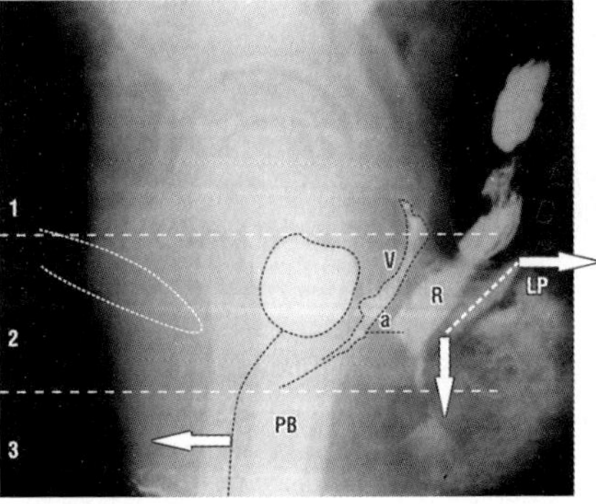

Fig. 6-40 Straining

Abnormal Middle and Posterior Zone Anatomy X-rays

There is failure to convert the abnormal vertical position of the vagina at rest (fig 6-39) to a horizontal position during straining (fig 6-40). The intra-abdominal and pelvic floor forces distend an already weakened vagina.

In figure 6-40 there is normal movement downwards and backwards of the Foley balloon, and the three directional forces (arrows) appear to be working adequately. However, there is little change in the angle 'a', and there is obvious distortion downwards of the central wall of vagina 'V', indicating also a middle zone defect.

There is no compression of level 2. Given the apparent normal functioning of the three muscle forces, the anatomical defect appears to be in the connective tissue insertions of the system, between muscle (LP) and vagina and perhaps perineal body also.

Clearly, weakness in the uterosacral ligaments (USL), rectovaginal fascia (RVF) and perineal body (PB) may all contribute to such dysfunction.

6.2.4 Dynamic Mapping with 'Simulated Operations': A Clinical Example

In the Integral Theory framework, diagnosis seeks to test the predictions of damage derived from the Clinical Assessment or Structured Assessment pathways. Diagnosis testing by means of 'simulated operations' is especially useful in patients with urgency symptoms as these are not 'zone specific'. As the 'trampoline analogy' demonstrates, any ligament, if loose, may cause urgency symptoms. With 'simulated operations' methodology, the patient herself is used as the 'urodynamic machine'; that is, the reference point to determine by how much urgency symptoms are diminished while a particular structure is being mechanically supported.

The following case report is presented as an example of the extent to which this method can assist the diagnostic process. It is emphasized that only the *changes* in stress or urge (table in fig 6-41) are used in clinical decision making. The changes in ultrasound and urodynamics simply reinforce the fact that restoration of anatomy also restores function.

Background to the Clinical Example

The patient, a 32 year old, stated that she had suffered from both stress and urge incontinence all her life, but these symptoms had worsened since childbirth. Symptomatically, she had stress incontinence, urge incontinence, frequency 13-20 times per day, nocturia 4-5 times per night, difficulty in emptying her bladder, and low abdominal and sacral backache. On examination, there was obvious laxity in her external urethral ligaments, and suburethral vagina (hammock). She had second degree uterovaginal prolapse, second degree enterocele, and second degree paravaginal defect. Referring to the Pictorial Diagnostic Algorithm, it was clear she had anatomical defects in all three zones of the vagina. On urodynamic testing, there was sensory urgency but no detrusor instability. Her bladder capacity was 356 ml, emptying time

26 seconds, her maximum flow rate was 50 ml/sec and residual 170 ml. On cough stress testing (10 coughs), she lost a total of 5.1gm and she lost 26 gm of urine on 24 hour pad testing.

The algorithm indicated there was connective tissue laxity in all three zones of vagina. The patient was assessed with a full bladder and described strong feelings of urgency in the supine position.

The Intervention - 'Simulated Operation'

The structures 1-6, (6-41) in three zones of vagina were anchored seriatim. All results recorded were as agreed by two observers. A haemostat was unilaterally applied to the external urethral ligaments '1' and pubourethral ligaments '2'. The sub urethral vaginal hammock '3' was tightened unilaterally by taking up a fold of the vagina. Ring forceps were applied paravaginally '5', in both sulci, just behind the bladder neck, and also to anchor the cervix (the uterosacral ligaments '6') and to support the bladder base '4'. Care was taken not to obstruct the urethra during the anchoring process. The pressure applied was firm, but not sufficient to elicit pain. The reference points for the objective tests were the funnelling observed during straining on perineal ultrasound, and the zero closure pressure observed during coughing. The same 6 interventions were applied:

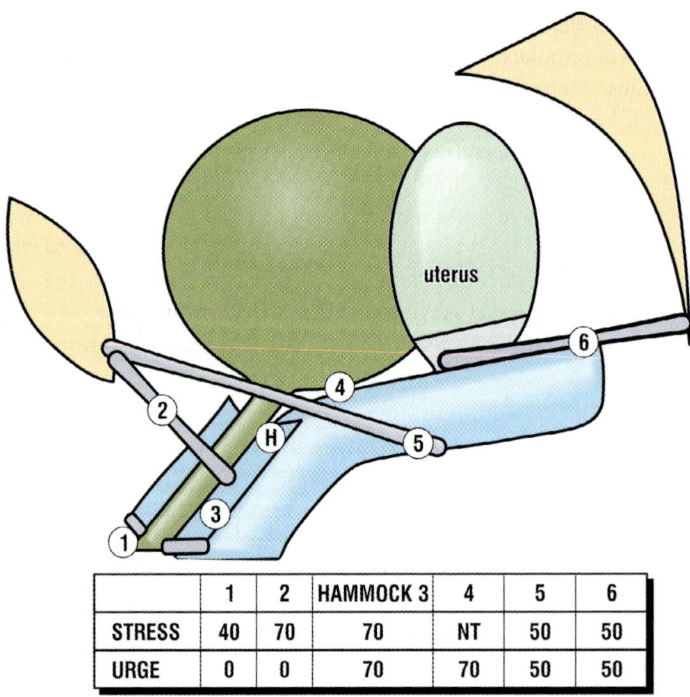

	1	2	HAMMOCK 3	4	5	6
STRESS	40	70	70	NT	50	50
URGE	0	0	70	70	50	50

Fig. 6-41 Changes in stress and urge incontinence. The figures represent the percentage diminution in observed urine loss on coughing ('stress') and percentage diminution in urge symptoms ('urge') following the anchoring, in turn, of each structure 1-6.

a) in the supine resting position. Percentage subjective diminution of urge symptoms with interventions 1 through 6 was recorded (fig 6-41);
b) in the supine position during repeated vigorous coughing (minimum 8 times). The percentage diminution in urine loss with interventions 1-6 was agreed upon by two observers (fig 6-41);
c) in the supine position during a single straining episode with simultaneous perineal ultrasound monitoring, the changes in urethrovesical geometry with interventions 1-6 were observed and recorded on film;
d) in the supine position during repeated vigorous coughing (minimum 8 times) simultaneous bladder and urethral pressures were recorded with interventions 1-6 using dual Gaeltec mictrotip transducers spaced 6 cm apart drawn through the urethra with an electric puller.

Note: the clinical, urodynamic and ultrasound tests were not performed simultaneously, but within a few minutes of each other.

The Post-Intervention Results – Anchoring One Structure at a Time

The post-intervention results are summarized collectively in figure 6-41 (clinical), the ultrasound results in figures 6-43 to 6-48 inclusive, and the closure pressure results in figures 6-49 to 6-55 inclusive.

Figure 6-41 is a schematic sagittal representation of the supporting structures of the vagina, bladder base and urethra. '1' is the external urethral ligament (EUL), '2' the pubourethral ligament (PUL), 'H' or '3' is the hammock, '4' the bladder base, '5' is the arcus tendineus fasciae pelvis (ATFP) and '6' is the uterosacral (USL). These were anchored seriatim, and the percentage diminution of symptoms of stress and urgency on supporting each structure is indicated.

Post intervention Results – Two Structures Anchored Simultaneously

This patient presented an ideal opportunity to directly challenge one aspect of the Integral Theory, that all structural components of the pelvic floor may play a synergistic role in maintaining continence for urge and stress. With reference to figure 6-41, tightening the hammock '3' plus midurethral anchoring '2' simultaneously gave 100% control of urine loss during coughing. Anchoring the cervix '6' plus both ATFP's '5' simultaneously diminished urgency symptoms to zero.

Figures 6-42 to 6-48 (inclusive) show the impact of support during ultrasound observations. These examples are presented to emphasize the potential of 'simulated operations' when applied to verifying tests such as ultrasound and urodynamics. The same techniques have also been applied during filling cystometry ('detrusor instability') and to determine the effect on tissue stiffness using a piezo-electric probe.

Comment

The morphological changes in the urethrovesical angle, bladder base descent, and the anterior and posterior shelf of the bladder (figs 6-43 to 6-48 inclusive) are of special interest. The 'shelf' is formed by the bladder trigone. The urethral pressure results are presented in terms of closure pressure change in the proximal and distal parts of the urethra. The functional urethral length is obviously lengthened during anchoring of

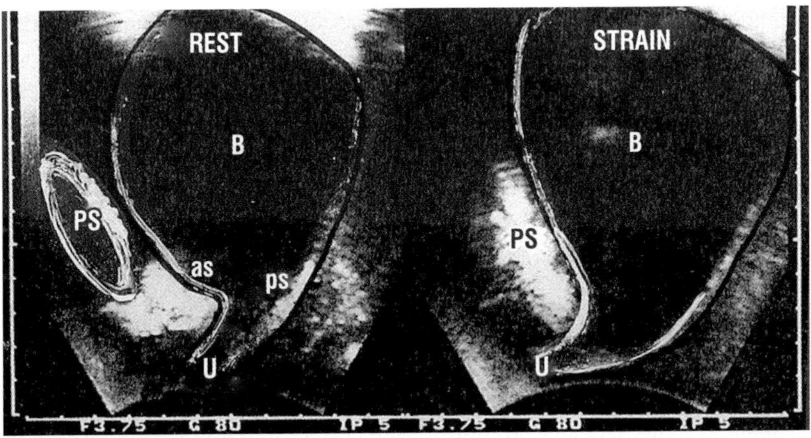

Fig. 6-42 (above) Ultrasound at rest
B = bladder; PS=pubic symphysis;
U = urethra; as = anterior bladder shelf;
ps = posterior bladder shelf.
Same labelling for all figures.

Fig. 6-43 (above) Ultrasound during straining
– This figure is the reference point for all
interventions. Note descent of bladder base and
funnelling of proximal urethra and associated
urine leakage on straining. Note absence of ps.

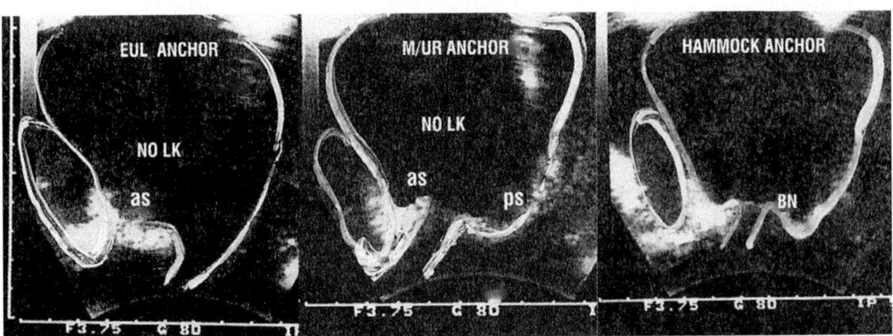

Fig. 6-44 EUL – During
straining with EUL anchor.
Note bladder base still
descends and funnels, but
there has been a restitution
of the anterior bladder shelf,
and no leakage on straining.

Fig. 6-45 PUL – During
straining with PUL anchor.
There is no bladder base
descent or funnelling. Note
restitution of anterior and
posterior bladder shelf, with
no leakage on straining.

Fig. 6-46 Hammock – During
straining with hammock
tightening. There is no bladder
base descent or funnelling.
Note restitution of anterior
and posterior bladder shelf,
with no leakage on straining.

the hammock, ATFP and cervix. With repeated vigorous coughing, control of urine loss with single anchoring was incomplete, 70% with either PUL ('2') or hammock ('3') anchoring (fig 6-41). Complete control of urine loss was achieved by combining two or more anchorings. For stress incontinence, combined tightening of the hammock plus PUL gave complete control of urine loss even with strong repetitive coughing. When both ATFP and cervical anchoring were combined, control of urge was total. *Combining two such 'simulated operations' directly demonstrates the synergistic action of structures in maintaining urinary continence.*

The change in closure pressure can be explained with reference to the formula Pressure = Force/Area (of the urethral tube). Improved closure as evidenced by

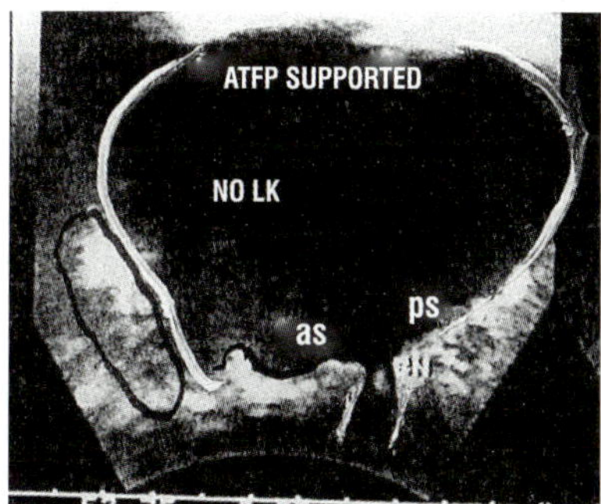

Fig. 6-47 (above) ATFP During straining with ATFP support. There is no bladder base descent or funnelling. Note restitution of anterior and posterior bladder shelf, with no leakage on straining.

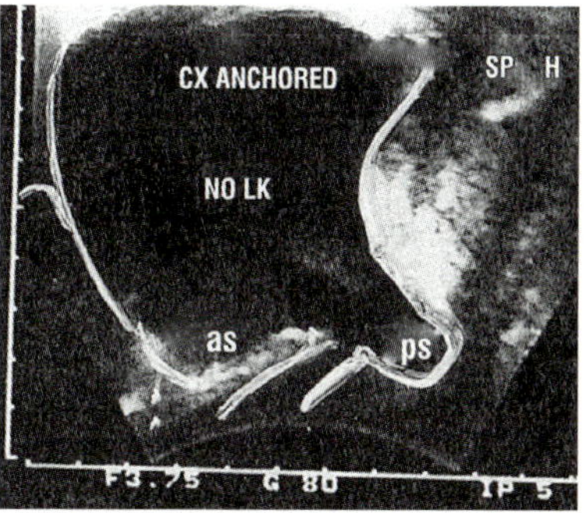

Fig. 6-48 (above) USL – During straining with anchoring of cervix. There is no bladder base descent or funnelling. Note restitution of anterior and posterior bladder shelf, with no leakage on straining.

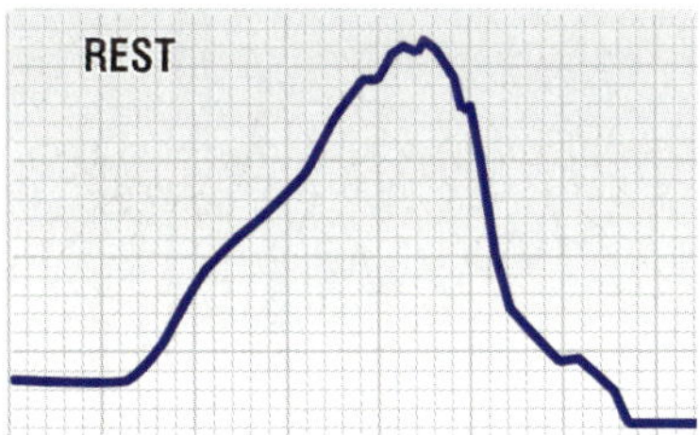

Fig. 6-49 (above) Urethral pressure at rest.

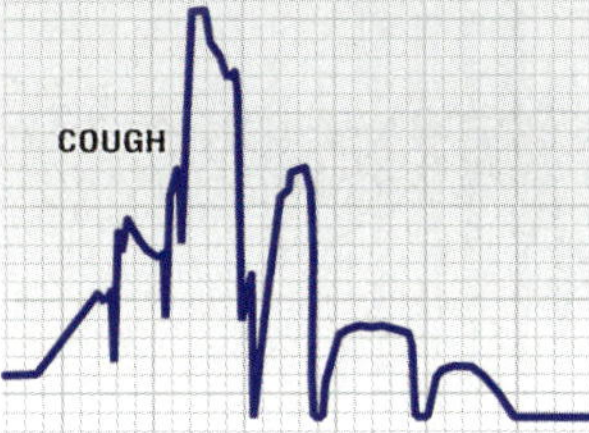

Fig. 6-50 (above) Urethral closure pressure (UCP) during coughing – The closure pressure is diminished in the proximal urethra, falling to zero in the distal urethra. This is the reference point for all subsequent interventions.

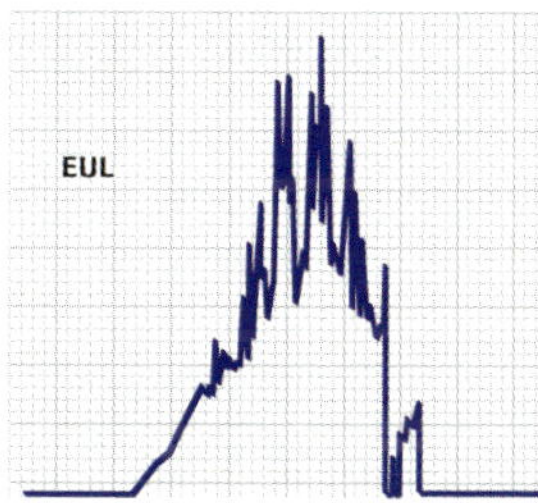

Fig. 6-51 (left) UCP during coughing with EUL anchor – The closure pressure is significantly increased in all parts of the urethra.

decreased urine loss with stress indicates the intra-urethral area was narrowed, also causing the intra-urethral pressure to rise.

Anchoring the insertion points of the muscles may work much like a trampoline: even one loose spring may prevent the membrane being tensioned. Restoring damaged ligaments (springs) allows the three muscle forces to stretch the vaginal membrane (trampoline). This supports the bladder base, preventing premature activation of the stretch receptors and consequently, the micturition reflex (sensation of urgency).

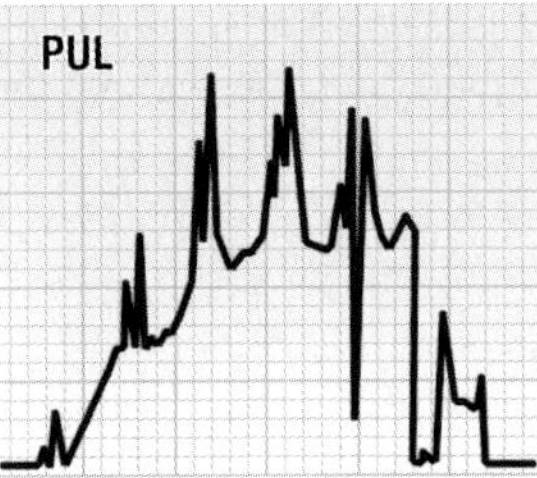

Fig. 6-52 (above) UCP during coughing with PUL anchor – The closure pressure is significantly increased in all parts of the urethra.

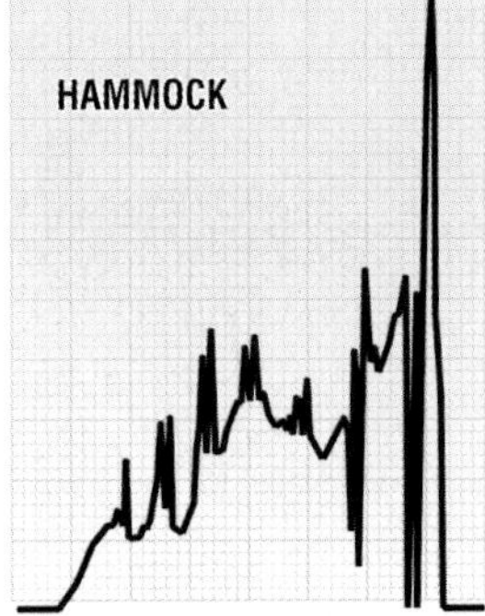

Fig. 6-53 (above) UCP during coughing with hammock tightening. The closure pressure is significantly increased in all parts of the urethra, as is functional urethral length (FUL).

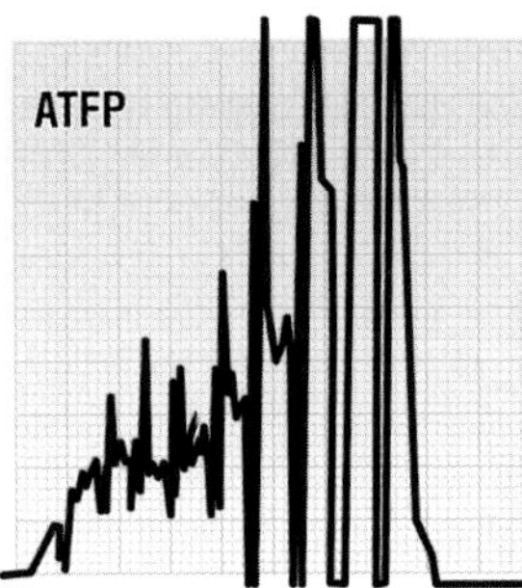

Fig. 6-54 (left) UCP during coughing with ATFP anchor. There is no significant improvement in closure pressure in any part of the urethra. This is an increase in PUL.

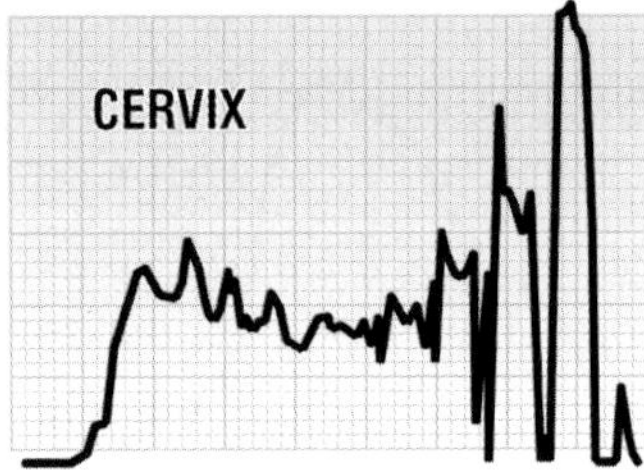

Fig. 6-55 (right) UCP during coughing with cervical anchoring. The closure pressure is significantly increased in the proximal urethra, but not distal urethra.

Acknowledgement: The author is grateful to Pr. Dr. Med B. Abendstein from Hall, Austria for his assistance with the test procedures.

Conclusion

These are coarse tests, but they do give an insight into the synergistic action of different structures. It is highly likely that pressure applied at one site (hammock) may have also partly anchored an adjacent site (PUL). As both belong to the anterior zone, and as both should be repaired during surgery, precise differentiation is not a practical concern.

Even with this limitation, the results emphasize the collective contributions of individual structures to the whole system thereby supporting the Integral Theory. Each of the six interventions created a symptomatic or objective change, while two simultaneous anchoring points were required to achieve total control of stress and urge.

This study gives a brief insight into the synergism of multiple structures in continence control. 'Simulated operations' appear to be a useful technique in determining more precisely which ligamentous/connective tissue defects may be contributing to stress and urge symptoms.

6.3   Summary Chapter 6

Urethral resistance, and especially how it changes exponentially (to the 4th power) with the changes in diameter enacted by the opening and closure mechanisms, is presented as the very basis for urodynamics, both as concerns intra-urethral pressure measurement and, flow. A prematurely activated micturition reflex explains both detrusor instability (DI) and the 'low compliance' bladder.

The concept of non-linear control of the opening and closure mechanisms, and the role of Chaos Theory in explaining symptom variability and inconsistency is introduced. The anatomical basis for DI is explained with reference to an actual urodynamic graph.

'Dynamic mapping' of the three zones of the vagina using ultrasound, urethral pressure and the patient's own perception of her symptoms as the reference point' in an individual patient demonstrate the synergistic nature of the three zones of the vagina in control of urgency symptoms and urine loss during coughing.

Current and Emerging Research Issues

7.1   Introduction

The muscles, nerves and ligaments of the pelvic floor work synergistically to maintain the *structure* of the pelvic floor and the proper *functioning* (opening and closure) of the pelvic organs. In terms of structure and function, connective tissue is the most vulnerable component of the pelvic floor. Two key precepts of the Integral Theory are:

1. Even a minor degree of ligamentous laxity has the potential to cause major pelvic floor symptoms;
2. These symptoms are potentially curable by reinforcing the pelvic ligaments using polypropylene tapes.

The validity of this simple surgical concept has been substantiated already by more than 500,000 anterior sling operations for cure of stress incontinence. There is also a rapidly growing validation of posterior zone symptom cure following the posterior sling. Therefore, it can no longer be stated that these conditions are surgically incurable. The minimalist surgical approach postulated by the theory and the excellent results, have facilitated a rapid evolution in surgical technique, as well as a plethora of delivery instruments and tapes. All this activity in surgical methods is a healthy sign of growth and it is to be encouraged.

Surgical techniques developed within the Integral Theory framework have been significantly refined and minimized, but some important questions remain, especially concerning the long term effects of interventions and materials. Individual clinicians must decide which technique, which tape, which material, (homologous, heterologous or synthetic) to use, according to their training and experience. All options have their risks and benefits. The solutions will only come from well-planned statistically relevant clinical trials, not from anecdotal descriptions. Any scientific comparisons must examine all risks and benefits, not focus on a single particular issue. The most significant challenges facing the proponents of the theory are:

1. To develop a reliable and accurate diagnostic system to find which structures have been damaged;
2. To accurately define the relationship of each structural component to a particular dysfunction.

The sections which follow are devoted to current and emerging research issues. They are presented under separate headings. Some, such as the cure of idiopathic faecal incontinence, have been significantly documented. Others, such as interstitial cystitis and vulvar vestibulitis, having only a few case reports and associations with other symptoms specific to a particular zone of the pelvis, are merely postulated.

A third, more fundamental issue, is the development of an understanding at the micro level. This involves issues about changes in the biochemistry of the tissue, the collagen cross links, etc. At present, it is not possible to assess a particular structure in this way. There is clinical and experimental evidence of genetically defective connective tissue in certain families. This helps to explain the occurrence of abnormal symptoms in nulliparous women.

Although oestrogen has little therapeutic impact on symptoms, there is evidence that oestrogen may prevent collagen degradation after the menopause.

Surgically, being able to assess subclinical damage in an apparently normal structure, is of considerable importance. Shull (1992) reported greater than 30% 'blowout' in other parts of the vagina following a site-specific repair. Up to 20% such herniations, in particular cystocoele, may occur after posterior IVS surgery. The reinforcing of one subsystem is likely to concentrate (or shift) the pelvic floor forces onto another weak part of the system and thereby cause another 'blowout' of the vaginal membrane. For example, the author has seen several cases of stress incontinence developing *de novo*, months after vault prolapse repair by Posterior IVS. Much work is needed at the micro level to determine hormonal and the other factors that influence connective tissue, genetics, effects of childbirth and ageing.

Currently, there are no reliable objective methods for gauging strength and elasticity of connective tissue. Improvements to diagnosis and management will come from a better assessment of connective tissue strength, and a better understanding of the interaction of structures within the pelvic floor.

A major obstacle in this endeavour is the non-linearity of the interactions between pelvic floor structures. In particular, how even minor variations in the degree of damage may result in quite different symptom expression in individual patients. The variation may be as extreme as from no symptoms with major damage, to major symptoms with minor damage. The symptomatic manifestations depend entirely on the balance of all the elements (nerves, muscle forces, and connective tissues) within the pelvic floor system. (see Chapter 3).

Constructing an elastometer which can 'map' the physical characteristics, strength and elasticity of the organs of the pelvic floor and their suspensory ligaments will be an important step towards assessing the biomechanical characteristics of connective tissue. Muscle size can be assessed using MRI and ultra sound techniques. From these it is possible to infer muscle forces. The biomechanical characteristics of the tissue, and the forces which act on them, are key components in the quest to develop a mathematical model of bladder neck opening and closure. It is hoped that successful mathematical modelling - a 'finite element model' - will allow analysis of pelvic floor functions in the same way that structural engineers use mathematical models to analyse potential stresses on structures.

An example of this methodology is the non-linear mathematical model of micturition created at the University of Western Australia by Professor Bush and his team using ABAQUS software. This model examined (and confirmed) some of the Integral Theory's predictions as regards micturition. The approach used in this model has potential application for unravelling the anatomical causation of specific symptoms in the individual patient. It may also help predict how surgical reinforcement of one part of the system may cause decompensation in other subclinically damaged structures[1]. Such sophisticated analysis will be based on improved applications of urodynamics and ultrasound, and will also require instruments which can accurately assess various structural aspects of the pelvic floor, such as tissue structure (strength and elasticity), strength of muscle force contraction, and effectiveness of the ligamentous anchoring points. The analysis will be enhanced by the development of an extensive and relevant data base to correlate specific symptoms with clinical outcomes following surgical repair of specific structures. This will allow more accurate probability factors to be calculated for each condition (figs1-11, 3-09). The computational power required even for the micturition model is very large and time consuming. However, improved methodology, and improved computer software and hardware will make "Finite Element Modelling' a reality in future clinical management.

7.2   Improvements in the Diagnostic Decision Path

The Integral Theory divides diagnosis into three zones of potential damage. This is a simple and efficient starting point, but it requires continuous refinement and adaptation in practice. How variations and error in the diagnostic process can be reduced or eliminated is of particular interest.

Diagnosing the 'zone of damage' involves a decision path based on a probability distribution of the occurrence of a symptom or test result. Refinement of the probability analysis is an ideal application for computer-assisted diagnosis. A significant decrease in pre-operative diagnostic error was demonstrated by the author in application of the Integral Theory Diagnostic Support (ITDS) system. The ITDS system has been planned as a dynamic tool which will improve in diagnostic accuracy as the data base increases over time. As the data base grows, feedback diagnosis will allow the clinician to more accurately define the weighting to be applied to each existing parameter, as well as providing the ability to add new parameters. For this to occur, data from many thousands of cases will be needed. The strategy is to develop a system whereby hundreds of clinicians can post anonymous data via the internet.

---

[1] 'Mechanical Model For the Opening of the Female Urethra', by Messner-Pellenc L. and Moron from the Departement de Mecanique, Ecole Polytechnique France and Professor Mark Bush from The University of Western Australia, School of Mechanical Engineering. The urethra was initially modelled using only the inflation from bladder contraction. Using material data of urethral properties from other studies, the characteristic funnelling observed during micturition could not be obtained. Furthermore, a force much greater than 60cm H_2O was required to inflate the urethra, suggesting that the internal pressure generated from the bladder may not have been sufficient to inflate the urethra. The funnelled shape was obtained by fixing the distal urethra, and applying external downward and backward forces to the proximal urethra. Even here, stiffening to the anterior and posterior urethral wall nodes was needed to obtain the funnelling: anteriorly, consistent with the ligament of Gilvernet, and, posteriorly, with the trigonal extension along the posterior wall of the urethra. The complete dissertation is available on the internet at: www.integraltheory.org.

7.3   The Integral Theory Diagnosis Support System (ITDS)

The Integral Theory Diagnosis Support System (ITDS) is a computerized version of the Structured Diagnostic system. It also has a data base function. With data from the questionnaire put into the computer, it pictorially presents anatomical defects in the three zones of vagina. The diagnosis is modified after input from the vaginal examination, and again after the ultrasound and urodynamics examinations.

The necessary resources for ITDS are contained on a compact disc which can be ordered from the website developed to accompany this book (www.integraltheory.org). The questionnaire, examination and urodynamics sheets are bar-coded for ease of use. It is emphasized that the diagnostic part of the ITDS is only a support tool. The ultimate responsibility for diagnosis and management rests, as always, with the attending surgeon.

7.4   Possible Clinical Associations

Many discoveries from the Integral Theory were made by a process of listing possible associations of symptoms and then following them up with a more deductive approach. The association of symptoms and anatomical defects presented in the Pictorial Diagnostic Algorithm are sufficiently documented to be used in diagnosis. There are other conditions based on associations that are not so well documented and these are potentially important research targets.

7.4.1 Vulvar Vestibulitis (Vulvodynia)

Vulvar vestibulitis is a symptom of the posterior zone. It is a disabling condition which occurs in up to 15% of women aged between 18 and 64. It is characterized by extreme entry dyspareunia. It is diagnosed by using a cotton bud applicator to gently touch the vestibule around the hymenal ring and the external urethral meatus. This gentle touching causes extreme discomfort for the patient.

Women with vestibulitis experience an intolerable pain sensation. Currently, the most efficacious treatment involves vestibulectomy or pelvic floor muscles exercises. Such treatment leads to cure rates of 85% and 50%, respectively (Marinoff 1991). The aetiology of vulvar vestibulitis has not yet been elucidated. In association with Professor Jacob Bornstein, of Haifa, Israel, the author has observed three consecutive patients who experienced complete cure of their vulvar vestibulitis by inserting a posterior sling to reinforce the posterior zone.

Other symptoms of the posterior fornix syndrome, urgency, frequency, nocturia and abnormal bladder emptying were also improved in these patients. This has given rise to a hypothesis that vulvar vestibulitis could be a referred pain caused by insufficient ligament support for the afferent unmyelinated nerve fibres carried in the uterosacral ligaments. Although only three women have been assessed so far, and the follow up six months only, the results are promising.

This hypothesis has been tested further. Two cc of 2% Xylocaine was injected into each of the uterosacral ligaments at the posterior fornix of the vagina of 10 consecutive patients who had been diagnosed with vulvodynia. The 10 patients were retested after five minutes. Eight patients reported complete disappearance of introital sensitivity, to two separate examiners. In the other two patients, direct testing confirmed that the allodynia (exaggerated sensitivity) had disappeared on one side, but remained on the other side. Retesting the patients showed that the blocking effects disappeared after 30 minutes.

The short-term disappearance of introital pain especially on one side is an important step in further substantiating the hypothesis that vulvodynia may be a referred pain originating from failure of lax uterosacral ligaments to support the afferent pain fibres within them.

7.4.2 Interstitial Cystitis

Three patients with Interstitial Cystitis (IC) have been observed with more than an 80% improvement of symptoms following posterior ligament reconstruction with polypropylene tapes. Although the results from these three cases were not in themselves sufficient to draw conclusions, they were instrumental in initiating a survey of known IC cases. With the assistance of Sandy McNicol, secretary of the Canadian Interstitial Cystitis Society, the structured Integral Theory Questionnaire (Appendix 1) was distributed to members. Of 136 questionnaires completed in the year 2000, 130 had two or more parameters consistent with posterior ligamentous laxity (Petros PE, unpublished data). It is known that vulvar vestibulitis and interstitial cystitis are related. Furthermore, urgency and pelvic pain are key symptoms in patients with posterior zone defect. Although any causal relationship is hypothetical at this stage, the association does require further investigation.

7.4.3 Unresolved Nocturnal Enuresis and Daytime Incontinence

In 1992 two young women, aged 14 and 17 years were assessed. Both were post-pubertal, both had unresolved nocturnal enuresis and daytime incontinence since they were babies. The 17 year old also had faecal incontinence. Standing x-ray assessment with dye in a Foley balloon catheter and vagina demonstrated excessive rotation and descent of the Foley balloon similar to that shown in figure 6-36 (page 167). Both patients were entirely cured of their nocturnal enuresis following an IVS operation to reconstruct the pubourethral ligament. Post-operative x-ray demonstrated the restoration of normal urethrovesical geometry at straining. It is emphasized that these patients had daytime urge and stress incontinence as well, a pattern different to that seen in most cases of nocturnal enuresis. Over the next ten years patients were asked specifically about nocturnal enuresis clearing or improving at puberty. More than 50 such patients were found. In many, the bed wetting improved at puberty, but they continued to be incontinent until cured by an anterior sling. Almost invariably there was a family history of this condition through the generations, both male and female.

The anatomical explanations given here for conditions such as nocturnal enuresis and vesico-uretic reflux intersect with those of paediatric urology. The anatomy and function in children cannot be very different to adults and it may be useful to re-examine some long-held concepts of female paediatric urology in the light of connective tissue anchoring points and muscle forces.

7.4.3 Vesico-Ureteric Reflux

A 42 year old patient presented with classical symptoms and radiological evidence of vesico-ureteric reflux. She was clinically cured of her symptoms with an anterior midurethral sling. It is possible to explain this patient's improvement by reference to the musculoelastic model for urethrovesical closure (fig 2-12). The ureters travel through the bladder wall before reaching the trigone. Because the bladder trigone relies on firm ligamentous attachments (which allow it to be stretched by the striated muscles of the pelvic floor), ligamentous laxity may loosen the trigone sufficiently to cause reflux.

Although only one case has been reported, its analysis may lead to new research and treatment directions for this condition.

7.5 Faecal Incontinence

In 1985, evidence of delayed pudendal nerve conduction times was presented (Swash et al. 1985). Attention was drawn to the coincidence of urinary and faecal incontinence (FI) and the role of damaged muscle in causation. Although this was an important scientific observation, it did not explain why FI occurred in nulliparas, or in patients without evidence of pelvic muscle damage. From the very first IVS operations for stress incontinence (SI) in 1988, the simultaneous cure of FI was observed in 90% of patients. Later, cure of FI following posterior IVS operation was also observed in situations where FI was associated with posterior zone symptoms but with no significant SI symptoms. Because these operations correct connective tissue only, it was concluded that damaged connective tissue was, most likely, an important cause of FI.

In 1993 Sultan et al. demonstrated a relationship between damaged internal anal sphincter (IAS) and FI in ten out of eleven patients who had evidence of damaged IAS on endoanal ultrasound. The implication of this study was that a damaged IAS may be an important cause of FI. As this concept was contrary to the data obtained by the author and other colleagues who were using the Integral Theory system, further studies were undertaken.

By this time, a musculo-elastic hypothesis for anorectal function and dysfunction had been conceptualized within the Integral Theory framework (Petros 1999). The sequence of observational experiments that is described in the section that follows were planned to test these different hypotheses seriatim.

First, a series of radiological and ultrasound studies were performed. Then a case report was presented demonstrating control of cough FI with midurethral anchoring.

To assess the relationship between FI and damaged IAS, a prospective endoanal ultrasound study was undertaken in 50 consecutive patients. Then endoanal pressure studies following reflex stimulation of the levator plate (LP) were made to prove whether or not LP contraction occurred during anorectal closure. This was followed by a case report which demonstrated the role of connective tissue in maintaining balance between the anorectal closure muscles in a patient with 'paradoxical contraction'. Finally, the muscle damage hypothesis was tested directly with pre and post operative pudendal nerve conduction times and anal manometry following surgery which reconstructed the anterior or posterior ligaments.

This section consists of data presented at scientific fora but as yet unpublished. It is included here to illustrate and support the concepts of anorectal function and dysfunction presented earlier in this book.

The Nerve-Damage and Connective Tissue Hypotheses for Causation of Faecal Incontinence in Context

The Integral Theory hypothesis emphasizes the role of connective tissue in FI causation and relies on the pelvic muscles to create the anorectal closure forces. Therefore, a damaged muscle *must* compromise closure. However, it is difficult to attribute nerve damage due to obstetric trauma as the major aetiological factor in faecal incontinence (Swash, et al. 1985) when 30% of a surgical series of 25 patients, had never been pregnant (Parks 1977).

Excessive straining was a feature in 65% of these patients (Parks 1977). This finding is consistent with a loose anterior rectal wall collapsing inwards. The anus can be characterised as a hollow tube which needs to be stretched to the limit of its elasticity so that it becomes sufficiently rigid to allow the smooth passage of faeces, and so that it may close efficiently.

Obstetric trauma may cause both connective tissue and nerve damage. This may explain findings of delayed conduction times in patients with stress incontinence (Swash et al. 1985), but also, in patients with uterovaginal prolapse, and no stress incontinence whatsoever (Smith 1989).

The apparent contradiction caused by surgical cure of FI in patients with nerve damage (Study No. 6) is easily resolved by the understanding that the pelvic floor muscles work as a diaphragm to contain the intra-abdominal contents. Much greater strength is required for this function than anorectal closure. Restoring the anchoring point of these muscles allows them to contract even more efficiently to close off the anal canal.

With regard to FI in nulliparous patients, connective tissue laxity may be congenital, and this, in turn is consistent with a lax anterior ligament inactivating the backward and downward closure forces.

Study No. 1 - Observational Videomyogram Data During Anorectal Closure and Defaecation

Two matched groups one with double faecal (FI) and urinary incontinence (n=27), and another with urinary incontinence only (n=20), and 4 patients continent for urine and faeces were studied with x-ray video myo-vagino-proctogram, perineal ultrasound, surface EMG, and digital palpation of the pelvic floor during rest and straining. Endoanal ultrasound and evacuating myoproctogram studies were performed in the FI patients. Urethral pressure studies, with dual sensor Gaeltec catheters (2.7 mm diameter) positioned in midurethra and bladder were performed simultaneously with EMG during straining and 'squeezing'.

Results

No patients had external anal sphincter defects. Internal anal sphincter thinning was found in 26% of FI patients. Surface EMG demonstrated changes at the introitus and posterior fornix on straining. The x-ray observations are presented below. Transperineal ultrasound examinations confirmed the three directional movements seen in figure 7-03. In some patients, there appeared to be an exaggerated backward and upward movement of levator plate accompanied with only a mere flicker of downward angulation of the anterior border of levator plate. Anchoring of the perineal body appeared to limit the former, and restore the latter. 'Squeezing' produced a reasonably equivalent bladder pressure rise (mean 24.5 cm H_2O, range 4-92 cm), to straining (mean 29.75 cm H_2O, range 0-72 cm).

Conclusions - Study No. 1

Both the video x-ray and ultrasound studies appear to confirm the presence of the same three directional muscle forces acting in both urethral and anorectal closure. The pubourethral ligament is the effective insertion point for all three forces. The lower 3 cm (or so) of urethra is densely bound to vagina with connective tissue, figure 7-01. The vagina, in turn, is densely bound to the perineal body and anus. Therefore any suspensory structure (e.g. the pubourethral ligament) attached to urethra and vagina, will also anchor the anus. The dynamics of the downward LMA force in anorectal closure are complex. LMA pulls down the anterior border of levator plate (LP). In doing so it also pulls down the already stretched recto-vaginal fascia (RVF) which inserts into LP. RVF is densely attached to the uterosacral ligament (USL). Therefore USL becomes the effective anchoring point for the downward force. The concept of the hypothesized musculoelastic mechanism is visually evident on comparing figure 7-02 with 7-04. Like a rubber hose, a hollow organ can only be closed by this mechanism if it can be adequately stretched to its limit of elasticity. Inability to adequately stretch the anorectal 'hose' is evident in figure 7-04. On straining, the anus is very narrow in the normal patient (fig 7-02), but opens out in the faecally incontinent patient (fig 7-04). Connective tissue laxity may cause a weaker muscle contraction, and this, in turn, may lead to inadequate anorectal closure. This concept is also consistent with the symptomatic classification: wind, liquid, and solid, in increasing order of severity. Clearly, wind would escape before fluid, and fluid before solid, depending on how

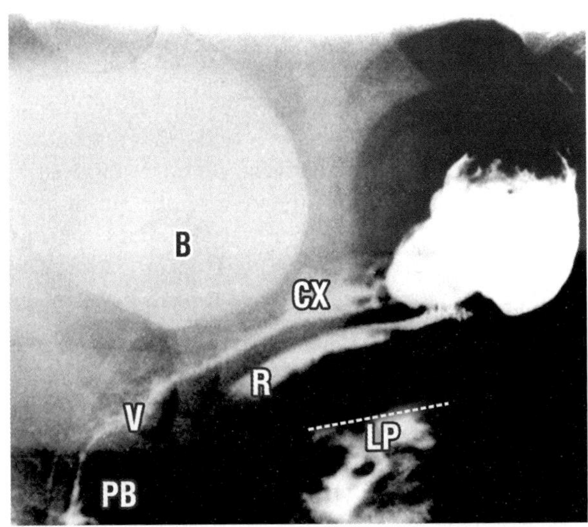

Fig. 7-01 Resting position of pelvic organs – Asymptomatic nulliparous patient. Sitting lateral X-Ray in the resting position with 10 ml of radio-opaque dye injected into a Foley catheter balloon (B), vagina (V), rectum (R) and levator plate (LP). PB = perineal body; CX = cervix. The bony opacity to the left of 'V' is the femur which acts as a reference point for organ movement.

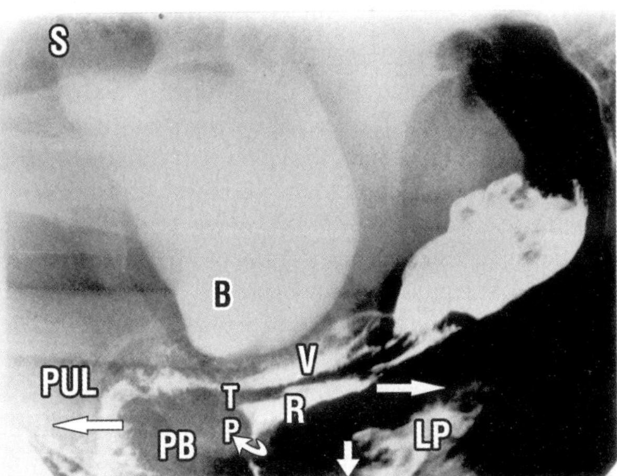

Fig. 7-02 Anorectal closure – Same patient as fig 7-01, straining position. The proximal vagina and rectum have been stretched backwards by LP (backward arrow), and rotated downwards in a plane against PUL and PB by a downward vector (downward arrow), associated with downward angulation of anterior portion of LP. The curved arrow 'p' indicates the plane of action of the puborectalis muscle. T = presumed anchoring point of the deep transversus perinei muscle.

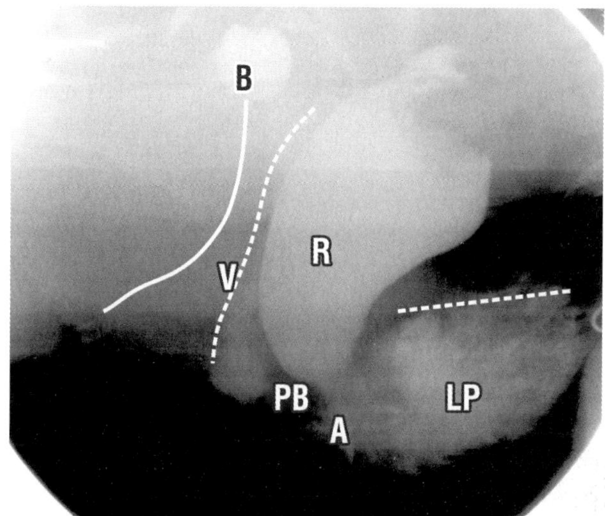

Fig. 7-03 Resting position defaecating proctogram – Faecal incontinence patient, sitting position. R = rectum; V = vagina; A = anus; PB = perineal body; LP = levator plate; B = Foley catheter balloon. With reference to figures 7-01 and 7-02, there is a vertical orientation of both V and R.

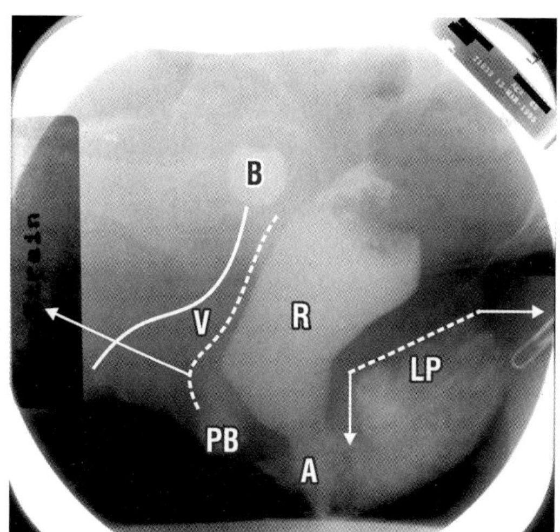

Fig. 7-04 Anorectal closure – Same patient as figure 7-04, straining. The same three vectors as in figures 7-01 and 7-02, appear to operate, but not so tightly.
Note the apparent 'anchoring' of posterior wall of anus, probably by puborectalis contraction. The distal part of the vagina and anterior anal wall appear to have been pulled forwards. Also note the apparent backward stretching of rectum and the downward angulation of anterior border of LP. Relative to the situations shown in figures 7-01 and 7-02, the anus is distended, suggesting inadequate closure.

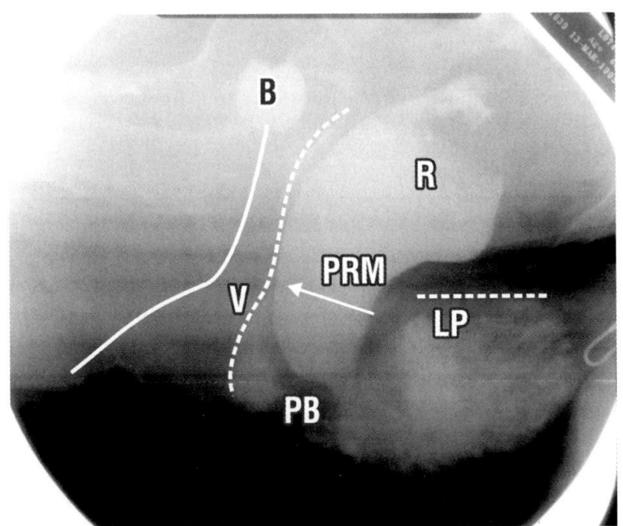

Fig. 7-05 'Squeezing' (same patient as in fig. 7-03) – Both LP and anorectal angle have been pulled upwards and forwards (arrow) from below, probably by contraction of puborectalis (PRM). Relative to figure 7-04, the anus is narrowed, and the anorectal junction becomes more angulated. All this appears to demonstrate the vital role of PRM in anorectal closure.

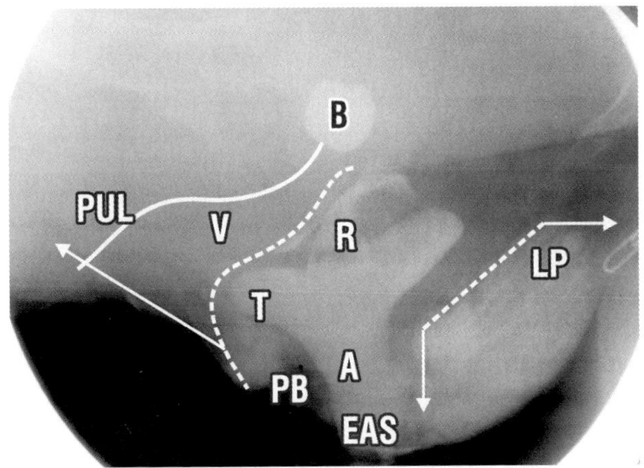

Fig. 7-06 Defaecation (same patient) – Relative to figures 7-02 and 7-01, the anterior and posterior rectal walls appear to have been pulled outwards; the anorectal angle has been opened out, apparently by backward stretching (posterior arrow) and angulation downwards of the anterior border of LP; rectum appears anchored at T (deep transverse perinei insertion) and the distal part of vagina and anterior anal wall appear to have been stretched forwards (forward arrow). As PRM has to relax, only contraction of PCM can account for this stretching. There appears to be a rectocoele above 'T'. The backward vector (backward arrow) appears to act against the midurethral insertion of PUL. Note that there are the same 3 vectors as in figures 7-02 and 7-04.

tightly the muscle forces can close off the anorectal cavity. According to the hypothesis, postanal repair and gracilis muscle transposition work by immobilizing the anus, much like 'squeezing' does in figure 7-05. An immobilised anus would be a necessary precondition for the anorectal closure by the downward and backward stretching of rectum as proposed. It was demonstrated that the pelvic organs are elevated during squeezing, and depressed during straining. Yet similar bladder pressure rises were observed during these manoeuvres. This observation would appear to remove raised intra-abdominal pressure as a primary factor in organ closure. Intra-abdominal pressure cannot elevate and depress the pelvic organs at the same time. The hypothesis predicts that the external anal sphincter would contract at initiation of defaecation, so as to anchor the insertion of LMA, but would need to relax as the bolus descends to distend the anus. Age-related degeneration of connective tissue superimposed on childbirth damage explains the late onset of faecal incontinence.

Study No. 2 - Prevention of Cough Stress FI with Midurethral Anchoring (A Case Report)

One patient presented with a long history of involuntary leakage of solid faeces on coughing or straining. Faecal leakage during coughing and straining was controlled immediately on application of unilateral pressure at midurethra with a ring forceps. On removing the forceps, leakage was noted again on straining. The faecal bolus was pushed back into the rectum. On reapplying the forceps, leakage ceased immediately.

This procedure was repeated several times, and the same result reproduced on each occasion. This case report demonstrated directly the role of competent PUL in the control of faecal incontinence in its role as an anchoring point for LP contraction.

Study No. 3 - The Role of the Levator Plate in Anorectal Closure

The aim of Study No. 3 was to test whether the anal pressure rises during reflex levator contraction. Observations from Study No. 1 indicated that the levator plate (LP) may have an important role in anorectal closure. Anatomically, the levator plate inserts into the posterior wall of the rectum. However, existing knowledge assigns no role for LP in ano-rectal closure.

The anatomical basis for this study is that the levator plate is attached to the posterior wall of the rectum, and that vaginal stimulation causes reflex levator muscle contraction (Shafik 1995). The study was to test the prediction that any stretching of the vagina would cause raised intra-anal pressure.

Ten patients with FI and ten matched control patients with no FI were tested. Mean ages were 65 (FI) and 61.5 years (no-FI). Patients were matched for age, menopause and hormonal status. Forward digital pressure was applied to the anterior vaginal wall in the region of midurethra. Gaeltec microtransducers in the anal canal measured pressures before and after stretching.

Anal pressure differences between the 10 FI and 10 controls were significant (Student's 't' test, $p = 0.034$). Forward digital pressure on the anterior vaginal wall caused a mean 47 cm water rise in endoanal pressure in the control group, and a mean 30 cm rise in the FI group.

Conclusions - Study No. 3

The results supported the musculoelastic hypothesis that LP/LMA contraction is an essential element in anorectal closure (fig 7-02).

Study No. 4 - The Role of the Internal Anal Sphincter in the Causation of Faecal Incontinence

The exact role of the internal anal sphincter (IAS) in the maintenance of faecal continence (FI) is not well understood. Controversy exists as concerns whether a damaged IAS can cause faecal incontinence. Shafik (1990) suggested that the internal anal sphincter's role was confined to maintaining resting anal tone, and that a damaged IAS per se could not cause faecal incontinence. Sultan et al. (1993) implied that a damaged IAS may be an important cause of FI. This was based on their endoanal ultrasound studies which demonstrated an association between childbirth and damaged IAS in 49 of 127 patients after vaginal delivery. Sphincteric damage was associated with FI in 10 out of 11 patients, implying causation of FI, the exact proportion of IAS to EAS damage not being specified. As these data did not fit with our previous experience (Petros 1999), we set out to prospectively examine the relationship between FI and damaged IAS in a group of patients presenting with double incontinence faecal and urinary, who presented to a tertiary referral pelvic floor clinic. The faecal incontinence described in this study was mainly of the 'idiopathic' type.

The EAS was intact on direct and ultrasonic assessment in all patients. IAS damage was defined as complete rupture or attenuation, less than 2mm thickness in some part of the sphincter. Complete rupture was found in one patient, and damage in a further 17 (total 36%). The remaining 64% had normal IAS. All 3 nulliparous patients had normal IAS and EAS. Only 36% of the patients had evidence of IAS damage. On further analysis, even Sultan's 1993 ultrasound study is more consistent with IAS being a factor associated with FI, rather than a major cause thereof, as of the 49 patients with reported IAS defects in Sultan's study, only 11 actually had faecal incontinence. One patient from this group had no IAS or EAS damage at all.

The occurrence of FI in 3 nulliparous females in our study confirms previous reports of FI in 7 nulliparous patients (Parks et al. 1977). Damage to IAS or striated muscle cannot cause FI in nulliparas. A congenital connective tissue hypothesis explains such data. The connective tissue hypothesis is further validated by report of 90% surgical cure in patients presenting with double incontinence, faecal and urinary, who also had a suburethral sling for stress incontinence (Petros 1999).

Conclusions - Study Number 4

IAS damage, *per se*, is unlikely to be a major direct cause of FI, at least in the 'idiopathic' group of patients. Shafik's suggestion that the internal anal sphincter's role is to maintain resting anal tone, is attractive. Such a role is analogous to mucosal sealing by the horseshoe shaped periurethral striated muscle sphincter.

Study No. 5 - Paradoxical Contraction of the Puborectalis Muscle

Introduction

The anorectal closure muscles LP, LMA and puborectalis muscle (PRM) act in a balanced way. Imbalance due to connective tissue laxity may cause what has been described as 'paradoxical contractions' of the PRM.

In figure 2-36 it was shown that, because LP/LMA rely on firm PUL and USL insertion points to pull the rectum backwards and downwards, lax PUL and USL could weaken the muscle forces sufficiently to unbalance the system *structurally* such that even a PRM contraction may create the very acute ano-rectal angle shown in figure 7-07.

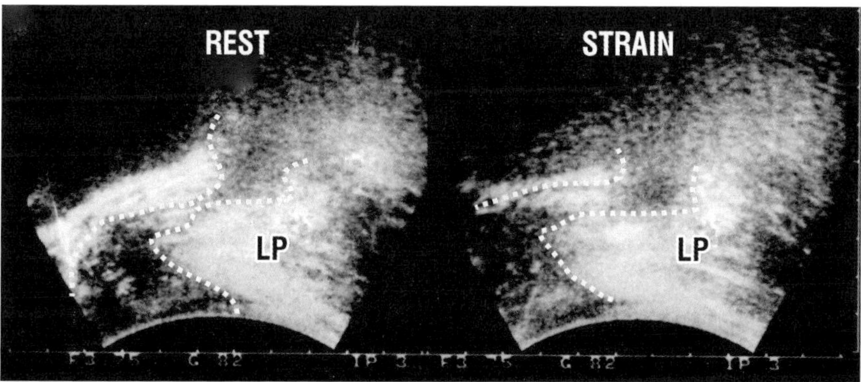

Fig. 7-07 Perineal ultrasound of 'Paradoxical contraction' of puborectalis muscle

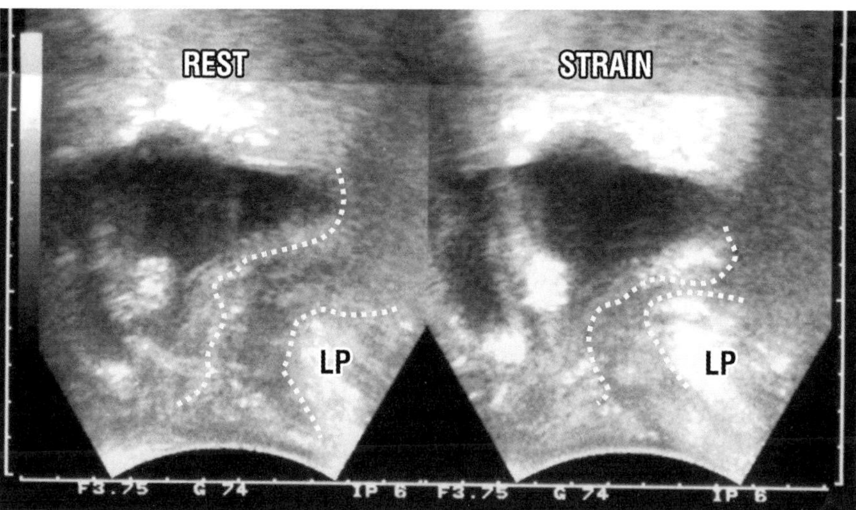

Fig. 7-08 Post-operative perineal ultrasound, at rest and straining, following reconstruction of pubourethral ligament, uterosacral ligament and rectovaginal fascia and perineal body with 8mm polypropylene tapes. (Same patient as figure 7-07.)

Clinical picture

The patient in figure 7-07 experienced difficulty with defaecation and also had faecal incontinence. Defaecating proctogram suggested spasm of the puborectalis muscle. Note the acute anorectal angle at rest and especially on straining (fig 7-07). The patient had second degree vault prolapse, lax rectovaginal fascia and a very deficient perineal body.

Surgery

The patient underwent Posterior IVS to reconstruct the uterosacral ligaments with a polypropylene tape, repair of rectovaginal fascia and perineal body, plus anterior IVS to reconstruct the pubourethral ligament. These three connective tissue structures form critical anchoring points for the optimal contraction of the closure muscles, PCM, LP and LMA, evident on inspecting figure 7-07.

Results

Post-operatively, the patient was cured of faecal incontinence and was able to defaecate normally. With reference to the post-operative perineal ultrasound examination (fig 7-08), there is apparent absence of 'paradoxical contraction' of puborectalis at rest. The anorectal angle is now essentially normal.

Conclusions

The restoration of anatomy shown in figure 7-08 is consistent with the concept of balance between the forward (puborectalis muscle (PRM)) and backwards (levator plate (LP) muscle forces. With reference to figure 7-07, it could be hypothesized that these three defects could prevent LP stretching the rectum backwards. This could unbalance the system sufficiently for PRM to stretch the rectum excessively forwards, producing an acute angulation even at rest (fig 7-07). This process is exaggerated during straining.

Study No. 6 - Pelvic Ligament Reconstruction and Cure of Faecal Incontinence without Changes in Anal Pressure or Pudendal Nerve Conduction Times

Introduction

Although the initial report (Petros 1999) concerned FI mainly associated with stress urinary incontinence, three of that group of patients subsequently presented with recurrence of FI associated with posterior zone symptoms. All three were cured by a Posterior IVS. Study number 6 was designed to establish the importance of competent pubourethral and uterosacral ligaments for the maintenance of faecal continence. The hypothesis for FI in this study is essentially the same as that for urinary incontinence. Hence the guidance as to where (i.e. in which zone) to operate was taken from the Pictorial Diagnostic Algorithm (fig 1-11).

This study was carried out with the participation of the Department of Colorectal Surgery, Royal Perth Hospital. Results (n = 27) below are as presented at the IUGA Melbourne, 2001. The Department of Colorecctal Surgery performed the pudendal nerve conduction times, anal pressure manometry and independently assessed the patients post-operatively.

Twenty-seven patients, mean age 59.5 years presented with symptoms of both urinary and faecal incontinence (FI). All had endoanal ultrasound, anorectal manometry, and pudendal nerve conduction times (PNCT) performed.

Surgery

Surgery was guided by the same anatomical classification used to guide urinary dysfunction. Anterior IVS operation replaced damaged ligaments anteriorly (n = 2) and the Posterior IVS posteriorly (n = 9). Sixteen patients had both operations performed simultaneously. Fifteen patients returned for postoperative manometry and PNCT.

Results

Only FI results are reported. Mean assessment time was 16 months (range 6-24 months). Post-operatively there were no statistically significant changes in mean anal pressure, squeeze pressures, or PNCT.

Twenty patients were entirely cured of FI, 2 >80% cured, and five were not cured. No correlation was found between low anal pressures, damaged pudendal nerves, damaged IAS and surgical results. Of the five patients with failed surgery, two were cured of both FI and urinary incontinence by further surgery, all to the posterior ligaments. Of the cured patients two began to deteriorate after 12 months. Generally speaking, although the urinary and faecal incontinence seemed to be cured, or to recur simultaneously, two patients were cured of urinary, but not faecal incontinence.

Table 3	
Pre-operative Tests: 27 FI patients	
Nerve damage	n = 16
Low resting pressure (<40cm H_2O)	n = 14
Low 'squeeze' pressure (<100cm H_2O)	n = 19
Partly damaged IAS	n = 13

Conclusions - Study No. 6

Overall, 81% of patients were more than 85% cured. Only connective tissue was reconstructed and there were no statistically significant changes in anal pressures or nerve conduction times. Incidence of urinary and faecal incontinence seemed to be linked. Cure is explained by restoration of the ligamentous insertion points of the same three directional muscle forces which stretch the bladder base backwards and downwards to close off the urethra.

It was concluded that connective tissue damage is most likely a major cause of idiopathic faecal incontinence. That patients with damaged muscles could be cured may be explained by the fact that the pelvic muscles require far more strength to contain the intra-abdominal organs than to close an organ. Thus, even a damaged muscle may be strong enough to work satisfactorily if this insertion point is restored.

Appendix 1 – Patient Questionnaires and Other Diagnostic Resource Tools

Patient Questionnaire

Self administered patient questionnaire

Part I Personal Details

Date: ____________

Name: Date of birth :
Address: Telephone:
Weight : ________ kg
Number of vaginal deliveries   ( )
Number of caesarean sections   ( )

Part II Symptoms

Describe in your own words your main urinary symptoms and duration:

— —

— —

— —

— —

All sections: tick appropriate square . ⬚ *Write extra details if you wish.*

A. Stress Incontinence (SI) Symptoms	No	Yes some-times	Yes 50% or more
Do you lose urine during:			
(A) Sneezing	☐	☐	☐ *
(A) Coughing	☐	☐	☐ *
(A) Exercise	☐	☐	☐ *
(1) Walking			
(A) (2) Stooping, squatting or getting up from a chair	☐	☐	☐
(P,M) *Symptoms of deficient emptying*			
(3) Do you feel that your bladder isn't emptying properly?	☐	☐	☐
(3) Do you ever have difficulty starting off your stream?	☐	☐	☐
(3) Is it a slow stream?	☐	☐	☐
(3) Does it stop and start involuntarily?	☐	☐	☐

*   Note to physician: the filter '50% or more' (column 3) has a proven correlation for SI being caused by anterior zone defect. For all other symptoms a 'sometimes' notation is sufficient to attribute a symptom to a particular zone. 'A', 'M' and 'P' indicate the zone of causation and where the symptoms should be transcribed on the Diagnostic Summary Sheet (fig 3-03). Numbers in parentheses refer to notes at the end of the questionnaire.

A1

	No	Yes some- times	Yes 50% or more
Urge symptoms:			
Do you ever have an uncontrollable desire to pass urine?	☐	☐	☐
If so, do you wet before arriving at toilet?	☐	☐	☐
If so, how many times a day do you wet? (Write number)			
Good day	— — —		
Bad day	— — —		
How much? A few drops	No	Yes	
A teaspoon full	No	Yes	
A tablespoon or more	No	Yes	
(4) Do you have pain while passing urine?	No	Yes	
(P) How many times during the night do you get up to pass urine?	— — —		
How many times do you pass urine during the day? (Write number)	— — — —		
(A, M)(5) In the morning do you wet immediately on getting out of bed?	☐	☐	☐
(A) (5a) Did you wet the bed as a child but not after puberty?	No	Yes	
(P) (5b) Did your problems begin soon after puberty?	No	Yes	
(P) (5c) Are your symptoms worse before a period ?	No	Yes	

Bowel symptoms:		
(A,P) (6a) Do you have difficulty evacuating your bowels?	No	Yes
(A,P) (6b) Do you ever soil yourself (faeces)?	No	Yes
wind	No	Yes
liquid faeces	No	Yes
solid faeces	No	Yes

Social inconvenience:		
(A,P) (7) Are you 'moist' with urine much of the time?	No	Yes
(8) Do you leave puddles on the floor?	No	Yes
Do you lose urine in bed at night?	No	Yes
Do you wear a pad or liner on going out? (Circle) Never /sometimes /always		
If so, how many pads/liners per day? (Write number) — — — —		

Previous operations: (circle the answer which matches)		
(P) (9) Have you had a hysterectomy?	No	Yes
If so, when? (write date) — — — —		
(10) Have you had previous surgery for incontinence?	No	Yes
If so, when? (write date) — — — —		
Are you <u>better</u> or <u>worse</u> since? (Circle)	Worse	Better
(10) Have you had previous vaginal surgery?	No	Yes
If so, when? (write date) — — — —		

	No	Yes some-times	Yes 50% or more
(P)(11) *Pelvic pain*			
Do you have deep pain on intercourse?	☐	☐	☐
Do you have a pain down at the bottom of your spine?	☐	☐	☐
Do you have a pain down at the bottom of your abdomen?	☐	☐	☐
(12) Do you have pain at the entrance to your vagina?	☐	☐	☐

Quality of life grading

Please circle a grading between 1 and 5 to describe the effect that incontinence has on your normal activities. 1 is low impact, 5 is high impact.
1 = normal
2 = mild, no effect on lifestyle
3 = can't drink, must locate toilets on going out
4 = always wears pads, very restricted social life
5 = totally housebound.

Explanatory Code for Physicians - Significance of '50% filter' (column 3)

Symptoms vary because control is a non-linear interaction of 'mechanical' and 'neurological' phenomena. Therefore when transcribing the response data to the Diagnostic Summary Sheet (figure 3-03), a 'sometimes' response is taken as a positive indication. The exception is stress incontinence (column 3). A tick in column 3 is required for a positive response because of proven correlation of the 50% filter with pad test results. The significance of the 50% filter for the other symptoms has yet to be tested statistically.

Explanatory Notes for the Numbers Preceding the Questionnaire Responses

(1)   This is usually caused by low urethral pressure (ISD) but may be from lax posterior zone.

(2)   If there is minimal SI with coughing, it is termed 'paradoxical leakage'. In age group >70 yrs generally due to PUL (pubourethral ligament) defect. Exclude tethered vagina syndrome in patients with previous vaginal surgery if a tight scar at bladder neck.

 (3)   USL (uterosacral ligament) cystocoele, but also after excessive bladder neck elevation, or tight suburethral sling.

(4)   Exclude UTI, chlamydia, etc.

(5)   Generally PUL defect even with previous operation, but exclude tethered vagina if tight scar at bladder neck.

(5a) This condition runs in families. It indicates congenital PUL weakness.

(5b) & (5c) The cervix softens to allow menstruation to pass, weakening the anchoring point of USL.

(6a) Posterior zone defect (perineal body/ rectocoele/USL) and sometimes PUL.

(6b) Defective PUL/USL and /or anal mucosal prolapse (descending perineal syndrome).

(7)   Low urethral pressure - usually with lax suburethral vagina (80%), but can be caused by lax posterior zone (20%).

(8)   This may be defective PUL, but may be also due to USL defect.

(9)   Suspect posterior zone defect especially in age group > 60 years.

(10) Think of tethered vagina syndrome in patients with positive answers for '5' and '2' who have scarring or tightness at bladder neck.

(11) Posterior zone defect.

(12) Vulvar vestibulitis which may also be caused by posterior zone defect.

Comprehensive 24 Hour Urinary Diary*

Name __ __ __ __ __ __ __ __ __ __ __ __ __ __ __   Date __ __ __ __

This chart is a 24 hour record of your fluid intake, voiding and leakage (incontinence). Please complete prior to your visit. Begin with the first toilet visit on arising. You will need a plastic measuring jug.

   1. Record time of all intake voidings and leakage
   2. Measure amount of fluid taken in (intake)
   3. Measure amounts voided
   4. Describe what you were doing at the time of leakage_
   5. Estimate amount of leakage according to the scale in column 5 (1,2,or 3)
   6. If the urge to urinate preceded the urine leakage write YES

If you felt no urge when the leakage occurred, write NO.

Indicate good day ( ) average day ( ) bad day ( )

1. Time	2. Intake	3. Output Amount voided (ml)	4. Activity e.g toilet, cough,...	5. Amount of Leakage 1 - damp (few drops only 2 - wet underwear or pad 3 - soaked pad ran down leg	Urge Present? No / Yes

Note: The Urinary Diary is used to verify the consistency of the patient's questionnaire responses. It has no direct contribution to the decision tree. It should be done at the same time as the 24 hour pad test.

* Author: David Browne, Queensland, Australia. By permission.

'Objective' Tests

Pad tests

(A)   Cough X 10   (   ) gm
      Handwashing Test (30 Seconds)   (   ) gm
      *24 Hr Pad Test   (   ) gm
      *indicate with a tick: good day ( ) average day ( ) bad day ( )

Perineal Ultrasound

(A)   Bladder neck descent   (   ) mm
(A)   Funnelling   No / Yes
(A)   Prevention of funnelling with midurethral anchor Test: No / Yes

Urodynamics

Bladder capacity   (   ) ml
(M) (P) Emptying time (>60 seconds)   (   ) secs
(M) (P) Residual urine (>30 ml)   (   ) ml
Detrusor instability   No / Yes
(A) Maximal urethral closure pressure (MUCP)   (   )
A = anterior zone; M = middle zone; P = posterior zone

Pad Test Methodology Explanatory Notes

Pads are weighed on a 1000 gm digital scale.

24 Hour Pad Tests

This test measures the severity of the problem and includes urine loss from both stress and instability. Preweighed pads are worn continuously and collected over a 24 hour period.

Ask the patient to purchase a packet of menstrual pads and to set aside one dry pad. Weigh the dry pad.

Once a pad is wet it is placed in a sealed plastic bag. Because there is very little weight variation between the same type of menstrual pad when dry, the wet pads can be weighed in toto and the weight of equivalent number of dry pads subtracted to yield the weight of urine. Unless SI is very severe, a large 24 hour loss generally points to instability as the major problem.

Rapid Provocative Pad Tests

10 coughs are specific for stress incontinence (anterior zone defect). 'Cough activated instability' is easily diagnosed by asking the patient to observe if urine loss continues after cessation of coughing.

Handwashing during 30 seconds objectively tests for bladder instability by activating the micturition reflex, urine leakage associated with urgency.

Variability

With all objective tests, the loss may vary significantly from day to day. This is because the control mechanisms of the body are complex and non-linear. More reliability is obtained by asking whether day of testing is a 'good', 'average' or 'bad' day.

Post-Treatment Questionnaire

Name: ____

Date: _____ / _____ / _______   Date of Birth: _____ / _____ / _______

Instructions

Tick the box corresponding to the appropriate answer.
Select only one answer to each question, unless otherwise indicated.

Section 1 -Symptoms You Had Before Your Last Surgery

What were your main symptoms before surgery? Tick one or more in the brackets.
Important: If any of the symptoms below began ***after*** the surgery, write "new" inside the brackets.

Q1 [   ] Urine loss during exertion or coughing
Q2 [   ] "Can't hold on" - Wet before arriving at toilet
Q3 [   ] "Going to toilet frequently to pass urine"
Q4 [   ] "Getting up at night to pass urine"
Q5 [   ] "Can't empty bladder properly"
Q6 [   ] Lower abdominal or pelvic pain
Q7 [   ] "Prolapse" (Lump in the vagina)
Q8 [   ] Bowel emptying
Q9 [   ] Bowel soiling

Section 2 -Symptoms After Surgery

The aim of this section is to assess if symptoms have improved since the surgery. Only answer the questions that are relevant to your condition.

Q1: Urine loss during exertion or coughing
Has this improved since surgery?
Better   Worse   Unchanged   Estimate % improvement.
 [ ]   [ ]   [ ]   [ ]

Q2 "Can't hold on" - Wet before arriving at toilet
Has this improved since surgery?
Better   Worse   Unchanged   Estimate % improvement.
 [ ]   [ ]   [ ]   [ ]

Q3 "Going to toilet frequently to pass urine"
Has this improved since surgery?
Better   Worse   Unchanged
 [ ]   [ ]   [ ]
 How many hours can you "hold on" during the day now?   [ ] (write number)

Q4 "Getting up at night to pass urine"
Has this improved since surgery?
Better   Worse   Unchanged
 [ ]   [ ]   [ ]
How many times a night do you get out of bed to pass urine now?   [   ](write number)

Q5 " Can't empty bladder properly"
Has this improved since surgery?
Better   Worse   Unchanged   Estimate % improvement.
 [ ]   [ ]   [ ]   [ ]

Q6 Lower abdominal or pelvic pain
Has this improved since surgery?
Better   Worse   Unchanged   Estimate % improvement.
 [ ]   [ ]   [ ]   [ ]

Q7 "Prolapse" (Lump in the vagina)
Has this improved since surgery?
Better   Worse   Unchanged   Estimate % improvement.
 [ ]   [ ]   [ ]   [ ]

Q8 Bowel emptying
Has this improved since surgery?
Better   Worse   Unchanged   Estimate % improvement.
 [ ]   [ ]   [ ]   [ ]

Q9 Bowel soiling
Has this improved since surgery?
Better   Worse   Unchanged   Estimate % improvement.
 [ ]   [ ]   [ ]   [ ]

Q10 Overall, how would you rate the results of your operation?
          More than 90% improved [ ]
          More than 70% improved [ ]
          50% improved   [ ]
          No change   [ ]
          Worse than before   [ ]

Q11 Knowing what you know now, would you have such an operation again?
          Yes [ ]   No [ ]

Q12 Would you recommend such an operation to a friend?
          Yes [ ]   No [ ]   Not sure [ ]

Further Comments

Please feel free to add any further comments below.

Example of a Completed Diagnostic Summary Sheet

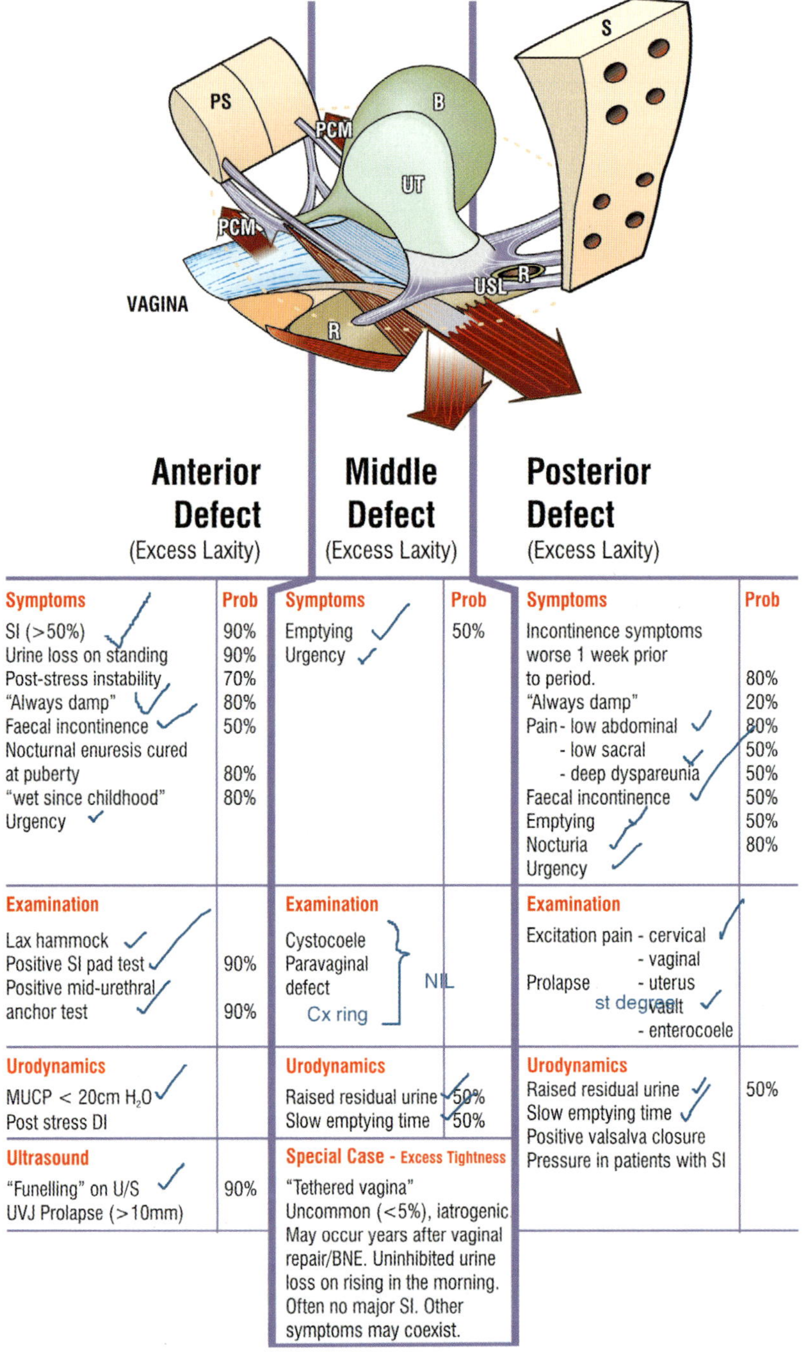

Fig 3-03 example: An example of a completed Diagnostic Summary Sheet (See page 59)

Example of a Completed Examination Sheet

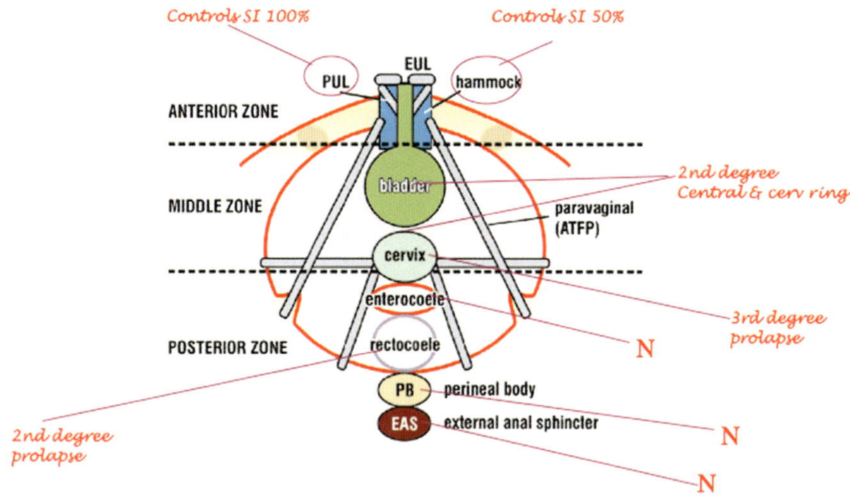

Fig 304 example: An example of a completed examination sheet (see page 61), in this case showing the anatomical defects found in a patient with stress incontinence and vaginal prolapse.

Appendix 2 – References and Further Reading

The references listed below are organised in parts corresponding to how they appear in this book. They are classified in two sections for each Chapter: 'text references' and 'further reading'. The works of authors mentioned in the text are listed under 'text references', and those relevant to aspects of the topic are listed under 'further reading'.

Chapter 2: The Anatomy and Dynamics of Pelvic Floor Function and Dysfunction

Brown JS, Sawaya G, Thorn DH Grady D Hysterectomy and urinary incontinence: a systematic review, *Lancet* (2000) 356:535-539

Bush MB, Petros PEP, Barrett- Lennard BR On the flow through the human urethra *Biomechanics* (1997) 30: 967-969.

Courtney H Anatomy of the pelvic diaphragm and ano-rectal musculature as related to sphincter preservation in ano-rectal surgery. *American Journal Surgery*, (1950), 79:155-173.

Creed K. Functional diversity of smooth muscle. *British Med. Bulletin,* (1979), 3:243-247

De Lancey J O L Structural support of the urethra as it relates to stress incontinence: the hammock hypothesis *Am J Obst Gynecol* (1994) 170: 1713-1723.

Huisman AB. Aspects on the anatomy of the female urethra with special relation to urinary continence. *Contr Gynecol & Obstets.,* (1983) 10:1-31.

Ingelman-Sundberg A The pubovesical ligament in stress incontinence. *Acta Obstets & Gynecol Scandinavica,* (1949), 28:183-188.

Jeffcoate TNA *Principles of Gynaecology.* (1962), (2nd Ed.) Butterworths, London.

Lose G and Colstrup H, Mechanical properties of the urethra in healthy and stress incontinent females: dynamic measurements in the resting urethra, *J Urol.,* (1990) 144: 1258-1262.

Netter F *Atlas of Human Anatomy* (1989) CIBA-Geigy Corp Ardsley USA

Nichols DH & Randall CL *Vaginal Surgery.* (1989), 3rd Ed, Williams Wilkins, Baltimore. 1-46.

Parks AG, Swash M and Urich H Sphincter Denervation in ano-rectal incontinence and rectal prolapse. *Gut*; (1977) ;18: 656-665.

Petros PE and Ulmsten U. Urethral pressure increase on effort originates from within the urethra, and continence from musculovaginal closure, *Neurourology and Urodynamics,* (1995), 14:337-350

Petros PE and Ulmsten U 'Urethral and bladder neck closure mechanisms' *Am J Obst Gynecol.* (1995) 173: 346-347

Petros PE and Ulmsten U Role of the pelvic floor in bladder neck opening and closure: I muscle forces, *Int J Urogynecol and Pelvic Floor,* (1997) 8: 74-80

Petros PE and Ulmsten U Role of the pelvic floor in bladder neck opening and closure: II vagina. *Int J Urogynecol and Pelvic Floor,* (1997) 8: 69-73

Petros PE The pubourethral ligaments-an anatomical and histological study in the live patient, *Int J Urogynecology* (1998) 9: 154-157.

Petros PE, Von Konsky B Anchoring the midurethra restores bladder neck anatomy and continence, *Lancet* (1999) 354:997-998

Petros PE Cure of urinary and fecal incontinence by pelvic ligament reconstruction suggests a connective tissue etiology for both. *International Journal of Urogynecology* (1999);10:356-360

Petros PE ltr Influence of hysterectomy on pelvic floor dysfunction *Lancet* (2000), 356 :1275.

Petros PE The anatomy of the perineal membrane: its relationship to injury in childbirth and episiotomy, *Aust. NZ J Obstet.Gynaecol* (2002) 42:577-8

Swash M, Henry MM, Snooks SJ Unifying concept of pelvic floor disorders and incontinence. *Journal of the Royal Society of Medicine*, (1985),78: 906-911.

Yamada H. Aging rate for the strength of human organs and tissues. *Strength of Biological Materials*, Williams & Wilkins Co, Balt. (Ed) Evans FG. (1970); 272-280.

Zacharin RF A suspensory mechanism of the female urethra. *Journal of Anatomy*, (1963), 97:423-427.

Chapter 2: Further Reading

Ayoub SF Anterior fibres of the levator ani muscle in man. *Journal of Anatomy*, (1979), 128:571-580.

Berglas B & Rubin IC Study of the supportive structures of the uterus by levator myography. *Surgery Gynecol & Obstets.*, (1953), 97:667-692.

DeLancey J Correlative Study of Paraurethral Anatomy. *Obstet. Gynecol.*(1986); 68:91-97.

Denny-Brown D & Robertson E Physiology of micturition. *Brain*, (1933), 56:149-191.

Dickinson RL The vagina as a hernial canal. *American Journal Obstets Dis Women & Child.* (1889), 22:692-697.

Dickinson RL Studies of the levator ani muscle. *American Journal Obstets Dis Women & Child.* (1889), 22:898-917.

Downing SJ & Sherwood OD The physiological role of relaxin in the pregnant rat 1V The influence of relaxin on cervical collagen and glycosaminoglycans, *Endocrinology.* (1986), 118:471-479

Falconer C, Ekman-Orderberg G, Malmstrom A and Ulmsten U Clinical outcome and changes in connective tissue metabolism after Intravaginal Slingplasty in stress incontinent women, *Int Urogynecol J* (1996) 7: 133-137.

Fothergill WE Pathology & the operative treatment of displacements of the pelvic viscera. *Journal of Obstets & Gynaecol of the British Empire*, (1907), 13:410-419.

Gosling JA Dickson JS & Humpherson JR Gross & microscopic anatomy of the urethra II. *Functional Anatomy of the Urinary Tract*, (1983), Churchill Livingstone, Edinburgh. 5.1-5.20.

Gosling JH, Dixon JS & Critchley HOD A comparative study of the human external sphincter & periurethral ani muscles. *British Journal Urol*ogy, (1981), 53:35-41.

Gosling JA Structure of the lower urinary tract and pelvic floor. *Gynaecological Urology*, (1985), 12: 285-294.Ed Raz S, WB Saunders & Co London.

Kovanen V, Suominen H, Risteli J & Risteli L Type IV collagen and laminin in slow and fast skeletal muscle in rats - effects of age and life-time endurance training. *Collagen Rel Res.* (1988), 8:145-153.

Milley PS & Nicholls DH The relationship between the pubourethral ligaments and the urogenital diaphragm in the human female. *Anat Rec.* (1971), 170:281-283.

Nichols DH & Randall CL Massive eversion of the vagina, in *Vaginal Surgery.* (1989), 3rd Ed, Eds Nichols DH & Randall CL, Williams Wilkins, Baltimore. 328-357.

Nordin M Biomechanics of collagenous tissues, in *Basic Biomechanics of the Skeletal System.* (1980), Eds, Frankel VH & Nordin M., Lee & Febiger, Philadelphia. P87-110.

Olesen KP & Walter S Bladder base insufficiency. *Acta Obstets & Gynecol Scandinavica*, (1978), 57:463-468.

Paramore RH Some further considerations on the supports of the female pelvic viscera, in which the intra-abdominal pressure is still further defined. *Journal of Obstets & Gynaecol of the British Empire*, (1908), 14:172-187.

Paramore RH The supports in chief of the female pelvic viscera. *Journal of Obstets & Gynaecol of the British Empire*, (1908), 30: 391-409.

Peacock EE Structure, synthesis and interaction of fibrous protein and matrix. *Wound Repair.* (1984), 3rd Edition, Publishers WB Saunders Co, Philadelphia. 56-101.

Petros PE A cystocele may compensate for latent stress incontinence by stretching the vaginal hammock, *Gynecol and Obst Investigation* (1998); 46: 206-209.

Petros PE Vault prolapse 1: dynamic supports of the vagina, *Int J Urogynecol and pelvic floor* (2001) 12:292-295.

Porter NH A physiological study of the pelvic floor in rectal prolapse. *Journ R. Coll.of Surg England*, (1962). 31: 379-404.

Power RM Embryological development of the levator ani muscle. *American Journal of Obstets & Gynecol.*, (1948), 55:367-381

Rud T, Asmussen M, Andersson KE, Hunting A & Ulmsten U Factors maintaining the intra-urethral pressure in women. *Investigative Urology,* (1980), 17: 4, 343-347.

Sultan AH, Kamm MA, Hudson CN, Thomas JM and Bartram CI Anal-sphincter disruption during vaginal delivery, *N Eng J Med* (1993); 329: 1905-11

Tanagho EA The anatomy & physiology of micturition. *Clinics in Obstets & Gynecol,* (1978), 5: 1:3-26.

Tanagho EA & Miller ER Initiation of voiding. *British Journal of Urology,* (1970), 42:175-180.

Tanagho EA, Myers FH, Smith DR Urethral resistance: its components and implications, No 2. striated muscle component. *Investigative Urology,* (1969), 7:195

Wendell-Smith, CP & Ulsen PM The musculature of the pelvic floor. *Scientific Foundation of Obstets & Gynaecol.* (Eds) Philipp EE, Barnes J & Newton M, William Heinemann Medical Books Ltd, London, (1977), 78-84.

Walter JB & Israel MS (Eds) Inflammatory Reaction, in *Walter & Israel Pathology*, 5th Ed., Churchill and Livingstone, Edin, (1979) 71-85.

Wilson PD Posterior pubourethral ligaments in normal and genuine stress incontinent women. *Journal of Urology* (1982), 130:802-805.

Woodburne RT Structure and function of the urinary bladder. *Journal of Urology,* (1960), 84:79-85.

Zacharin RF Pelvic floor anatomy and cure of pulsion enterocoele. Springer-Verlag, Wien, (1985).

Chapter 3: The Diagnosis of Connective Tissue Damage

Abrams P, Blaivas J, Stanton S and Andersen J Standardisation of Terminology of Lower Urinary Tract Function. *Scand J. Urol Nephrol.* (1988), Suppl. 114.

Bates P, Bradley WE, Glen E, Hansjorg M, Rowan D, Sterling A and Hald T *International Continence Society First Report on the Standardisation of Terminology of Lower Urinary Tract Function* –(1975)

Bates CP The unstable bladder, *Clinics in Obstetrics and Gynaecology* (1978) 5: 1:109 - 122.

Black N, Griffiths J, Pope C, Bowling A and Abel P Impact of surgery for stress incontinence on morbidity: cohort study. *Brit. Med J* (1997), 315: 1493-8.

Creed K Functional diversity of smooth muscle. *British Med. Bulletin*, (1979), 3:243-247

Kelly HA & Dumm WM Urinary incontinence in women without manifest injury to the bladder. *Surgery Gynecol & Obstets.*, (1914), 18:444-450.

Mayer R, Wells T, Brink C, Diokno A and Cockett A Handwashing in the cystometric evaluation of detrusor instability, *Neurourology and urodynamics*, (1991). 10: 563-569

Petros PE and Ulmsten U An Integral Theory of Female Urinary Incontinence. *Acta Obstetricia et Gynecologica Scandinavica* (1990), 69: Suppl 153 :1-79.

Petros PE and Ulmsten U Pinch test for diagnosis of stress urinary incontinence. *Acta Obstetricia et Gynecologica Scandinavica*, (1990), 69: Suppl 153:33-35.

Petros PE and Ulmsten U Urge incontinence history is an accurate predictor of urge incontinence. *Acta Obstetricia et Gynecologica Scandinavica*, (1992) 71: 537-539.

Petros PE and Ulmsten U An analysis of rapid pad testing and the history for the diagnosis of stress incontinence. *Acta Obstetricia et Gynecologica Scandinavica*, (1992), 71: 529-536.

Petros PE and Ulmsten U Bladder instability in women: A premature activation of the micturition reflex. *Neurourology and Urodynamics* (1993);12: 235-239

Petros PE and Ulmsten U. An Integral Theory and its method for the diagnosis and management of female urinary incontinence. *Scand J Urol Nephrol*, (1993). 27: Suppl 153, 1-93

Petros PE and Ulmsten U *The posterior fornix syndrome: a multiple symptom complex of pelvic pain and abnormal urinary symptoms deriving from laxity in the posterior fornix.* Scand. J Urol. and Nephrol., (1993), 27: Supp. No 153 89-93.

Petros PE (letter) Is detrusor instability a premature variant of a normal micturition reflex? *Lancet* (1997) 349: 1255-6.

Petros PE and Ulmsten U "Urethral pressure increase on effort originates from within the urethra, and continence from musculovaginal closure", *Neurourology and Urodynamics*, (1995).14:337-350

Petros PE and Ulmsten U An anatomical classification- a new paradigm for management of lower female urinary dysfunction, *European Journal of Obstetrics & Gynecology and Reproductive Biology* (1998) 80:87-94.

Petros PE Symptoms of defective emptying and raised residual urine may arise from ligamentous laxity in the posterior vaginal fornix, *Gynecol and Obst Investigation*, (1998), 45: 105-108.

Petros PE and Ulmsten U An anatomical classification- a new paradigm for management of urinary dysfunction in the female *Int J Urogynecology* (1999) 10: 29-35.

Petros PE, Von Konsky B Anchoring the midurethra restores bladder neck anatomy and continence, *Lancet* (1999) 354:997-998

Petros PE Application of Theory to the management of pelvic floor dysfunction, *Pelvic Floor* (2001) Eds. Swash

Petros PE Changes in bladder neck geometry and closure pressure following midurethral anchoring suggest a musculoelastic mechanism activates closure, *Neurourol. and Urodynamics* (2003) 22:191-197

Richardson AC, Edmonds PB & Williams NL Treatment of stress urinary incontinence due to paravaginal fascial defect. *Obstets & Gynecol*, (1980), 57: 357

Zacharin RF & Gleadell LW Abdominoperineal urethral suspension. *American Journal Obstets & Gynecol.*, (1963), 86: 981.

Chapter 3: Further Reading

Farnsworth BN Posterior Intravaginal Slingplasty (infraccocygeal sacropexy) for severe posthysterectomy vaginal vault prolapse- a preliminary report, *Int J Urogynecol* (2002)13:4-8

Hukins WL & Aspden R Composition and properties of connective tissues. *Trends in Biochemical Sciences*, (1985) 7,10: 260-264.

Krantz KE Anatomy of the urethra and anterior vaginal wall. *American Journal Obstets & Gynecol.*, (1950), 62:374-386.

Lose LG Study of urethral closure function in healthy and stress incontinent women. *Neurology and Urodynamics,* (1992) ;11:55-8.

Pilsgaard K. Mouritsen L Follow-up after repair of vaginal vault prolapse with abdominal colposacropexy. *Acta Obstetricia et Gynecologica Scandinavica.* (1999) 78:66-70,

Rechberger T, Uldbjerg N & Oxlund H Connective tissue changes in the cervix during normal pregnancy and pregnancy complicated by a cervical incompetence *Obstets & Gynecol.,* (1988), 71:563-567.

Thonar EJMA & Kuettner KE Biochemical basis of age related changes in proteoglycans. *Biology of Protoeglycans.* (1987), Editors Wight TN & Mecham RP, Academic Press Inc. 211-246.

Uldbjerg N and Ulmsten U The physiology of cervical ripening and cervical dilatation and the effect of abortifaciunt drugs, in *Induction of abortion,* Bailliere's *Clinical Obst and Gynaecol,*(1990) Ed Bygdeman M, Baillere Tindall Lond. 263-281.

Yamauchi M, Woodley DT & Mechanic GL Aging and cross-linking of skin collagen. *Biochemical and Biophysical Research Communications,* (1988), 152:898-901.

Chapter 4: Reconstructive Pelvic Floor Surgery

Amid, PK Classification of biomaterials and their related complications in abdominal wall hernia surgery, *Hernia* (1997) 1: 15-21

Black N, Griffiths J, Pope C, Bowling A and Abel P Impact of surgery for stress incontinence on morbidity: cohort study. *Brit. Med J* (1997), 315: 1493-8.

Brown J, Seeley D, Grady D, Ensrud K & Cummings S Hysterectomy: The effect on prevalence of urinary incontinence. *International Urogynecology Journal,* (1994), 5: 370.

De Lancey J O L Structural support of the urethra as it relates to stress incontinence: the hammock hypothesis *Am J Obst Gynecol* (1994) 170: 1713-1723.

Delorme E, La Bandelette transobturatrice: un procede mininvasif pour traiter l'incontinence urinaire d'effort de la femme. *Progres en Urologie,* 11; 1306-1313, 2001.

Falconer C, Ekman-Orderberg G, Malmstrom A and Ulmsten U Clinical outcome and changes in connective tissue metabolism after Intravaginal Slingplasty in stress incontinent women, *Int Urogynecol J* (1996) 7: 133-137.

Farnsworth BN Posterior Intravaginal Slingplasty (infraccocygeal sacropexy) for severe posthysterectomy vaginal vault prolapse - a preliminary report, *Int J Urogynecol* (2002) 13 :4-8.

Gleick J "Inner Rhythms" in *Chaos- making a new science,*(1987) Cardinal, Penguin, England, 275-300.

Harrison JH, Swanson DS & Lincoln AF. A comparison of tissue reactions to plastic materials. *AMA Archives of Surgery,* (1956), 139-143.

Iglesia CB, Fenner DE and Brubaker L The use of mesh in gynaecologic surgery, *Int Urogyne Surgery* (1997) 8:105-115

Jeffcoate TNA Genital Prolapse, in *Principles of Gynaecology.,* Ed Jeffcoate TNA, (1962), (2nd Ed.) Butterworths, London, 282-30

Kelly HA & Dumm WM Urinary incontinence in women without manifest injury to the bladder. *Surgery Gynecol & Obstets.,* (1914), 18:444-450.

Koelbl H, Stoerer S, Seliger G, Wolters M Transurethral penetration of a tension-free vaginal tape, *BJOG:* (2001) 108; 7 763

Lim YN, Rane A Suburethral vaginal erosion and pyogenic granuloma formation: an unusual complication of intravaginal slingplasty (IVS)., *Int Urogynecol J Pelvic Floor Dysfunct.* (2004);15(1):56-8.

Lim YN, Muller R, Corstiaans A, Dietz HP, Barry C, Rane A. Suburethral slingplasty evaluation study in North Queensland, Australia: the SUSPEND trial. *Aust N Z J Obstet Gynaecol.* (2005); 45(1):52-9

Milani R, Salvatore S, Soligo S,a Pifarotti P, Meschia M, Cortese M, Functional and anatomical outcome of anterior and posterior vaginal prolapse repair with prolene mesh *BJOG: An International Journal of Obstetrics & Gynaecology* 112 (1), 107-111.

Nichols DH & Randall CL *Vaginal Surgery.* (1989), 3rd Ed, Williams Wilkins, Baltimore.

Papadimitriou JM, Ashman RB (1989) Macrophages: current views on their differentiation, structure and function, *Ultrastruct Path* 13: 343-358

Papadimitriou J and Petros PEP, Histological studies of monofilament and multifilament polypropylene mesh implants demonstrate equivalent penetration of macrophages between fibrils, *Hernia*,(2005) 9: 75-78.

Peacock EE *Structure, synthesis and interaction of fibrous protein and matrix. Wound Repair.* (1984), 3rd Edition, Publishers WB Saunders Co, Philadelphia. 56-101.

Petros PEP, Richardson PA, Midurethral Tissue Fixation System sling – a 'micromethod' for cure of stress incontinence – preliminary report, *ANZJOG*, (2005); 45: 372–375

Petros PEP, Richardson PA, Tissue Fixation System posterior sling for repair of uterine/vault prolapse – A preliminary report. *ANZJOG*, (2005); 45: 376–379

Petros PE, Ulmsten U And Papadimitriou J The Autogenic Neoligament procedure: A technique for planned formation of an artificial neo-ligament. *Acta Obstetricia et Gynecologica Scandinavica*, (1990), 69: Suppl.153: 43-51.

Petros PE and Ulmsten U Pinch test for diagnosis of stress urinary incontinence. *Acta Obstetricia et Gynecologica Scandinavica*, (1990), 69: Suppl 153:33-35.

Petros PE & Ulmsten U The tethered vagina syndrome, post surgical incontinence and I-plasty operation for cure. *Acta Obstetricia et Gynecologica Scandinavica*, (1990) 69: Suppl. 153, 63-67.

Petros PE and Ulmsten U The development of the Intravaginal Slingplasty procedure: IVS II- VI *Scandinavian Journal of Urology and Nephrology* (1993); 27: Suppl. 153 ; 61-84

Petros PE & Ulmsten U The free graft procedure for cure of the tethered vagina syndrome, *Scandinavian Journal of Urology and Nephrology* (1993) 27: Suppl. 153 ; 85-87

Petros PE The Intravaginal Slingplasty Operation, a minimally invasive technique for cure of urinary incontinence in the female, *Aust NZ J Obst and Gyn* (1996); 36: 463-461

Petros PE New ambulatory surgical methods using an anatomical classification of urinary dysfunction improve stress, urge, and abnormal emptying, *Int J Urogynecology* (1997) 8: 270-278.

Petros PE Development of generic models for ambulatory vaginal surgery: a preliminary report, *Int J Urogynecology* (1998) 9:19-27.

Petros PE 'Development of the Intravaginal Slingplasty, and other ambulatory vaginal procedures' Doctor of Surgery thesis University of Western Australia (1999)

Petros PE Medium-term follow up of the Intravaginal Slingplasty operation indicates minimal deteroration of continence with time. *Aust. NZ J Obstet.Gynaecol.* (1999) 39:354-356.

Petros PE Cure of urinary and fecal incontinence by pelvic ligament reconstruction suggests a connective tissue etiology for both. *International Journal of Urogynecology* (1999);10:356-360

Petros PE ltr Influence of hysterectomy on pelvic floor dysfunction *Lancet* (2000), 356 :1275.

Petros PE Vault prolapse II: Restoration of dynamic vaginal supports by the infracoccygeal sacropexy, an axial day-care vaginal procedure, *Int J Urogynecol and pelvic floor* (2001) 12:296-303

Petros PE The split labium minus flap graft technique, *Int J Urogyne* (2004) (in press)

Rechberger,T Rzezniczuk K, Skorupski P, Adamiak A,Tomaszewski J et al. A randomized comparison between monofilament and multifilament tapes for stress incontinence surgery. *Int J Urogyne* (2003) 14; 432-436

Richardson AC, Edmonds PB & Williams NL Treatment of stress urinary incontinence due to paravaginal fascial defect. *Obstet & Gynaecol.* (1981), 57: 357-362

Shull BL, Capen CV, Riggs MW and Kuehl TJ Preoperative and postoperative analysis of site-specific pelvic support defects in 81 women treated with sacrospinous ligament suspension and pelvic reconstruction, *J Obstet Gynecol* (1992); 166; 1764-71.

Ulmsten U, Johnson P, and Petros P Intravaginal Slingplasty, *Zentralblatt fur Gynakologie,* (1994);116: 398-404.

Ulmsten U, Henriksson L, Johnson P, and Varhos G An ambulatory surgical procedure under local anesthesia for treatment of female urinary incontinence, *Int Urogynecol* J (1996); 7: 81-86.

Van Winkle W & Salthouse TN Biological response to sutures and principles of suture selection monograph. *Ethicon,* (1976).

White GR An anatomical operation for cure of cystocele *JAMA* (1909) 53: 113

Yamada H Ageing rate for the strength of human organs and tissues. *Strength of Biological Materials,* (1970) Williams & Wilkins Co, Balt. (Ed) Evans F. 272-280.

Zacharin RF A suspensory mechanism of the female urethra. *Journal of Anatomy,* (1963), 97:423-427.

Chapter 4: Further Reading

Bailey AJ, Bazin S & De Launey A Changes in the nature of collagen during development and restoration of granulation tissue. *Biochemica et Biophysica Acta,* (1973), 328:383-390.

Bailey AJ, Sims TJ, Le Lous M & Bazin S Collagen polymorphism in experimental granulation tissue. *Biochem & Biophysical Research Communications,* (1975), 66:1160-1165.

Douglas DM The healing of aponeurotic incisions. *British Journal of Surgery,* (1952), 40:79-84.

Farnsworth BN A multicentre trial of the Intravaginal Slingplasty procedure with critical analysis of results, surgical methodology and complications thereof, *Int J Urogynecol* (2001)12 –16.

Goff BH Secondary reconstruction of damaged pelvic floor, practical consideration of the damaged pelvic floor with the technique for its secondary reconstruction. *Surgery Gynecol & Obstets.,*(1928), 46:855-866.

Harrison JH et al. Synthetic Materials as vascular prosthesis. *American Journal of Surgery,* (1958), 95:16-24.

Leibovich SJ & Ross R The role of the macrophage in wound repair. A study with hydrocortisone and antimacrophage serum. *American Journal of Pathology,* (1975), 78:71-91.

Madden JW & Peacock EE Dynamic metabolism of scar collagen and re-modelling of dermal wounds. *Annals of Surgery,* (1971), 174:p511.

Muller HK Mechanism of clearing injured tissue. *Handbook of Inflammation No 3 Tissue Regeneration and Repair,* (1981), 145-175.

Osterburg D Influence of capillary multifilament sutures on the antibacterial action of inflamatory cells in infected wounds. *Acta Chir Scandinavica,* (1983), 149:751-57.

Peacock EE Structure, synthesis and interaction of fibrous protein and matrix. *Wound Repair.* (1984), 3rd Edition, Publishers WB Saunders Co, Philadelphia. 56-101.

Petros PE and Ulmsten U The combined intravaginal sling and tuck operation. An ambulatory procedure for stress and urge incontinence. *Acta Obstetricia et Gynecologica Scandinavica,* (1990); 69: Suppl.153:53-59.

Petros PE and Ulmsten U The tuck procedure: A simplified vaginal repair for treatment of female urinary incontinence. *Acta Obstetricia et Gynecologica Scandinavica*, (1990), 69: Suppl 153: 41-42.

Petros PE and Ulmsten U Cure of urge incontinence by the combined intravaginal sling and tuck operation. *Acta Obstetricia et Gynecologica Scandinavica*, (1990), 69: Suppl 153: 61-62.

Petros PE and Ulmsten U Non-stress non-urge incontinence- diagnosis and cure- preliminary report. *Acta Obstetricia et Gynecologica Scandinavica*, (1990), 69: Suppl 153: 69-70.

Petros PE and Ulmsten U The combined intravaginal sling and tuck operation. An ambulatory procedure for stress and urge incontinence *Acta Obstetricia et Gynecologica Scandinavica*, (1990), 69: Suppl 153: 53-59.

Petros PE and Ulmsten U Surgical principles deriving from the Integral Theory, *Scandinavian Journal of Urology and Nephrology* (1993) – 27: Suppl. 153 - PART III: 41-49.

Petros PE and Ulmsten U An anatomical basis for success and failure of female incontinence surgery, *Scandinavian Journal of Urology and Nephrology* (1993) 27: Suppl. 153 - PART IV: 53-60.

Petros PE Tissue reaction to implanted foreign materials for cure of stress incontinence (letter) *American Journal of Obstetrics and Gynecology* (1994); 171: 1159

Petros PE Ambulatory incontinence and vaginal surgery. *Aust Med J* (1994) 161: 171-172.

Postlethwaite RW, Schauble JF, Dillon ML & Morgan J Wound healing. II An evaluation of surgical suture material. *Surgery Gynaecol & Obstets*, (1959), 555-566.

Postlethwaite RW Longterm comparative study of non-absorbable sutures. *Archives of Surgery*, (1970), 101:489.

Postlethwaite RW, Willigan DVM & Ulin AW Human tissue reaction to sutures. *Annals of Surgery*, (1975), 181:144-152.

Richardson DA, Bent EA, Ostergard D et al. Delayed reaction to the dacron buttress suture used in urethropexy. *Journal of Reproductive Medicine*, (1984), 29:689-692.

Salthouse TM Biological response to sutures. *Otolaryngol Head Neck Surgery*, (1980), 88:658-664.

Salthouse T Some aspects of macrophage behaviour at the implant interface. *Journal of Biomed Material Res.*, (1984), 18:395-401

Shull BL, Capen CV, Riggs MW, Kuehl TJ. Preoperative and postoperative analysis of site-specific pelvic support defects in 81 women treated with sacrospinous ligament suspension and pelvic reconstruction. *J Obstet Gynecol.* 1992; 166: 1764–1771.

Ulmsten U and Petros PE Surgery for female urinary incontinence. in *Current Science* (1992).4:456-462

Van Winkle W &Hastings JC Considerations in the choice of suture material for various tissues, *Surgery, Gynecology and Obstetrics*, (1972) 135: 113-126.

Chapter 5: Pelvic Floor Rehabilitation

Appell RA, Bourcier A La Torre F (1998) Eds *Textbook of Pelvic Floor Dysfunction*

Bo, K Pelvic floor muscle exercise for the treatment of female stress urinary incontinence: III. Effects of two different degrees of pelvic floor muscles exercises. *Neurourol Urod,,* (1990). 9: 489-502.

Kegel AH *Progressive resistant exercise in the functional restoration of the perineal muscles.* Am.J. Obstets & Gynecol., (1948), 56:238-248.

Petros PE and Skilling PM The physiological basis of pelvic floor exercises in the treatment of stress urinary incontinence. *Br J Obstet Gynaecol* (1999) 106:615-616

Petros PE and Skilling PM Pelvic floor rehabilitation according to the Integral Theory of Female Urinary Incontinence- First report, *European Journal of Obstetric s& Gynecology and Reproductive Biology* (2001) 94: 264-269.

Skilling PM and Petros PE Synergistic non-surgical management of pelvic floor dysfunction: second report, *Int J Urogyne* (in press)

Chapter 6: Mapping the Dynamics of Connective Tissue Dysfunction

Abrams P, Blaivas J, Stanton S and Andersen J Standardisation of Terminology o Lower Urinary Tract Function. *Scand J. Urol Nephrol.* (1988), Suppl. 114.

Bates CP The unstable bladder, *Clinics in Obstetrics and Gynaecology* (1978) 5: 1: 109 - 122.

Bates P, Bradley WE, Glen E, Hansjorg M, Rowan D, Sterling A and Hald T*International Continence Society First Report on the Standardisation of Terminology of Lower Urinary Tract Function* –(1975)

Bush MB, Petros PEP, Barrett- Lennard BR On the flow through the human urethra *Biomechanics* (1997) 30: 967-969.

Constantinou CE and Govan DE Contribution and timing of transmitted and generated pressure components in the female urethra. *Female Incontinence,* (1981), Alan R Liss New York, 113-120.

Constantinou CE Resting and stress urethral pressures as a clinical guide to the mechanism of continence,in *Clinics in Obstetrics and Gynaecology* Ed Raz S, WB Saunders Co London (1985), 12: 343-356.

Creed K Functional diversity of smooth muscle. *British Med. Bulletin,* (1979), 3:243-247

Enhorning G Simultaneous recording of intravesical and intraurethral pressure. *Acta Chir Scandinavica,* (1961), Supplement No 27:61-68

Farnsworth BN Posterior Intravaginal Slingplasty (infraccocygeal sacropexy) for severe posthysterectomy vaginal vault prolapse- a preliminary report, *Int J Urogynecol* (2002) 13 :4-8.

Gleick J "Inner Rhythms" in *Chaos- making a new science,*(1987) Cardinal, Penguin, England, 275-300.

Jeffcoate TNA *Principles of Gynaecology.* (1962), (2nd Ed.) Butterworths, London.

Lose G Impact of changes in posture and bladder filling on the mechanical properties of the urethra in healthy and stress incontinent women, *Neurourology and Urodynamics* (1990). 9:459-469

Lose G Simultaneous recording of pressure and cross-sectional area in the female urethra. A study of urethral closure function in healthy and stress incontinent women *Neurourol Urodyn* (1992);11: 55-89

Lose G and Colstrup H Mechanical properties of the urethra in healthy and stress incontinent females: dynamic measurements in the resting urethra, *J Urol.,* (1990) 1258-1262.

Marinoff, SC, Turner, MLC Vuvar vestibulitis syndrome: an overview. *Am J Obstet Gynecol* (1991); 165:1228-33.

Mayer R, Wells T, Brink C, Diokno A and Cockett A Handwashing in the cystometric evaluation of detrusor instability, *Neurourology and urodynamics,* (1991). 10: 563-569

Power RM Embryological development of the levator ani muscle. *American Journal of Obstets & Gynecol.,* (1948), 55:367-381.

Petros PE and Ulmsten U Bladder instability in women: A premature activation of the micturition reflex. *Neurourology and Urodynamics* (1993). 12, 235-239

Petros PE and Ulmsten U "Urethral pressure increase on effort originates from within the urethra, and continence from musculovaginal closure", *Neurourology and Urodynamics,* (1995).14:337-350

Petros PE The effect of urethral pressure variation in women (letter) *Int Urogynecol J and Pelvic Floor* (1996) 7: 274.

Petros PE *Severe chronic pelvic pain in women may be caused by ligamentous laxity in the posterior fornix of the vagina,* Aust NZ J Obstet Gynaecol. 1996; 36:3: 351-354.

Petros PE New ambulatory surgical methods using an anatomical classification of urinary dysfunction improve stress, urge, and abnormal emptying, *Int J Urogynecology* (1997) 8: 270-278.

Petros PE A cystocele may compensate for latent stress incontinence by stretching the vaginal hammock.*Gynecol and Obst Investigation* (1998); 46; 206-209

Petros PE Change in urethral pressure during voluntary pelvic floor muscle contraction and vaginal stimulation *Int J urogynecology* (1998) 8:318.

Petros PE and Bush MB A mathematical model of micturition gives new insights into pressure measurement and function, *Int J urogynecology* (1998) 9: 103-107.

Petros PE The sign of stress incontinence, should we believe what we see? *Aust NZ J Obstet Gynaecol.* (1998);38:352-353

Petros PE Detrusor instability and low compliance may represent different levels of disturbance in peripheral feedback control of the micturition reflex. *Neurourol and Urod* (1999) 18:81-91.

Petros PE, Von Konsky B Anchoring the midurethra restores bladder neck anatomy and continence, *Lancet* (1999) 354: 997-998

Petros PE Finite element models – a template for future urodynamics. *Neurourol &Urodynamics* (2001) 20: 231-233

van Doorn, van Waalwijk ESC, Remmers A, Jaknegt RA Conventional and extramural ambulatory urodynamic testing of the lower urinary tract in the female, *J Urol* (1992), 147: 1319-1325

Chapter 6: Further Reading

Kauffman SA The Origins of Order, Oxford Uni Press, NY (1993), 173-235.

May RM Simple mathematical models with very complicated dynamics. *Nature* (1976)261:459-467.

Molloy WBM Targeted treatment of female urinary dysfunction, Lancet (2002)vol 358;9308, p800

Petros PE and Ulmsten U Cough transmission ratio: An indicator of suburethral vaginal wall tension rather than urethral closure? *Acta Obstetricia et Gynecologica Scandinavica,* (1990), 69:Suppl. 153: 37-39.

Petros PE Doctoral thesis University of Uppsala, Sweden,(1993) 'Detrusor Instability - a Critical Analysis'

Petros PE and Ulmsten U Tests for detrusor instability in women. These mainly measure the urethral resistance created by pelvic floor contraction acting against a premature activation of the micturition reflex. *Acta Obstetricia et Gynecologica Scandinavica,* (1993): 72: 661-667.

Petros PE and Ulmsten U Natural volume handwashing urethrocystometry - a physiological technique for the objective diagnosis of the unstable detrusor. *Gynecol Obstet Investigation,* (1993), 36 : 42-46.

Petros PE A cystocele may compensate for latent stress incontinence by stretching the vaginal hammock, (1998) Gynecol and Obst Investigation (1998); 46; 206-209.

Petros PE The Art and Science of Medicine, *Lancet* (2001) 358:1818-1819
Petros PE Non-linearity in Clinical Practice, *Journal for Evaluation in Clinical Practice* (2002) (in press)
Popper KR Th*eories. Falsifiability.* The Logic of Scientific Discovery. (1980), Unwin, Hyman, London, 27-146
Schaer GN, Koechli OR, Schuessler B, Haller U Perineal ultrasound for evaluating the bladder neck in urinary stress incontinence. *Obstet Gynecol* (1995);85:224-229.
Shafik A A new concept of the anatomy of the anal sphincter mechanism and the physiology of defecation, Acta Anat (1990); 138:359-363.
Swash M, Henry MM,Snooks SJ Unifying concept of pelvic floor disorders and incontinence. Journal of the Royal Society of Medicine,(1985),78:906-911.

Chapter 7: Current and Emerging Issues

Bornstein J, Petros PEP, 'Vulvodynia- a referred neuropathic pain originating within the uterosacral ligaments' ANZJOG 2005,in press
Parks AG, Swash M and Urich H Sphincter Denervation in ano-rectal incontinence and rectal prolapse. *Gut;* (1977) ;18: 656-665.
Petros PE 'Development of the Intravaginal Slingplasty, and other ambulatory vaginal procedures' Doctor of Surgery thesis University of Western Australia (1999)
Petros PE Medium-term follow up of the Intravaginal Slingplasty operation indicates minimal deteroration of continence with time. *Aust. NZ J Obstet.Gynaecol.* (1999) 39:354-356.
Petros PE Cure of urinary and fecal incontinence by pelvic ligament reconstruction suggests a connective tissue etiology for both. *International Journal of Urogynecology* (1999);10:356-360
Petros PE, Bornsetin J, *Vulvodynia may be a referred pain originating from laxity in the uterosacral ligaments,* Aust NZ J Obstet Gynaecol (2004) 44: 483–486
Shafik A *A new concept of the anatomy of the anal sphincter mechanism and the physiology of defecation,* Acta Anat (1990), 138:359-363.
Shafik A Vagino-levator reflex: description of a reflex and its role in sexual performance, *European J Obstet &Gynecol and Reprod Biology* (1995); 60: 161-164.
Smith ARB, Hosker GL & Warrell DW The role of partial denervation of the pelvic floor in the aetiology of genito-urinary prolapse and stress incontinence of urine: a neurophysiological study. *British Journal of Obstets & Gynaecol.,* (1989a), 96:24-28.
Smith A, Hosker G and Warrell D The role of pudendal nerve damage in the aetiology of genuine stress incontinence in women. *British Journal Obstet. and Gynaecol.,* (1989b), 96: 29-32.
Sultan AH, Kamm MA, Hudson CN, Thomas JM and Bartram CI Anal-sphincter disruption during vaginal delivery, *N Eng J Med* (1993); 329: 1905-11

Chapter 7: Further Reading

Bergeron S, Binik YM, Khalife S, Pagidas K, Glazer HI, Meana M, Amsel R A randomized comparison of group cognitive-behavioral therapy, surface electromyographic biofeedback, and vestibulectomy in the treatment of dyspareunia resulitng from vulvar vestibulitis. *Pain* (2001);91;297-306.
Duthie GS, Bartolo DCC, faecal continence and defaecation, in *Coloproctology and the Pelvic Floor,* (1992), 2nd Ed, Eds Henry MM and Swash M, Butterworth Heinemann Oxford, 86-97.

Henry MM and Swash M (Eds) *Coloproctology and the Pelvic Floor* (1992) 2nd Edn. Butterworth Heineman Oxford.

Lotery HE, McClure N, Galask RP *Vulvodynia*. Lancet 2004; 363: 1058-60

Marinoff, SC, Turner, MLC Vuvar vestibulitis syndrome: an overview. *Am J Obstet Gynecol* (1991); 165:1228-33.

Shull BL, Capen CV, Riggs MW and Kuehl TJ Preoperative and postoperative analysis of site-specific pelvic support defects in 81 women treated with sacrospinous ligament suspension and pelvic reconstruction, *J Obstet Gynecol* (1992); 166; 1764-71.

Shafik A A new concept of the anatomy of the anal sphincter mechanism and the physiology of defaecation IV, Colo-proctology (1982),1: 49-54.

Snooks SJ Badernock DF, Tiptaft RC & Swash M. Perineal nerve damage in genuine stress urinary incontinence: an electrophysiological study. *British Journal of Urology,* (1985), 57:422-426.

Swash M, Henry MM, Snooks SJ Unifying concept of pelvic floor disorders and incontinence. *Journal of the Royal Society of Medicine,* (1985),78: 906-911.

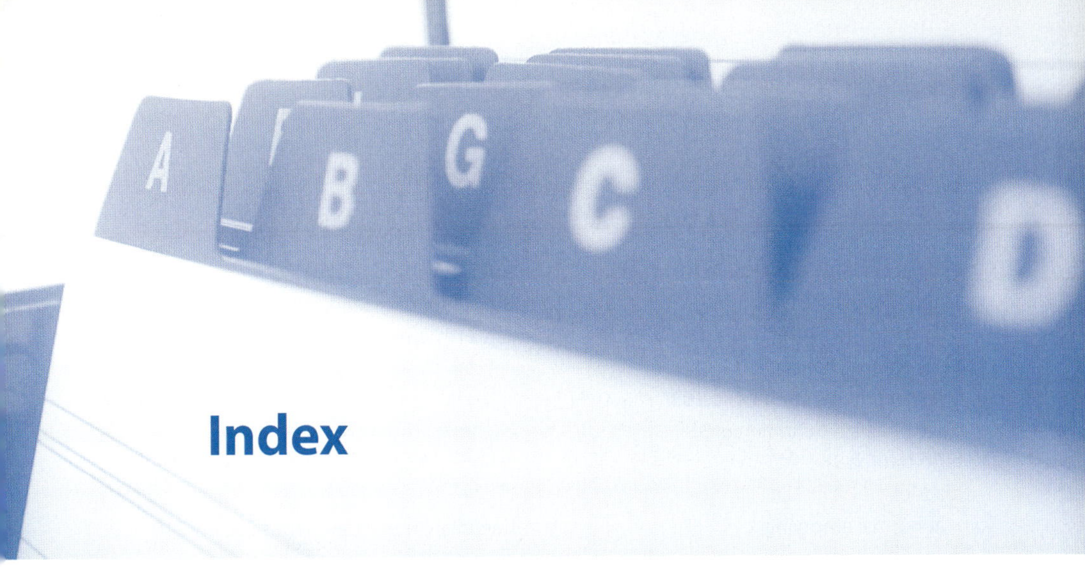

Index

B

C

D

E

N

 Q

R

 S

T

Z